T0263333

Early Childhood Mental Health: Empirical Assessment and Intervention from Conception through Preschool

Editor

MINI TANDON

CHILD AND ADOLESCENT PSYCHIATRIC CLINICS OF NORTH AMERICA

www.childpsych.theclinics.com

Consulting Editor
HARSH K. TRIVEDI

July 2017 • Volume 26 • Number 3

ELSEVIER

1600 John F. Kennedy Boulevard • Suite 1800 • Philadelphia, Pennsylvania, 19103-2899

http://www.theclinics.com

CHILD AND ADOLESCENT PSYCHIATRIC CLINICS OF NORTH AMERICA Volume 26, Number 3
July 2017 ISSN 1056–4993, ISBN-13: 978-0-323-53124-5

Editor: Lauren Boyle
Developmental Editor: Kristen Helm

Child and Adolescent Psychiatric Clinics of North America (ISSN 1056-4993) is published quarterly by Elsevier Inc., 360 Park Avenue South, New York, NY 10010-1710. Months of issue are January, April, July, and October. Business and Editorial Offices: 1600 John F. Kennedy Boulevard, Suite 1800, Philadelphia, PA 19103-2899. Periodicals postage paid at New York, NY and additional mailing offices. Subscription prices are $316.00 per year (US individuals), $566.00 per year (US institutions), $100.00 per year (US students), $367.00 per year (Canadian individuals), $688.00 per year (Canadian institutions), $200.00 per year (Canadian students), $439.00 per year (international individuals), $688.00 per year (international institutions), and $200.00 per year (international students). International air speed delivery is included in all *Clinics* subscription prices. All prices are subject to change without notice. **POSTMASTER:** Send address changes to *Child and Adolescent Psychiatric Clinics of North America*, Elsevier Health Sciences Division, Subscription Customer Service, 3251 Riverport Lane, Maryland Heights, MO 63043. **Customer Service: 1-800-654-2452 (U.S. and Canada); 314-447-8871 (outside U.S. and Canada). Fax: 314-447-8029. E-mail:** JournalsCustomer Service-usa@elsevier.com **(for print support) or** journalsonlinesupport-usa@elsevier.com **(for online support).**

Reprints. For copies of 100 or more of articles in this publication, please contact the Commercial Reprints Department, Elsevier Inc., 360 Park Avenue South, New York, New York 10010-1710 Tel.: 212-633-3874; Fax: 212-633-3820, E-mail: reprints@elsevier.com

Child and Adolescent Psychiatric Clinics of North America is covered in *MEDLINE/PubMed (Index Medicus), ISI, SSCI, Research Alert, Social Search, Current Contents,* and *EMBASE/Excerpta Medica.*

Contributors

CONSULTING EDITOR

HARSH K. TRIVEDI, MD, MBA
President and Chief Executive Officer, Sheppard Pratt Health System, Clinical Professor
and Vice Chair of Psychiatry, University of Maryland School of Medicine, Baltimore,
Maryland

CONSULTING EDITOR EMERITUS

ANDRÉS MARTIN, MD, MPH

FOUNDING CONSULTING EDITOR

MELVIN LEWIS, MBBS, FRCPSYCH, DCH

EDITOR

MINI TANDON, DO
Assistant Professor, Child Psychiatry, Division of Child and Adolescent Psychiatry,
Washington University School of Medicine in St Louis, Director, Preschool Age Clinic, BJC
Behavioral Health, St Louis, Missouri

AUTHORS

CHRISTOPHER ARCHANGELI, MD
Child and Adolescent Psychiatry Fellow, Division of Child Psychiatry, University of
Vermont Medical Center, University of Vermont College of Medicine, Burlington, Vermont

NEIL W. BORIS, MD
Center for Prevention and Early Intervention Policy, Florida State University, Tallahassee,
Florida

TERYN BRUNI, PhD
Post-Doctoral Fellow, Department of Pediatrics, C.S. Mott Children's Hospital, University
of Michigan Medical School, Ann Arbor, Michigan

JOHN N. CONSTANTINO, MD
Psychiatrist-In-Chief, St Louis Children's Hospital, Blanche F. Ittleson Professor of
Psychiatry and Pediatrics, Director, William Greenleaf Eliot Division of Child Psychiatry,
Co-Director, Intellectual and Developmental Disabilities Research Center, Departments of
Psychiatry and Pediatrics, Washington University School of Medicine in St Louis, St Louis,
Missouri

AMY DRAYTON, PhD
Assistant Professor, Department of Pediatrics, C.S. Mott Children's Hospital, University of Michigan Medical School, Ann Arbor, Michigan

ANDREA GIEDINGHAGEN, MD
Division of Child and Adolescent Psychiatry, Washington University School of Medicine in St Louis, St Louis, Missouri

MARY MARGARET GLEASON, MD
Associate Professor, Department of Psychiatry and Behavioral Sciences, Tulane University School of Medicine, New Orleans, Louisiana

LACEY HALL, MS
Department of Psychology, St. Jude Children's Research Hospital, Memphis, Tennessee

JIM HUDZIAK, MD
Professor of Psychiatry, Medicine, Pediatrics and Communication Sciences & Disorders, Director of the Vermont Center for Children, Youth, and Families, Division of Child Psychiatry, University of Vermont Medical Center, Thomas M Achenbach Endowed Chair of Developmental Psychopathology, University of Vermont College of Medicine, Burlington, Vermont

MELISSA JONSON-REID, MSW, PhD
Ralph and Muriel Pumphrey Professor of Social Work, George Warren Brown School of Social Work, Washington University, St Louis, Missouri

ANNA KELLEY, PsyD
Post-Doctoral Fellow, Department of Psychiatry and Behavioral Sciences, Tulane University School of Medicine, New Orleans, Louisiana

RACHEL M. KNIGHT, PhD
Assistant Professor, Department of Pediatrics, C.S. Mott Children's Hospital, University of Michigan Medical School, Ann Arbor, Michigan

RACHEL E. LEAN, PhD
Post-Doctoral Research Associate, Department of Psychiatry, Washington University School of Medicine in St Louis, St Louis, Missouri

SHANNON N. LENZE, PhD
Assistant Professor of Psychiatry, Washington University School of Medicine in St Louis, St Louis, Missouri

DAYNA J. LePLATTE-OGINI, MD
Clinical Instructor, Department of Psychiatry, University of Michigan, Ann Arbor, Michigan

AMY LICIS, MD, MSCI
Assistant Professor of Neurology, Washington University School of Medicine in St Louis, St Louis, Missouri

JOAN L. LUBY, MD
Samuel and Mae S. Ludwig Professor of Child Psychiatry, Department of Psychiatry, Washington University School of Medicine in St Louis, St Louis, Missouri

NASUH M. MALAS, MD, MPH
Clinical Assistant Professor, Department of Psychiatry, University of Michigan, Ann Arbor, Michigan

SHEILA M. MARCUS, MD
Clinical Professor, Department of Psychiatry, University of Michigan, Ann Arbor, Michigan

NATASHA MARRUS, MD, PhD
Assistant Professor, Department of Psychiatry, Division of Child and Adolescent Psychiatry, Washington University School of Medicine in St Louis, St Louis, Missouri

MELISSA MIDDLETON, PhD
Assistant Professor, Department of Psychiatry and Behavioral Sciences, Tulane University School of Medicine, New Orleans, Louisiana

NATALIE MORRIS, MS
Doctoral Fellow, Department of Pediatrics, C.S. Mott Children's Hospital, University of Michigan, Ann Arbor, Michigan

MARIA MUZIK, MD, MS
Assistant Professor, Department of Psychiatry, University of Michigan, Ann Arbor, Michigan

PARESH D. PATEL, MD, PhD
Clinical Associate Professor, Department of Psychiatry, University of Michigan, Ann Arbor, Michigan

ALBA PERGJIKA, MD, MPH
Division of Child and Adolescent Psychiatry, Washington University School of Medicine in St Louis, St Louis, Missouri

JOANNA M. QUIGLEY, MD
Clinical Assistant Professor, Department of Psychiatry, University of Michigan, Ann Arbor, Michigan

KIMBERLY RENK, PhD
Department of Psychology, University of Central Florida, Orlando, Florida

CYNTHIA E. ROGERS, MD
Assistant Professor, Departments of Psychiatry and Pediatrics, Washington University School of Medicine in St Louis, St Louis, Missouri

KATHERINE L. ROSENBLUM, PhD
Clinical Associate Professor, Department of Psychiatry, University of Michigan, Ann Arbor, Michigan

LAURA SAYERS, MA, CCC-SLP
Senior Speech-Language Pathologist, Department of Speech-Language Pathology, C.S. Mott Children's Hospital, University of Michigan, Ann Arbor, Michigan

CHRIS D. SMYSER, MD
Assistant Professor, Departments of Neurology, Radiology, and Pediatrics, Washington University School of Medicine in St Louis, St Louis, Missouri

CHAD M. SYLVESTER, MD, PhD
Instructor, Department of Psychiatry, Washington University School of Medicine in St Louis, St Louis, Missouri

MINI TANDON, DO
Assistant Professor, Child Psychiatry, Division of Child and Adolescent Psychiatry, Washington University School of Medicine in St Louis, Director, Preschool Age Clinic, BJC Behavioral Health, St Louis, Missouri

DIANA J. WHALEN, PhD
Post-Doctoral Fellow, Department of Psychiatry, Washington University School of Medicine in St Louis, St Louis, Missouri

ELLIE WIDEMAN, MSW
Doctoral Student, George Warren Brown School of Social Work, Washington University, St Louis, Missouri

Contents

Preface: Early Childhood Mental Health: Empirical Assessment and Intervention from Conception Through Preschool   xiii

Mini Tandon

Early and Comprehensive Assessment

Early Childhood Mental Health: Starting Early with the Pregnant Mother   411

Shannon N. Lenze

> Perinatal mental health has important implications for maternal and child outcomes. Most women with psychiatric disorders during pregnancy go undiagnosed and untreated, despite widespread initiatives for early identification. Universal screening for psychiatric disorders, particularly depression and anxiety, has been implemented in obstetric and primary care settings. However, there is little evidence regarding the effectiveness on psychiatric symptom reduction or prevention of adverse outcomes in children. Recently, comprehensive screening and follow-up programs integrated within obstetric or primary care settings have shown promising results in improving maternal mental health outcomes. Further work is needed to determine best clinical and most cost-effective practices.

Assessment: The Newborn   427

Rachel E. Lean, Chris D. Smyser, and Cynthia E. Rogers

> Neonatal neurobehavioral assessment has become a standardized component of clinical care provided to newborn infants, guiding neonatal clinical care and subsequent access to early interventions and services. Links between neonatal assessment and neurosensory and motor impairments in high-risk infants have been relatively well established. In contrast, the extent to which newborn neurobehavioral assessment might also facilitate the early identification of infants susceptible to socioemotional impairments in early childhood is less well documented. This review examines longitudinal links between the neonatal neurobehavioral assessment, temperament, and socioemotional outcomes in early childhood.

Clinical Assessment of Young Children   441

Melissa Middleton, Anna Kelley, and Mary Margaret Gleason

> Mental health assessment of young children provides valuable information to shape a formulation and guide treatment. Early childhood mental health assessment can occur in an increasing number of settings beyond traditional mental health practices, including childcare settings, primary care settings, and other settings where children and family are regularly seen. Although many of the components of an early childhood mental health assessment are included in the assessment of older children, assessment of very young children requires some specific developmental adjustments and additional considerations including attention to the parent-child relationship and caregiving context and rapid development.

Psychopathology and Intervention

Beyond Reactive Attachment Disorder: How Might Attachment Research Inform Child Psychiatry Practice?   455

Neil W. Boris and Kimberly Renk

 Video content accompanies this article at www.childpsych. theclinics.com.

This article provides an updated review of attachment research with a focus on how comprehensive clinical assessment and intervention informs the care of young children. Child psychiatrists can serve as an important part of care coordination teams working with young children who have histories of early maltreatment and/or disruption in caregiving whether or not the children they are seeing meet criteria for an attachment disorder. Child psychiatrists should be familiar with both comprehensive assessment and the recent attachment-based interventions and appreciate how pharmacotherapy can be a useful adjunctive intervention when intensive therapy alone is ineffective.

Trauma and Very Young Children   477

Melissa Jonson-Reid and Ellie Wideman

This article examines the intersection of early childhood mental health and trauma. Working definitions, incidence, and prevalence of trauma events for this population are outlined with an emphasis on children younger than age 4 years. Trauma impacts on early childhood development are reviewed, with attention to clinical consequences, protective factors, and resilience. Best practices for assessment, screening tools, and treatment methods are presented based on the current research. Future implications include clinician and researcher partnerships to increase the number of effective screening and intervention tools for addressing trauma in very young children.

Disruptive Behavior Disorders in Children 0 to 6 Years Old   491

Mini Tandon and Andrea Giedinghagen

Disruptive behavior disorders (DBDs), specifically oppositional defiant disorder and conduct disorder, are common, serious, and treatable conditions among preschoolers. DBDs are marked by frequent aggression, deceitfulness, and defiance, and often persist through the lifespan. Exposure to harsh or inconsistent parenting, as frequently seen with parental depression and stress, increases DBD risk. Candidate genes that may increase DBD risk in the presence of childhood adversity have also been identified, but more research is needed. Neurophysiologic and structural correlates with DBD also exist. Parent management training programs, focusing on increasing parenting competence and confidence, are the gold standard treatment of preschool DBDs.

Depression and Anxiety in Preschoolers: A Review of the Past 7 Years   503

Diana J. Whalen, Chad M. Sylvester, and Joan L. Luby

This article reviews recent empirical literature on the prevalence, correlates, assessment, and treatment of preschool-onset internalizing disorders. Major advances in the acceptance and recognition of both preschool-onset depression and anxiety have occurred over the past decade. This work has been greatly enhanced by the discovery of genetic, neural, and physiologic indicators, which further validate these constellations of symptoms in young children. Despite this growth in research, much work still needs to be done to further elucidate the cause, risk, treatment, and protective factors for preschool-onset internalizing disorders.

Attention Deficit Hyperactivity Disorder in Preschool-Age Children   523

Mini Tandon and Alba Pergjika

Attention deficit hyperactivity disorder is a neurodevelopmental disorder marked by age-inappropriate deficits in attention or hyperactivity/impulsivity that interfere with functioning or development. It is highly correlated with other disorders, such as oppositional defiant disorder, conduct disorder, and mood symptoms. The etiology is multifactorial, and neuroimaging findings are nonspecific. Although assessment tools exist, there is variability among them, and historically, parent-teacher agreement has not been consistent. Treatment algorithm for attention deficit hyperactivity disorder in preschoolers includes behavioral interventions first followed by psychopharmacologic treatment when behavioral therapies fail. Other nonpharmacologic and nonbehavioral interventions are discussed including the role of exercise and nutrition.

Intellectual Disability and Language Disorder   539

Natasha Marrus and Lacey Hall

Intellectual disability (ID) and language disorders are neurodevelopmental conditions arising in early childhood. Child psychiatrists are likely to encounter children with ID and language disorders because both are strongly associated with challenging behaviors and mental disorder. Because early intervention is associated with optimal outcomes, child psychiatrists must be aware of their signs and symptoms, particularly as related to delays in cognitive and adaptive function. Optimal management of both ID and language disorders requires a multidisciplinary, team-based, and family centered approach. Child psychiatrists play an important role on this team, given their expertise with contextualizing and treating challenging behaviors.

The Early Origins of Autism   555

John N. Constantino and Natasha Marrus

Autism spectrum disorders (ASDs) are neurodevelopmental disorders whose core features of impaired social communication and atypical repetitive behaviors and/or restrictions in range of interests emerge in toddlerhood and carry significant implications at successive stages of development. The ability to reliably identify most cases of the condition far earlier than the average age of diagnosis presents a novel opportunity for early intervention, but the availability of such an intervention is disparate across US communities, and its impact is imperfectly understood. New research may transform the clinical approach to these conditions in early childhood.

Feeding Disorders   571

Natalie Morris, Rachel M. Knight, Teryn Bruni, Laura Sayers, and Amy Drayton

Feeding disorders often present in children with complex medical histories as well as those with neurodevelopmental disabilities. If untreated, feeding problems will likely persist and may lead to additional developmental and medical complications. Treatment of pediatric feeding disorders should involve an interdisciplinary team, but the core intervention should include behavioral feeding techniques as they are the only empirically supported therapy for feeding disorders.

Sleep Disorders: Assessment and Treatment in Preschool-Aged Children   587

Amy Licis

Sleep issues are common in preschoolers, defined in this article as ages 3 to 5 years. Sleep deprivation can cause behavioral and cognitive issues. Sleep issues seen in the preschool years include insomnia, obstructive sleep apnea, parasomnias, and restless legs syndrome. Sleep issues seem to exacerbate mood and attention disturbances. Conversely, children with psychiatric disorders are likely to have sleep problems. Treatment of sleep issues is important for long-term mental health and optimization of functioning.

Setting the Stage for Collaboration and Future Directions

Partnerships with Primary Care for the Treatment of Preschoolers   597

Sheila M. Marcus, Nasuh M. Malas, Joanna M. Quigley, Katherine L. Rosenblum, Maria Muzik, Dayna J. LePlatte-Ogini, and Paresh D. Patel

This article reviews mental health access issues relevant to preschool children and data on this population obtained through the Michigan Child Collaborative Care Program (MC3). The MC3 program provides telephonic consultation to primary care physicians (PCPs) in 40 counties in Michigan and video telepsychiatric consultation to patients and families. Attention-deficit/hyperactivity disorder and disruptive behavioral disorders are frequent initial presenting diagnoses, but autism spectrum disorders, parent-child relational issues, trauma, and posttraumatic stress disorder should also be considered. Collaborative care programs provide promising ways to promote access to child psychiatric services when these services are distant to local PCP offices.

The Future of Preschool Prevention, Assessment, and Intervention   611

Jim Hudziak and Christopher Archangeli

Preschoolers are in the most rapid period of brain development. Environment shapes the structure and function of the developing brain. Promoting brain health requires cultivation of healthy environments at home, school, and in the community. This improves the emotional-behavioral and physical health of all children, can prevent problems in children at risk, and can alter the trajectory of children already suffering. For clinicians, this starts with assessing and treating the entire family, equipping parents with the principles of parent management training, and incorporating wellness prescriptions for nutrition, physical activity, music, and mindfulness.

Index   625

CHILD AND ADOLESCENT PSYCHIATRIC CLINICS

FORTHCOMING ISSUES

October 2017
Pediatric Integrated Care
Gregory K. Fritz, Tami D. Benton, and
Gary Maslow, *Editors*

January 2018
**Co-occurring Medical Illnesses in Child
and Adolescent Psychiatry: Updates
and Treatment Considerations**
Matthew D. Willis, *Editor*

April 2018
Internet Habits and Youth Mental Health
Paul Weigle and Kristopher Kaliebe,
Editors

RECENT ISSUES

April 2017
**Transitional Age Youth and Mental Illness:
Influences on Young Adult Outcomes**
Adele Martel and D. Catherine Fuchs,
Editors

January 2017
**Health Information Technology for Child
and Adolescent Psychiatry**
Barry Sarvet and John Torous, *Editors*

October 2016
Substance Use Disorders, Part II
Ray Chih-Jui Hsiao and Paula D. Riggs,
Editors

Preface

Early Childhood Mental Health: Empirical Assessment and Intervention from Conception Through Preschool

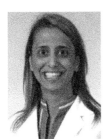

Mini Tandon, DO
Editor

The importance of early assessment and intervention cannot be overemphasized. Emerging data from a number of studies, such as noted for autism and language disorders among others, indicate that critical periods exist in which timely assessment and intervention may prove to enhance developmental trajectories and prevent or reduce severity of psychiatric sequelae. The field of child and adolescent psychiatry has capitalized on advances made in neuroimaging and genetics to further inform longitudinal trajectories of psychiatric illness with roots traceable to conception or early infancy and childhood. Given the morbidity and mortality associated with psychiatric illness, the focus of this issue is on early detection and assessment of the beginnings of such disorder, starting with conception. The issue then follows with a review of interventions for established disorders, emphasizing those with the most empirical investigation to date. While it is noteworthy that such advances in the understanding of assessment and intervention have been made, it remains that we are just beginning to scratch the surface. Given limited public health resources, it seems plausible that allocation of such resources to early assessment and preventive interventions may prove most beneficial.

This issue is organized into two major sections: Early and Comprehensive Assessment, followed by Psychopathology and Intervention. In this manner, it is hoped that the reader can readily digest the complexity and uniqueness of standardized assessment methods utilized for mothers who are pregnant, newborns, and pre-school-age children in general. Next, the issue delineates key disorders that often emerge as early as infancy and the preschool age. Toward the end of the issue, given the shortage of child psychiatrists in general, and early childhood providers more specifically, the issue

Child Adolesc Psychiatric Clin N Am 26 (2017) xiii–xiv
http://dx.doi.org/10.1016/j.chc.2017.04.001
1056-4993/17/© 2017 Published by Elsevier Inc.

childpsych.theclinics.com

incorporates an article that reflects a model for collaboration with primary care to address the needs of our youngest. Future directions and more novel approaches to mental health care are addressed in the final article. Several noteworthy authors with clinical and research expertise in these areas have generously contributed their time to develop this body of information and review. We hope you will find the issue informative and practical as you work with our most impressionable and youngest.

Mini Tandon, DO
Washington University School of Medicine
660 South Euclid Avenue
Campus Box 8504
St Louis, MO 63110, USA

E-mail address:
tandonm@wustl.edu

Early and Comprehensive Assessment

Early Childhood Mental Health

Starting Early with the Pregnant Mother

Shannon N. Lenze, PhD

KEYWORDS

- Pregnancy • Perinatal • Depression • Anxiety • Screening

KEY POINTS

- Psychiatric disorders commonly occur in pregnancy and postpartum.
- Psychiatric illness during pregnancy carries risk to mother and infant.
- Pregnant women are in increased contact with health care providers, providing a key window in which to identify psychosocial and psychiatric problems and initiate treatment.

INTRODUCTION

Maternal mental health during the perinatal period, defined as during pregnancy to 1 year postpartum, is increasingly recognized as a critical public health problem. Decades of research of maternal postpartum depression have shown adverse consequences for infant and child development.[1,2] More recently, attention has shifted toward examining the effects of antenatal exposure to psychiatric symptoms on infant and child outcomes. Fetal exposure to mental illness during pregnancy has been associated with adverse consequences to the developing infant and child.[1,3] Thus, early intervention is imperative to prevent negative health consequences for mothers and their offspring.[3]

Despite the implications of maternal psychiatric health during pregnancy and postpartum, most women go undiagnosed and untreated. A recent review of perinatal depression identification and screening estimated that more than 50% of women with antenatal and postnatal depression go unrecognized and untreated.[4] Furthermore, even among women identified as needing treatment, it is estimated that less than 10% receive an adequate trial of treatment and less than 5% of these women achieve remission of depressive symptoms.[4]

Screening for psychiatric disorders during postpartum, and more recently during pregnancy, has been widely encouraged. In 2016 the US Preventive Services Task

---

The author reports no conflicts of interest.

Department of Psychiatry, Washington University School of Medicine, Campus Box 8504, 660 South Euclid Avenue, St Louis, MO 63110, USA

E-mail address: slenze@wustl.edu

Force updated its position on screening for depression with the recommendation for universal screening for depression in adults, including pregnant and postpartum women.[5] These recommendations are not without controversy and even differ from other national and international guidelines.[6]

This article reviews screening for psychiatric disorders during the perinatal period. First, the prevalence and incidence of mental health disorders in pregnancy are reviewed. Second, the implications to maternal and child health are discussed. Third, details of why, who, and how to screen (including which instruments) are highlighted. Barriers to care and the role of psychosocial assessment beyond psychiatric assessment are also considered. Finally, we discuss future directions (fathers, alternative models, and using technology). Most evidence available pertains to perinatal depression and anxiety. Evidence for bipolar disorder, schizophrenia, and psychosis are highlighted as available. Although alcohol, drug, and tobacco use disorders during pregnancy and postpartum are also common and equally important, these disorders are not reviewed in this article (see Ref.[7] for review).

PREVALENCE AND INCIDENCE OF PSYCHIATRIC DISORDERS IN PREGNANCY

Depression and anxiety are the most common psychiatric symptoms reported during pregnancy. The onset of depressive symptoms during the perinatal period is not consistent for all women. For example, onset may occur during pregnancy and resolve postpartum; others are triggered by parturition, whereas others may develop during pregnancy and continue throughout the postpartum period. Given that at least 50% of women who are depressed antenatally remain depressed postpartum, detection of depression during pregnancy is imperative because it could decrease the burden of illness on mothers and their children.[8] Prevalence and incidence of depressive disorders are highlighted later. These estimates vary across studies because of different definitions of depression (ie, structured diagnostic interviews or symptoms above threshold on a screening measure), differing settings (low vs high incomes), and different definitions of the time period being studied[3]: approximately 18% of pregnant women experience depressive symptoms during pregnancy and early postpartum; 9% to 15% develop a new episode of depression during pregnancy through the first 3 months postpartum[9,10]; and incidence of perinatal depression is particularly high in low income, minority populations, with rates ranging from 24% to 47%.[11,12]

Perinatal anxiety is also commonly reported by pregnant women.[13] Perinatal depression and anxiety are frequently comorbid, and at least one-third of women report significant concurrent symptoms.[14,15] Although some studies have asserted that women are no more likely to experience psychiatric disorders during the perinatal period than at other times, others have suggested higher prevalence of depression, generalized anxiety disorder, and obsessive-compulsive disorder during the postpartum period.[10,13,14] Prevalence rates of anxiety disorders from a few nationally representative studies are listed next:

- Generalized anxiety disorder prevalence rate during pregnancy ranges from 1.9% to 8.5%[16,17]
- Increased generalized anxiety disorder rates 6-month postpartum at 6.1% to 8.2%[16,17]
- Panic disorder rates during pregnancy range from 1.4% to 9.1%[13]
- Panic disorder rates range from 0.5% to 2.9% early postpartum[13,16]
- Social anxiety disorder rates range from 0.2% to 6.5%[13,18]
- Obsessive-compulsive disorder rates range from 1.2% to 5.2% during pregnancy and about 4% postpartum[13,16,19]

- Posttraumatic stress disorder rates are estimated to be between 3% and 16% (4%–23% reporting subthreshold levels), with higher rates (around 19%) found in public-payer settings[20,21]

Prevalence of bipolar disorder during pregnancy seems to be similar to those of nonpregnant women at about 2.8%, although few studies have examined the epidemiology of severe mental illness during pregnancy.[13,22] It is unclear whether pregnancy is protective for recurrence of bipolar episodes or not, because studies to date have provided conflicting results.[22] What is clear, however, is that the immediate postpartum period (within the first 30 days) is an acute risk period for onset of mania or psychosis in women with history of bipolar illness.[3,22] The occurrence of postpartum psychosis is rare, 1 or 2 per 1000 births.[23]

There are several key risk factors associated with the development of perinatal psychiatric disorders including previous history of psychiatric disorder, life stress, poor social relationships or lack of partner support, history of trauma, and poverty.[3,24]

IMPLICATIONS FOR CHILD MENTAL HEALTH

A centrally held tenant for developmental science is predicated on early life experiences, including those in utero, which influence later development, perhaps best summed by Prechtl, "Neither health nor development commence at birth."[25,26]

Depression during pregnancy may lead to poor adherence to prenatal care; poor self-care; and other unhealthy lifestyle choices, including nicotine, alcohol, and drug use.[1,27–30] Depression, anxiety, and stress during pregnancy are associated with increased risk of miscarriage, preterm birth, low birth weight, small for gestational age babies, gestational hypertension, and preeclampsia.[31–34] Schizophrenia has also been associated with low birth weight and preterm delivery, although relevant confounds include smoking, poverty, and substance use.[35,36]

Several longitudinal studies have investigated the effects of antenatal depression and anxiety ranging from infancy through early adulthood.[1] Goodman and colleagues[37] found a dose-response relationship between severity and overall exposure to depressive symptoms experienced during pregnancy and the newborn's ability to regulate state and autonomic stability. Antenatal depression is associated with increased risk of childhood and adolescent emotional, behavioral, and cognitive problems.[38–42] Data from the South London Child Development Study, a longitudinal birth cohort first studied in the 1980s, demonstrated offspring exposed to depression during pregnancy were almost 3.5 times more likely to develop depression in adulthood as those without antenatal exposure.[43]

Antenatal anxiety may also be associated with childhood internalizing,[44,45] negative affectivity at 18 months,[44,45] attention, behavior problems, and impulsivity.[46,47] Perinatal-specific anxiety, such as uncontrollable worry about motherhood or the infant and severe fear of childbirth, is a robust predictor of adverse birth and developmental outcomes.[48–51] There is little consensus as to the timing of exposure of depressive or anxiety symptoms in terms of risk for adverse offspring outcomes. Glover[52] recently found later gestation to be most predictive, although other studies have suggested 24 to 26 weeks as a sensitive period.[53]

IMPLEMENTING SCREENING FOR MATERNAL PSYCHIATRIC DISORDER
What Is Screening?

A screening test has been defined as a test or inquiry used to divide people into high- or low-risk groups.[6] This should be distinguished from a screening program, which is designed to reduce risk and/or improve outcomes through early identification and management of disease. Milgrom and Gemmill[6] emphasize that screening programs should include at minimum a validated test, feedback about the results, diagnostic procedure for positive screens, management options for positive diagnoses with contextual consideration, and treatment options for those who want it. Implementation of screening programs often requires considerable modification of standard practice. For example, it often requires additional staff/provider training, increases provider workload, and mandates additional resources for follow-up of screening results, all of which add to costs of care.[54] To date, most of the evidence regarding the benefits and costs of screening pertain to postpartum depression. There are a few studies investigating antenatal screening for depression and prenatal or postnatal screening for anxiety.[55]

Several studies have shown that depression screening on its own does little to change treatment use.[55] Screening programs, particularly those that are integrated within obstetric care, have shown promising results.[56,57] For example, the TRIPPD (Translating Research into Practice for Postpartum Depression) study randomized 28 practices to either a collaborative care model or usual care.[56] Women in the collaborative care program were significantly more likely to achieve remission by 6 and 12 months postpartum. Similar programs are also showing good success with integrated screening and treatment within obstetric settings.[58,59]

When Should Screening Occur?

Women who screen positive during pregnancy are much more likely to be linked to and access care than those screened postpartum.[59] Women are in frequent contact with health care providers during pregnancy, which increases the ability to identify depression and initiate appropriate treatment referrals. The best time during pregnancy and postpartum in which to screen for anxiety is still unclear. However, Ayers and colleagues[60] recommend the following considerations to guide screening decisions: (1) choose a time when women are most in contact with health services; (2) if the aim of screening is to reduce impact of anxiety on the fetus, then earlier screening is preferred; and (3) repeat testing is recommended for those scoring high on the measure.

Who Should Be Screening?

Any provider that supports or provides services for women during the perinatal period has the potential to initiate mental health screening; however, many providers do not believe that they have the necessary training or resources to do so.[55] Obstetricians-gynecologists are often the primary health care providers for women, particularly during the childbearing years.[61] Other providers are also well positioned to implement screening programs, including pediatricians,[62,63] general health practitioners,[64] family practice,[65] and maternal and child health nurses.[66] Women, Infants, and Children nutrition programs or Head Start may also be potential avenues to reach women in need.[67,68]

Where Should Screening Take Place?

Several studies have indicated that screening is most effective when it takes place in the same location at which follow-up services are available.[56,69] Women are less likely to receive follow-up care when given a referral for off-site services and thus screening on its own is unlikely to improve outcome.[56,70–72] Collaborative care, in which mental health screening, diagnosis, and intervention is imbedded within a primary care provider site (eg, obstetricians-gynecologists or pediatrics practice) is a promising approach; however, studies of collaborative care for perinatal mental health are rare.[73–75]

Current Evidence Regarding Perinatal Screening Practices

O'Connor and colleagues[76] review of the perinatal depression screening literature highlighted that most research regarding screening for depression rarely investigated screening in isolation from more comprehensive treatment or intervention programs. They concluded that depression screening programs for pregnant and postpartum women reduces the prevalence of depression and increases treatment response or symptom remission, especially if treatment supports are available. However, they noted that there are still few quality studies, especially during pregnancy.[76] Similarly, Thombs and colleagues,[77] in their systematic review of depression screening during pregnancy and postpartum, found only one study that met their quality criteria.

WHICH SCREENING INSTRUMENTS SHOULD I USE?

O'Connor and colleagues[76] reviewed common instruments for depression screening during pregnancy and postpartum for the US Preventive Services Task Force report. Other investigators have also compared depression screening measures in terms of sensitivity and specificity during pregnancy and postpartum (for reviews see Refs.[78,79]). **Table 1** highlights some of the commonly used screening instruments validated for use during pregnancy or postpartum and general comments about pros and cons for their use in screening. Specificity and sensitivity estimates vary depending on when the measure is administered (pregnancy vs postpartum) and setting or population (ie, minority, low-income, other cultural groups).[95–97]

Perinatal depression screening is the most commonly administered. Screening for anxiety and other disorders presents with other challenges. First, providers must distinguish between transient versus enduring anxiety. Because of the transient nature of anxiety, it is recommended that anxiety should be measured twice over a period of a few weeks to identify persistent distress.[98] Furthermore, general anxiety symptoms and pregnancy or postpartum-related anxiety should also be distinguished because they have differing implications for intervention.[60] Typically, screening for posttraumatic stress disorder in obstetric settings is rare.[99] A recent study found screening for posttraumatic stress disorder feasible in obstetric settings, although availability of on-site follow-up with providers trained in trauma services is ideal.[99] Key guidelines for choosing screening measures are that the choice of the measure to be used in a specific setting needs careful attention, not all measures are feasible in all settings, and screening measures are not meant to be diagnostic (appropriate follow-up plans need to be in place).[6]

BARRIERS AND FACILITATORS TO SCREENING AND INTERVENTION

Although the importance of perinatal mental health screening is recognized as important and validated screening measures exist, recent studies have shown less than half of providers routinely conduct mental health screening[89] Kingston and colleagues[100–102] conducted a large series of studies with Canadian patients and providers regarding perinatal depression screening. They found more than 90% of women surveyed indicated they were comfortable with answering screening questions, especially when provider initiated. In this important series of reports, the investigators provide several insights into the harms, barriers, and facilitators of mental health screening. In terms of potential harms of screening, the investigators noted.[100]

Table 1
Commonly used and validated self-report screening instruments for psychiatric disorders during pregnancy

Symptoms	Measure	# Items	Comments
Depression	EPDS	10	Validated for use in antenatal and postnatal depression; somatic items removed; several languages available; more evidence to date for use in perinatal symptoms than any other measure
			Does not assess irritability
	PHQ-9	9	Summary scoring or diagnostic algorithm available; commonly used in other medical settings
	PDSS	35	Validated against diagnostic criteria; developed specifically for new mothers
			Longer than other measures
	BDI-II	21	Generally thought as a gold standard depression symptom measurement
			Contains somatic symptoms; must purchase forms to use; mixed evidence as to performance in perinatal populations
	CES-D	20	Validated against diagnostic criteria
Bipolar/mania	MDQ	13	One of the only screening measures for bipolar disorder
			Adequate sensitivity and specificity in postpartum
			More information needed about appropriate perinatal use
Anxiety	STAI	20 state and 20 trait	Widely used measure of anxiety; measures transient and enduring anxiety
			State scale may inflate transient anxiety symptoms during pregnancy
	HADS-A	7	Anxiety subscale
			Has often been found to be highly correlated with the EPDS
	EPDS-3A	3	Three items from depression scale indicate anxiety; brief
			Inconsistent accuracy reported, sensitivity and specificity still unclear
	GAD-7	7	Brief anxiety screening tool commonly used in primary care settings
	OCI-R	18	High sensitivity and specificity for obsessions subscale
			Limited data for performance during pregnancy
Pregnancy-specific anxiety	PRAQ	55	Good internal reliability, covers broad range of pregnancy-related concerns
			Limited psychometric data available
	PSAS	4	Similar to STAI in specific context of pregnancy
			Inconsistent results in predicting perinatal outcomes

(continued on next page)

Table 1
(continued)

Symptoms	Measure	# Items	Comments
Posttraumatic stress disorder	PC-PTSD	4	Developed for use in VA primary care settings Assesses intrusion, avoidance, arousal, and numbing Limited psychometric data available for perinatal period
	PCL-C	17	Widely used measure with good sensitivity and specificity

Abbreviations: BDI-II, Beck Depression Inventory-II[80]; CES-D, Center for Epidemiologic Studies Depression Scale[81]; EPDS, Edinburgh Postnatal Depression Scale[82]; EPDS-3A, Edinburgh Postpartum Depression Scale 3 Anxiety Items[83]; GAD-7, Generalized Anxiety Disorder–7 item[84]; HADS-A, Hospital Anxiety and Depression Scale–Anxiety[85]; MDQ, Mood Disorder Questionnaire[86]; OCI-R, Obsessive Compulsive Inventory-Revised[87]; PCL-C, PTSD Checklist–Civilian version[88,89]; PC-PTSD, Primary Care PTSD screen[90]; PDSS, Postpartum Depression Screening Scale[91]; PHQ-9, Patient Health Questionnaire-9 item[92]; PRAQ, Pregnancy Related Anxiety Questionnaire[93]; PSAS, Pregnancy Specific Anxiety Scale[51]; STAI, State Trait Anxiety Inventory.[94]

- The screening instrument is used as diagnostic and no follow-up is provided for positive screens
- False positives
- Limited or no resources for follow-up of positive screens
- Costs
- Only one study to date has specifically examined the harms of screening for psychiatric disorders during pregnancy or postpartum[103]; in this study, no harms were indicated

Four common barriers to accurate mental health screening include[100]:

- Partner, friends, family telling women their emotions are normal
- Want to handle emotions and problems on their own
- Prefer to discuss problems with their significant others rather than health care providers
- Unclear what signals normal versus nonnormal emotions in pregnancy

These factors can be facilitators to mental health screening[100]:

- Provider relationship (providers need to be nonjudgmental, sensitive, caring, and interested)
- Provider normalizing mental health problems
- Knowing help is available
- Understanding treatment options

THE ROLE OF PSYCHOSOCIAL ASSESSMENT DURING PREGNANCY

Psychosocial assessment refers to obtaining a multidimensional picture of a woman's psychosocial circumstances.[104] This can include current and past histories of cultural, social, and psychological risk factors for mental health problems.[24] Psychosocial risk factors for poor mental health outcomes include[104]

- Past history of mental health conditions
- Inadequate social support
- Poor quality relationship with partner

- Interpersonal violence
- Stressful life events
- Poverty
- Adverse childhood experiences (physical or sexual abuse or neglect)
- Substance abuse
- Personality vulnerabilities (eg, low self-esteem)

Studies have indicated that screening for depression is important but psychosocial assessment is also needed to be able to identify and manage psychosocial needs.[105] Failure to address psychosocial needs or adverse social circumstances results in poorer treatment adherence or response.[104] Furthermore, adverse psychosocial circumstances during the perinatal period are predictive of adverse infant and childhood outcomes.[106,107]

Similar to psychiatric screening during pregnancy or postpartum, it is recommended that psychosocial assessments should be part of integrated care rather than stand-alone evaluations.[108] Comprehensive guidelines have been published in Australia to guide using psychosocial assessments in clinical practice. Key points are summarized next[104]:

- Conduct assessment as early as practical during pregnancy and 6 to 12 weeks postpartum
- Assessments can be self-report or interview
- Psychoeducation should be provided before assessment to normalize commonly experienced challenges and availability of support
- After assessment, identify the level of support likely needed and preferences of the woman
- Assist women who deny further care with obtaining relevant community supports
- Arrange follow-up care or evaluation as needed
- Suggest involvement with significant support person

FUTURE DIRECTIONS
Including Fathers

Preliminary estimates suggest between 9% and 10% of fathers during the perinatal period experience major depression and between 4% and 18% suffer from anxiety.[109,110] Detection of depression or other mental health issues in fathers has important implications for his partner, child, and the family.[111] To date, little research has focused on best practices in psychosocial or mental health screening for expectant or new fathers.[110] Studies are underway to validate screening tools that can reliably detect depression and anxiety.[112] Others are examining father-inclusive models of care in obstetric settings,[113,114] modifications of existing treatment modalities to be better tailored to the needs of fathers (see Ref.[115] for a review), and SMS messaging to deliver informational and supportive text messages and interactive mood tracking.[116]

Technology

Innovative use of new technology to optimize screening and early intervention is promising.[117] Technology has the potential to overcome barriers to screening, such as accessibility, flexibility, and convenience.[117] Online administration of several depression screening measures (Edinburgh Postnatal Depression Scale, Postpartum Depression Screening Scale, and the Patient Health Questionnaire-9 item) have been validated,[118–120] although sample sizes were small and may not be generalizable. Benefits of using text or other mobile technologies include that they are[117] easier to administer repeatedly in a more cost-efficient manner, they may provide more sensitive screening because they may disclose more compared with face-to-face interaction,[121] and they limit human error in calculating results.[122]

Challenges remain in the ability to use technology that warrants further investigation, including the best way to provide feedback and follow-up of screening results.[117] Ecological momentary assessment, repeated assessment of emotions and behaviors in real-time, has also been shown to provide more accurate and high-resolution measurement of symptoms[123] and is a promising method of assessment. Internet-based interventions for perinatal depression and anxiety are also under development.[124–126]

Alternative Delivery Models

Centering Pregnancy is a model of prenatal care in which prenatal health care is delivered in a group format.[127] A standard curriculum of 10 sessions over the course of 6-months provides participants with information about health, nutrition, breastfeeding, and weight gain.[127] Incorporating mental health education is one potential way to help decrease stigma and improve identification and treatment initiation.[4] Other investigators are exploring ways to incorporate more preventative mental health interventions based on mindfulness and stress-reduction interventions (S. Kornfield, personal communication, 2016).

SUMMARY

Perinatal psychiatric disorders are common and have significant adverse effects on mothers and their offspring. Universal screening for psychiatric disorders, particularly depression and anxiety, has been implemented in obstetric and primary care settings. However, there is little evidence regarding the effectiveness of screening on psychiatric symptom reduction or prevention of adverse outcomes in children. Recently, comprehensive screening and follow-up programs integrated within obstetric or primary care settings have shown promising results in improving maternal mental health outcomes. Future work is needed to determine the most effective and efficient ways to identify and treat mental illness in pregnant women. Innovative use of technology and alternative health care settings also hold promise.

REFERENCES

1. Stein A, Pearson RM, Goodman SH, et al. Effects of perinatal mental disorders on the fetus and child. Lancet 2014;384(9956):1800–19.
2. Goodman SH, Rouse MH, Connell AM, et al. Maternal depression and child psychopathology: a meta-analytic review. Clin Child Fam Psychol Rev 2011;14(1):1–27.
3. O'Hara MW, Wisner KL. Perinatal mental illness: definition, description and aetiology. Best Pract Res Clin Obstet Gynaecol 2014;28(1):3–12.
4. Cox EQ, Sowa NA, Meltzer-Brody SE, et al. The perinatal depression treatment cascade: baby steps toward improving outcomes. J Clin Psychiatry 2016;1189–200. http://dx.doi.org/10.4088/JCP.15r10174.
5. Siu AL. US Preventive Services Task Force (USPSTF). Screening for depression in adults: us preventive services task force recommendation statement. JAMA 2016;315(4):380–7.
6. Milgrom J, Gemmill AW. Identifying perinatal depression and anxiety: evidence-based practice in screening, psychosocial assessment and management. West Sussex (UK): John Wiley & Sons; 2015.

7. Jones TB, Bailey BA, Sokol RJ. Alcohol use in pregnancy: insights in screening and intervention for the clinician. Clin Obstet Gynecol 2013;56(1):114–23.
8. Robertson E, Grace S, Wallington T, et al. Antenatal risk factors for postpartum depression: a synthesis of recent literature. Gen Hosp Psychiatry 2004;26(4): 289–95.
9. Kessler RC. The epidemiology of depression among women. In: Keyes CLM, Goodman SH, editors. Women and depression: a handbook for the social, behavioral, and biomedical sciences. London: Cambridge University Press; 2006. p. 22–37.
10. Gavin NI, Gaynes BN, Lohr KN, et al. Perinatal depression: a systematic review of prevalence and incidence. Obstet Gynecol 2005;106(5, Part 1):1071–83.
11. Beeghly M, Olson KL, Weinberg MK, et al. Prevalence, stability, and socio-demographic correlates of depressive symptoms in black mothers during the first 18 Months postpartum. Matern Child Health J 2003;7(3):157–68.
12. Bennett HA, Einarson A, Taddio A, et al. Prevalence of depression during pregnancy: systematic review. Obstet Gynecol 2004;103(4):698–709.
13. Vesga-López O, Blanco C, Keyes K, et al. Psychiatric disorders in pregnant and postpartum women in the United States. Arch Gen Psychiatry 2008;65(7): 805–15.
14. Wisner KL, Sit DY, McShea MC, et al. Onset timing, thoughts of self-harm, and diagnoses in postpartum women with screen-positive depression findings. JAMA Psychiatry 2013;70(5):490–8.
15. Austin M-PV, Hadzi-Pavlovic D, Priest SR, et al. Depressive and anxiety disorders in the postpartum period: how prevalent are they and can we improve their detection? Arch Womens Ment Health 2010;13(5):395–401.
16. Mota N, Cox BJ, Enns MW, et al. The relationship between mental disorders, quality of life, and pregnancy: findings from a nationally representative sample. J Affect Disord 2008;109(3):300–4.
17. Sutter-Dallay AL, Giaconne-Marcesche V, Glatigny-Dallay E, et al. Women with anxiety disorders during pregnancy are at increased risk of intense postnatal depressive symptoms: a prospective survey of the MATQUID cohort. Eur Psychiatry 2004;19(8):459–63.
18. Wenzel A, Stuart S. Anxiety in childbearing women: diagnosis and treatment, vol. viii. Washington, DC: American Psychological Association; 2011.
19. Grigoriadis S, de Meschino CD, Barrons E, et al. Mood and anxiety disorders in a sample of Canadian perinatal women referred for psychiatric care. Arch Womens Ment Health 2011;14(4):325–33.
20. Seng JS, Low LMK, Sperlich M, et al. Prevalence, trauma history, and risk for posttraumatic stress disorder among nulliparous women in maternity care. Obstet Gynecol 2009;114(4):839–47.
21. Kim HG, Harrison PA, Godecker AL, et al. Posttraumatic stress disorder among women receiving prenatal care at three federally qualified health care centers. Matern Child Health J 2013;18(5):1056–65.
22. Jones I, Chandra PS, Dazzan P, et al. Bipolar disorder, affective psychosis, and schizophrenia in pregnancy and the post-partum period. Lancet 2014; 384(9956):1789–99.
23. Sit D, Rothschild AJ, Wisner KL. A review of postpartum psychosis. J Womens Health 2006;15(4):352–68.
24. Austin M-P. Marcé International Society position statement on psychosocial assessment and depression screening in perinatal women. Best Pract Res Clin Obstet Gynaecol 2014;28(1):179–87.

25. Prechtl H. Continuity and change in early neural development. In: Prechtl H, editor. Continuity in neural functions from prenatal to postnatal life. London: Cambridge University Press; 1991. p. 1–15.

26. DiPietro JA. Maternal stress in pregnancy: considerations for fetal development. J Adolesc Health 2012;51(2, Supplement):S3–8.

27. Zuckerman B, Amaro H, Bauchner H, et al. Depressive symptoms during pregnancy: relationship to poor health behaviors. Am J Obstet Gynecol 1989;160(5): 1107–11.

28. Coverdale JH, Chervenak FA, McCullough LB, et al. Ethically justified clinically comprehensive guidelines for the management of the depressed pregnant patient. Am J Obstet Gynecol 1996;174(1, Part 1):169–73.

29. Kelly RH, Zatzick DF, Anders TF. The detection and treatment of psychiatric disorders and substance use among pregnant women cared for in obstetrics. Am J Psychiatry 2001;158(2):213–9.

30. Ludman EJ, McBride CM, Nelson JC, et al. Stress, depressive symptoms, and smoking cessation among pregnant women. Health Psychol 2000;19(1):21–7.

31. Grote NK, Bridge JA, Gavin AR, et al. A meta-analysis of depression during pregnancy and the risk of preterm birth, low birth weight, and intrauterine growth restriction. Arch Gen Psychiatry 2010;67(10):1012–24.

32. Grigoriadis S, VonderPorten EH, Mamisashvili L, et al. The impact of maternal depression during pregnancy on perinatal outcomes: a systematic review and meta-analysis. J Clin Psychiatry 2013;74(04):e321–41.

33. Ding X-X, Wu Y-L, Xu S-J, et al. Maternal anxiety during pregnancy and adverse birth outcomes: a systematic review and meta-analysis of prospective cohort studies. J Affect Disord 2014;159:103–10.

34. DiPietro JA. Psychological and psychophysiological considerations regarding the maternal–fetal relationship. Infant Child Dev 2010;19(1):27–38.

35. King-Hele S, Webb RT, Mortensen PB, et al. Risk of stillbirth and neonatal death linked with maternal mental illness: a national cohort study. Arch Dis Child Fetal Neonatal Ed 2009;94(2):F105–10.

36. Webb R, Abel K, Pickles A, et al. Mortality in offspring of parents with psychotic disorders: a critical review and meta-analysis. Am J Psychiatry 2005;162(6): 1045–56.

37. Goodman SH, Rouse MH, Long Q, et al. Deconstructing antenatal depression: what is it that matters for neonatal behavioral functioning? Infant Ment Health J 2011;32(3):339–61.

38. Pawlby S, Hay DF, Sharp D, et al. Antenatal depression predicts depression in adolescent offspring: prospective longitudinal community-based study. J Affect Disord 2009;113(3):236–43.

39. Pearson RM, Evans J, Kounali D, et al. Maternal depression during pregnancy and the postnatal period: risks and possible mechanisms for offspring depression at age 18 years. JAMA Psychiatry 2013;70(12):1312–9.

40. Velders FP, Dieleman G, Henrichs J, et al. Prenatal and postnatal psychological symptoms of parents and family functioning: the impact on child emotional and behavioural problems. Eur Child Adolesc Psychiatry 2011;20(7):341–50.

41. Davis EP, Sandman CA. Prenatal psychobiological predictors of anxiety risk in preadolescent children. Psychoneuroendocrinology 2012;37(8):1224–33.

42. Van Batenburg-Eddes T, Brion MJ, Henrichs J, et al. Parental depressive and anxiety symptoms during pregnancy and attention problems in children: a cross-cohort consistency study. J Child Psychol Psychiatry 2013;54(5):591–600.

43. Plant DT, Pariante CM, Sharp D, et al. Maternal depression during pregnancy and offspring depression in adulthood: role of child maltreatment. Br J Psychiatry 2015;207(3):213–20.
44. Reck C, Müller M, Tietz A, et al. Infant distress to novelty is associated with maternal anxiety disorder and especially with maternal avoidance behavior. J Anxiety Disord 2013;27(4):404–12.
45. Feldman R, Granat A, Pariente C, et al. Maternal depression and anxiety across the postpartum year and infant social engagement, fear regulation, and stress reactivity. J Am Acad Child Adolesc Psychiatry 2009;48(9):919–27.
46. O'Connor TG, Heron J, Golding J, et al, the AL SPAC Study Team. Maternal antenatal anxiety and behavioural/emotional problems in children: a test of a programming hypothesis. J Child Psychol Psychiatry 2003;44(7):1025–36.
47. Van den Bergh BR, Mennes M, Oosterlaan J, et al. High antenatal maternal anxiety is related to impulsivity during performance on cognitive tasks in 14- and 15-year-olds. Neurosci Biobehav Rev 2005;29(2):259–69.
48. Phillips J, Sharpe L, Matthey S, et al. Maternally focused worry. Arch Womens Ment Health 2009;12(6):409–18.
49. Hofberg K, Brockington IF. Tokophobia: an unreasoning dread of childbirth. Br J Psychiatry 2000;176(1):83–5.
50. Buss C, Davis EP, Muftuler LT, et al. High pregnancy anxiety during mid-gestation is associated with decreased gray matter density in 6–9-year-old children. Psychoneuroendocrinology 2010;35(1):141–53.
51. Roescha SC, Schetter CD, Woo G, et al. Modeling the types and timing of stress in pregnancy. Anxiety Stress Coping 2004;17(1):87–102.
52. Glover V. Maternal depression, anxiety and stress during pregnancy and child outcome; what needs to be done. Best Pract Res Clin Obstet Gynaecol 2014; 28(1):25–35.
53. Sandman CA, Buss C, Head K, et al. Fetal exposure to maternal depressive symptoms is associated with cortical thickness in late childhood. Biol Psychiatry 2015;77(4):324–34.
54. Gavin NI, Meltzer-Brody S, Glover V, et al. Is population-based identification of perinatal depression and anxiety desirable?. In: Milgrom J, Gemmill AW, editors. Identifying perinatal depression and anxiety. West Sussex (UK): John Wiley & Sons, Ltd; 2015. p. 11–31. Available at: http://onlinelibrary.wiley.com/doi/10.1002/9781118509722.ch1/summary. Accessed September 28, 2016.
55. Yawn BP, LaRusso EM, Bertram SL, et al. When screening is policy, how do we make it work?. In: Milgrom J, Gemmill AW, editors. Identifying perinatal depression and anxiety. West Sussex (UK): John Wiley & Sons, Ltd; 2015. p. 32–50. http://onlinelibrary.wiley.com/doi/10.1002/9781118509722.ch2/summary. Accessed September 28, 2016.
56. Yawn BP, Dietrich AJ, Wollan P, et al. TRIPPD: a practice-based network effectiveness study of postpartum depression screening and management. Ann Fam Med 2012;10(4):320–9.
57. Gjerdingen D, Katon W, Rich DE. Stepped care treatment of postpartum depression: a primary care-based management model. Womens Health Issues 2008; 18(1):44–52.
58. Flanagan T, Avalos LA. Perinatal obstetric office depression screening and treatment: implementation in a health care system. Obstet Gynecol 2016;127(5): 911–5.

59. Venkatesh KK, Nadel H, Blewett D, et al. Implementation of universal screening for depression during pregnancy: feasibility and impact on obstetric care. Am J Obstet Gynecol 2016;215(4):517.e1-8.
60. Ayers S, Coates R, Matthey S. Identifying perinatal anxiety. In: Milgrom J, Gemmill AW, editors. Identifying perinatal depression and anxiety. West Sussex (UK): John Wiley & Sons, Ltd; 2015. p. 93–107. http://onlinelibrary.wiley.com/doi/10.1002/9781118509722.ch6/summary. Accessed September 28, 2016.
61. Miranda J, Azocar F, Komaromy M, et al. Unmet mental health needs of women in public-sector gynecologic clinics. Am J Obstet Gynecol 1998;178(2):212–7.
62. Chaudron LH, Szilagyi PG, Kitzman HJ, et al. Detection of postpartum depressive symptoms by screening at well-child visits. Pediatrics 2004;113(3):551–8.
63. Earls MF, Health TC on PA of C and F. Incorporating recognition and management of perinatal and postpartum depression into pediatric practice. Pediatrics 2010;126(5):1032–9.
64. Buist A, Condon J, Brooks J, et al. Acceptability of routine screening for perinatal depression. J Affect Disord 2006;93(1–3):233–7.
65. Glasser S, Levinson D, Bina R, et al. Primary care physicians' attitudes toward postpartum depression is it part of their job? J Prim Care Community Health 2016;7(1):24–9.
66. Tandon SD. Addressing psychosocial risk factors among families enrolled in home visitation: issues and opportunities. In: Roggman L, Cardia N, editors. Home visitation programs. Switzerland: Springer International Publishing; 2016. p. 119–34.
67. Leijten P, Shaw DS, Gardner F, et al. The family check-up and service use in high-risk families of young children: a prevention strategy with a bridge to community-based treatment. Prev Sci 2014;16(3):397–406.
68. Beardslee WR, Ayoub C, Avery MW, et al. Family connections: an approach for strengthening early care systems in facing depression and adversity. Am J Orthopsychiatry 2010;80(4):482–95.
69. Katon WJ, Lin EHB, Von Korff M, et al. Collaborative care for patients with depression and chronic illnesses. N Engl J Med 2010;363(27):2611–20.
70. Segre LS, O'Hara MW, Brock RL, et al. Depression screening of perinatal women by the des Moines healthy Start project: program description and evaluation. Psychiatr Serv 2012;63(3):250–5.
71. Nelson DB, Freeman MP, Johnson NL, et al. A prospective study of postpartum depression in 17,648 parturients. J Matern Fetal Neonatal Med 2013;26(12): 1155–61.
72. Yawn BP, Olson AL, Bertram S, et al. Postpartum depression: screening, diagnosis, and management programs 2000 through 2010. Depress Res Treat 2012;2012:e363964.
73. Truitt FE, Pina BJ, Person-Rennell NH, et al. Outcomes for collaborative care versus routine care in the management of postpartum depression. Qual Prim Care 2013;21(3):171–7.
74. Katon W, Russo J, Reed SD, et al. A randomized trial of collaborative depression care in obstetrics and gynecology clinics: socioeconomic disadvantage and treatment response. Am J Psychiatry 2014;172(1):32–40.
75. Melville JL, Reed SD, Russo J, et al. Improving care for depression in obstetrics and gynecology: a randomized controlled trial. Obstet Gynecol 2014;123(6): 1237–46.
76. O'Connor E, Rossom RC, Henninger M, et al. Primary care screening for and treatment of depression in pregnant and postpartum women: evidence report

and systematic review for the us preventive services task force. JAMA 2016; 315(4):388–406.

77. Thombs BD, Arthurs E, Coronado-Montoya S, et al. Depression screening and patient outcomes in pregnancy or postpartum: a systematic review. J Psychosom Res 2014;76(6):433–46.

78. Mann R, Evans J. Screening tools and methods of identifying perinatal depression. In: Milgrom J, Gemmill AW, editors. Identifying perinatal depression and anxiety. West Sussex (UK): John Wiley & Sons, Ltd; 2015. p. 76–92. Available at: http://onlinelibrary.wiley.com/doi/10.1002/9781118509722.ch5/summary. Accessed September 28, 2016.

79. Meades R, Ayers S. Anxiety measures validated in perinatal populations: a systematic review. J Affect Disord 2011;133(1–2):1–15.

80. Beck AT, Steer RA, Brown GK. Manual for the Beck Depression Inventory-II, vol. 1. San Antonio (TX): Psychological Corporation; 1996.

81. Radloff LS. The CES-d scale a self-report depression scale for research in the general population. Appl Psychol Meas 1977;1(3):385–401.

82. Cox J, Holden J, Henshaw C. Perinatal mental health. The Edinburgh Postnatal Depression Scale (EPDS) manual. 2nd edition. London: RCPsych Publications; 2014.

83. Matthey S. Using the Edinburgh Postnatal Depression Scale to screen for anxiety disorders. Depress Anxiety 2008;25(11):926–31.

84. Spitzer RL, Kroenke K, Williams JBW, et al. A brief measure for assessing generalized anxiety disorder: the GAD-7. Arch Intern Med 2006;166(10):1092.

85. Zigmond AS, Snaith RP. The hospital anxiety and depression scale. Acta Psychiatr Scand 1983;67(6):361–70.

86. Hirschfeld RMA, Williams JBW, Spitzer RL, et al. Development and validation of a screening instrument for bipolar spectrum disorder: the mood disorder questionnaire. Am J Psychiatry 2000;157(11):1873–5.

87. Abramowitz JS, Deacon BJ. Psychometric properties and construct validity of the Obsessive–Compulsive Inventory—revised: replication and extension with a clinical sample. J Anxiety Disord 2006;20(8):1016–35.

88. Weathers FW, Litz BT, Herman D, et al. The PTSD checklist-civilian version (PCL-C). Boston: National Center for PTSD; 1994.

89. Buist A, O'Mahen H, Rooney R. Acceptability, attitudes, and overcoming stigma. In: Milgrom J, Gemmill AW, editors. Identifying perinatal depression and anxiety. West Sussex (UK): John Wiley & Sons, Ltd; 2015. p. 51–62. Available at: http://onlinelibrary.wiley.com/doi/10.1002/9781118509722.ch3/summary. Accessed September 28, 2016.

90. Prins A, Ouimette P, Kimering R, et al. The primary care PTSD screen (PC-PTSD): development and operating characteristics. Prim Care Psychiatry 2003;9(4):9–14.

91. Beck C, Gable R. Postpartum depression screening scale: development and psychometric testing. Nurs Res 2000;49(5):272–82.

92. Kroenke K, Spitzer RL, Williams JBW. The PHQ-9. J Gen Intern Med 2001;16(9): 606–13.

93. Van den Bergh BRH. The influence of maternal emotions during pregnancy on fetal and neonatal behavior. J Prenat Perinat Psychol Health 1990;5(2):119–30.

94. Spielberger CD, Gorsuch RL, Lushene RE. Manual for the state-TRait anxiety Inventory (STAI). Palo Alto (CA): Consulting Psychologists Press; 1970.

95. Chaudron LH, Szilagyi PG, Tang W, et al. Accuracy of depression screening tools for identifying postpartum depression among urban mothers. Pediatrics 2010;125(3):e609–17.

96. Hanusa BH, Scholle SH, Haskett RF, et al. Screening for depression in the postpartum period: a comparison of three instruments. J Womens Health 2008; 17(4):585–96.

97. Tandon SD, Cluxton-Keller F, Leis J, et al. A comparison of three screening tools to identify perinatal depression among low-income African American women. J Affect Disord 2012;136(1–2):155–62.

98. Matthey S, Ross-Hamid C. Repeat testing on the Edinburgh Depression Scale and the HADS-A in pregnancy: differentiating between transient and enduring distress. J Affect Disord 2012;141(2–3):213–21.

99. Wenz-Gross M, Weinreb L, Upshur C. Screening for post-traumatic stress disorder in prenatal care: prevalence and characteristics in a low-income population. Matern Child Health J 2016;20(10):1995–2002.

100. Kingston D, Austin M-P, Heaman M, et al. Barriers and facilitators of mental health screening in pregnancy. J Affect Disord 2015;186:350–7.

101. Kingston DE, Biringer A, Toosi A, et al. Disclosure during prenatal mental health screening. J Affect Disord 2015;186:90–4.

102. Kingston DE, Biringer A, McDonald SW, et al. Preferences for mental health screening among pregnant women: a cross-sectional study. Am J Prev Med 2015;49(4):e35–43.

103. Leung SSL, Leung C, Lam TH, et al. Outcome of a postnatal depression screening programme using the Edinburgh Postnatal Depression Scale: a randomized controlled trial. J Public Health (Oxf) 2010;fdq075. http://dx.doi.org/10. 1093/pubmed/fdq075.

104. Austin M-P, Fisher J, Reilly N. Psychosocial assessment and integrated perinatal care. In: Milgrom J, Gemmill AW, editors. Identifying perinatal depression and anxiety. West Sussex (UK): John Wiley & Sons, Ltd; 2015. p. 121–38. Available at: http://onlinelibrary.wiley.com/doi/10.1002/9781118509722.ch8/summary. Accessed September 28, 2016.

105. Connelly CD, Hazen AL, Baker-Ericzén MJ, et al. Is screening for depression in the perinatal period Enough? The Co-Occurrence of depression, substance abuse, and intimate partner violence in culturally diverse pregnant women. J Womens Health 2013;22(10):844–52.

106. Carter FA, Carter JD, Luty SE, et al. Screening and treatment for depression during pregnancy: a cautionary note. Aust N Z J Psychiatry 2005;39(4):255–61.

107. Nanni V, Uher R, Danese A. Childhood maltreatment predicts unfavorable course of illness and treatment outcome in depression: a meta-analysis. Am J Psychiatry 2012;169(2):141–51.

108. Barnett B. An integrated model of perinatal care. Eur Psychiatr Rev 2011;4(2): 71–4.

109. Giallo R, D'Esposito F, Christensen D, et al. Father mental health during the early parenting period: results of an Australian population based longitudinal study. Soc Psychiatry Psychiatr Epidemiol 2012;47(12):1907–16.

110. Leach LS, Poyser C, Cooklin AR, et al. Prevalence and course of anxiety disorders (and symptom levels) in men across the perinatal period: a systematic review. J Affect Disord 2016;190:675–86.

111. Fletcher R, Garfield CF, Matthey S. Fathers' perinatal mental health. In: Milgrom J, Gemmill AW, editors. Identifying perinatal depression and anxiety. West Sussex (UK): John Wiley & Sons, Ltd; 2015. p. 165–76. Available at:

http://onlinelibrary.wiley.com/doi/10.1002/9781118509722.ch10/summary. Accessed September 28, 2016.

112. Massoudi P, Hwang CP, Wickberg B. How well does the Edinburgh Postnatal Depression Scale identify depression and anxiety in fathers? A validation study in a population based Swedish sample. J Affect Disord 2013;149(1–3):67–74.

113. Ferguson H, Gates P. Early intervention and holistic, relationship-based practice with fathers: evidence from the work of the Family Nurse Partnership. Child Fam Soc Work 2015;20(1):96–105.

114. May FS, Mclean LA, Anderson A, et al. Father participation with mothers in the Signposts program: an initial investigation. J Intellect Dev Disabil 2013;38(1):39–47.

115. O'Brien AP, McNeil KA, Fletcher R, et al. New fathers' perinatal depression and anxiety—treatment options an integrative review. Am J Mens Health 2016. http://dx.doi.org/10.1177/1557988316669047.

116. Fletcher R, May C, Wroe J, et al. Development of a set of mobile phone text messages designed for new fathers. J Reprod Infant Psychol 2016;34(5):525–34.

117. Donker T, Cuijpers P, Stanley D, et al. The future of perinatal depression identification. In: Milgrom J, Gemmill AW, editors. Identifying perinatal depression and anxiety. West Sussex (UK): John Wiley & Sons, Ltd; 2015. p. 240–55. Available at: http://onlinelibrary.wiley.com/doi/10.1002/9781118509722.ch15/summary. Accessed September 28, 2016.

118. Drake E, Howard E, Kinsey E. Online screening and referral for postpartum depression: an exploratory study. Community Ment Health J 2013;50(3):305–11.

119. Flynn HA, Sexton M, Ratliff S, et al. Comparative performance of the Edinburgh Postnatal Depression Scale and the Patient Health Questionnaire-9 in pregnant and postpartum women seeking psychiatric services. Psychiatry Res 2011; 187(1–2):130–4.

120. Le H-N, Perry DF, Sheng X. Using the internet to screen for postpartum depression. Matern Child Health J 2008;13(2):213–21.

121. Donker T, van Straten A, Marks I, et al. Brief self-rated screening for depression on the Internet. J Affect Disord 2010;122(3):253–9.

122. Matthey S, Lee C, Črnčec R, et al. Errors in scoring the Edinburgh Postnatal Depression Scale. Arch Womens Ment Health 2012;16(2):117–22.

123. Ebner-Priemer UW, Trull TJ. Ecological momentary assessment of mood disorders and mood dysregulation. Psychol Assess 2009;21(4):463–75.

124. Danaher BG, Milgrom J, Seeley JR, et al. MomMoodBooster web-based intervention for postpartum depression: feasibility trial results. J Med Internet Res 2013;15(11):e242.

125. O'Mahen H, Himle JA, Fedock G, et al. A pilot randomized controlled trial of cognitive behavioral therapy for perinatal depression adapted for women with low incomes. Depress Anxiety 2013;30(7):679–87.

126. Logsdon MC, Barone M, Lynch T, et al. Testing of a prototype Web based intervention for adolescent mothers on postpartum depression. Appl Nurs Res 2013; 26(3):143–5.

127. Xaverius PK, Grady MA. Centering pregnancy in Missouri: a system level analysis. Sci World J 2014;2014:e285386.

Assessment: The Newborn

Rachel E. Lean, PhD[a],*, Chris D. Smyser, MD[b,c,d],
Cynthia E. Rogers, MD[a,e]

KEYWORDS

- Neonate • Assessment • Neurobehavioral • Temperament
- Socioemotional impairment

KEY POINTS

- Neonatal neurobehavioral assessment is a key mechanism by which neonates with central nervous system and neurobehavioral disturbances are identified.
- Neonates with highly reactive and dysregulated neurobehavioral profiles are at greater risk of temperamental difficulties by late infancy.
- The NICU Network Neurobehavioral Scale and the Neonatal Behavioral Assessment Scale show significant associations with externalizing, internalizing, and emotion-regulation problems in early-to-middle childhood, suggesting that neonatal screening measures capture early physiologic and neurobehavioral markers related to longer-term differences in early mental health.
- Psychiatric services should be embedded in wraparound longitudinal care for at-risk newborns to support socioemotional development in the context of the caregiver-infant relationship.

INTRODUCTION

Neonatal neurobehavioral assessment has become a standardized and common component of clinical care provided to newborn infants.[1] Early editions of neonatal neurobehavioral assessments date back to the 1900s[2] and primarily emphasized

Disclosure Statement: The authors have no commercial or financial conflicts of interest. Dr C.D. Smyser is funded by the National Institutes of Health K02NS089852, UL1TR000448, U54HD087011; Cerebral Palsy International Research Foundation; and The Dana Foundation. Dr C. Rogers is funded by the National Institutes of Health NICHD K23MH105179, and KL2TR000450.
 ^a Department of Psychiatry, Washington University School of Medicine, 660 South Euclid Avenue, Campus Box 8504, St Louis, MO 63110, USA; ^b Department of Neurology, Washington University School of Medicine, 660 South Euclid Avenue, Campus Box 8111, St Louis, MO 63110, USA; ^c Department of Radiology, Washington University School of Medicine, 660 South Euclid Avenue, Campus Box 8111, St Louis, MO 63110, USA; ^d Department of Pediatrics, Washington University School of Medicine, 660 South Euclid Avenue, Campus Box 8111, St Louis, MO 63110, USA; ^e Department of Pediatrics, Washington University School of Medicine, 660 South Euclid Avenue, Campus Box 8504, St Louis, MO 63110, USA
* Corresponding author.
E-mail address: leanr@psychiatry.wustl.edu

Child Adolesc Psychiatric Clin N Am 26 (2017) 427–440
http://dx.doi.org/10.1016/j.chc.2017.02.002
1056-4993/17/© 2017 Elsevier Inc. All rights reserved.

the evaluation of central nervous system (CNS) organization and maturation.[3–6] More recent assessments include items that focus on newborn neurobehavioral development, relating the developing nervous system to functional behavior in the postnatal environment.[2,7] Strength-based neurobehavioral measures highlight the importance of assessing infant capabilities according to the infant's developmental milieu.[2,4,8,9] Neonatal neurobehavioral assessments not only guide clinical decisions regarding care in the neonatal intensive care unit (NICU) but also help to determine which infants will need longer-term support via targeted therapeutic interventions and the early involvement of specialist developmental services following hospital discharge.[4,5,8,10,11]

To determine the clinical utility of neonatal screening measures, a growing body of evidence has begun to document the extent to which neonatal assessment predicts long-term cognitive and motor outcomes.[12–14] However, less is known regarding the utility of neonatal assessments for the identification infants at risk of socioemotional impairments. As such, this article provides an overview of empirical studies linking newborn neurobehavioral assessments to socioemotional outcomes in early childhood. Given that existing reviews have already highlighted strong associations between newborn neurologic assessments and later neurodevelopmental impairments,[12,15] this article focuses on neurobehavioral assessments only.

ASSESSMENT OF THE NEWBORN

The initial mechanism by which newborns, defined as infants in the first 28 days of life, are identified as having disturbances in CNS and neurobehavioral development is through routine clinical assessment in neonatal care units.[5] In addition to detailed physical and neurologic examinations, several standardized assessments are widely available to clinicians and researchers that provide a comprehensive evaluation of the newborn's neurobehavioral capabilities. Newborn assessments typically have at least 1 of 3 primary objectives:

1. To identify high-risk infants with CNS and neurobehavioral disturbances in need of treatment and/or intervention
2. To evaluate developmental progress in response to NICU interventions and family-centered therapies
3. To prognosticate longer-term neurodevelopmental outcomes.[5,8,16]

Due to the recent increase of family-centered approaches in neonatal care, an additional objective included in some assessments concerns the evaluation of the infant in the context of the parent-infant dyad to promote infant health and the caregiving relationship.[14,17]

Neonatal Neurobehavioral Assessments

Table 1 provides a general description of established neonatal neurobehavioral assessments. Variation exists across the assessments in terms of the domains examined, test construction, and differences in administration approaches regarding infant observation and/or manipulation or handling.[4,16] Most measures, however, have a dual emphasis on the assessment of CNS functions and the neurobehavioral profile.[2,6] Systematic assessment of neonatal CNS maturity and organization involves the evaluation of primitive reflexes, spontaneous or elicited movements, and sensory behaviors.[2,4,8] Reflexive and sensory behaviors undergo rapid sequential changes in the neonatal period[4,9] and, as such, they are useful neurophysiological constructs to discriminate compromised CNS function in high-risk versus healthy neonates. In addition to CNS function, assessment of the newborn neurobehavioral profile involves the evaluation of 3 key capacities:

1. Active or passive motor activity
2. State-organization or regulation of arousal
3. Attention or interactive abilities.

The assessment of newborn neurobehavior has proven useful for the prediction of general neurodevelopmental outcomes by age 2 years, with some research suggesting potentially to a greater extent than CNS abnormalities identified by cranial ultrasound.[5]

Recently developed and commonly used neonatal neurobehavioral screening measures include the Assessment of Preterm Infants' Behavior (APIB),[18] Neurobehavioral Assessment of the Preterm Infant (NAPI),[19] Neonatal Behavioral Assessment Scale (NBAS),[20] and the NICU Network Neurobehavioral Scale (NNNS).[1] Regarding test administration, the NBAS and NNNS are similar in terms of items being administered in clusters or packages but differ in that they were created to evaluate behavior in healthy versus high-risk infants,[12] respectively. A relative strength of the NNNS is its flexible administration that takes the arousal state of the infant into account.[8] Also, from an infant-centered perspective, the NBAS focuses on behavioral strengths and views the infant as an active participant who is capable of communicating through behavior.[2,12] Of the assessments, the NNNS is considered the most comprehensive because it integrates principals and components from the NBAS, NAPI, and APIB.[12] Furthermore, a recent review found that the NNNS and APIB have strong psychometric properties that make them ideal for research purposes, whereas the NAPI demonstrates stronger clinical usefulness.[16]

The APIB, Einstein Neonatal Neurobehavioral Assessment Scale (ENNAS), NAPI, NBAS, and NNNS provide an objective quantification of infant behavior observed during the clinician-infant interaction. As family-centered developmental approaches have become integrated in NICUs, the Newborn Behavioral Observations system (NBO)[17] and Newborn Individualized Developmental Care and Assessment Program (NIDCAP)[21] were developed to evaluate the infant in the context of the caregiver-infant relationship. The NBO is a strengths-based assessment that yields an individualized description of an infant's hierarchically organized neurobehavioral capabilites.[22] Throughout the NBO, the clinician involves the parent or parents in baby-led assessments, developing handling and caregiving techniques that parents can use in the home environment to sensitively respond to infant behavioral cues. Likewise, the NIDCAP is a family-centered systems-based protocol that focuses on newborn autonomic, motor, state-organization, attention or interaction, and self-regulation systems, observed before and after caregiving.[21] The unique aspect of the NIDCAP is to provide neonatal assessment or observation in a way that is developmentally sensitive and individualized, which includes adapting the postnatal environment to accommodate the infant's threshold for sensory input and/or neurobehavioral regulatory capacities.[14]

The Neurobiological Framework of Newborn Neurobehavior

The APIB, NBAS, and NIDCAP were developed based on the synactive framework,[14] which proposes that optimal biobehavioral development depends on the integration of mature of CNS and neurobehavioral systems. Specifically, the Synactive Theory of Neonatal Behavioral Organization[23] conceptualizes infant development as the progressive organization and integration of 5 systems or domains, including physiology, motor control, state-organization or arousal, attention or interaction capabilities, and self-regulation.[22] Integrated and synchronized systems help a mature infant to

Table 1
A general description of neonatal neurobehavioral assessments

Test	General Description	Components	Age Range	Administration Time (min)	Scoring
The Assessment of Preterm Infants Behavior (APIB)	Observation of infant's responses to handling & manipulation by the clinician, emphasis on newborn behavior during interaction with the environment	Autonomic movement, motor activity, state, self-regulation, attention, interaction	28 wk postmenstrual age to 1 mo	30–60	Unstandardized; 6 main system scores derived from 81 scores; 3 status scores available for 4 of the systems: baseline, response, postintervention; percentile used for clinical cut-offs
Neurobehavioral Assessment of the Preterm Infant (NAPI)	Observation of preterm infant's responses to handling & manipulation by the clinician, assessing the functional maturity of preterm infants Limited to medically stable preterm infants	Autonomic movement, reflexes, motor vigor, state attention, irritability	32-wk postmenstrual age to term age	30	Standardized; 7 clusters assessed using 41 items; item scores, observational state ratings, & summary ratings (least mature to most mature) available; centiles used for age-norms
Neonatal Behavioral Assessment Scale (NBAS)	Observation of infant's responses to handling & manipulation by the clinician to identify functional impairment & predict outcomes	Autonomic movement, reflexes, motor activity, state, attention or interaction capabilities	36 wk postmenstrual age to 6 wk	None specified, usually around 30	Unstandardized; 6 domains; 46 items & 7 supplementary items

Newborn Behavioral Observations system (NBO)	Nursing intervention, structured observations assessing infant competencies or vulnerabilities in the context of parent-infant dyad after care-giving sessions, encourages parent education & active caregiving	Motor tone, sensory capacities (visual & auditory), activity, habituation, self-regulation (crying & consolability), response to stress, interaction capabilities	Term to 3 mo	20–30	Unstandardized; 18 items; additional postintervention interview used to assess caregiver perceptions of the NBO as a learning tool
NICU Network Neurobehavioral Scale (NNNS)	Observation of infant's responses to handling & manipulation by the clinician, identifies functional impairments in preterm & at-risk term infants	Tone, reflexes, behavior, stress or abstinence signs	30 wk postmenstrual age to 4 mo	<30	Standardized; 45 items administered in 12 packages; item scores range 1–11; items can also be clustered into 13 domain summary scores; 7 stress packages available; stress items scored yes or no

manage sensory input and regulate behavior.[9] **Fig. 1** illustrates neonatal screening focuses on the developing CNS (ie, sensory functions and reflexes) and the integrated neurobehavioral profile (ie, motor control or regulation, state-organization, attention or orientation capabilities), impairments which relate to low sensitivity thresholds or high reactivity and poor regulation in the infant.[9,24] Given the interrelated nature of newborn neurobehavioral systems, and that neonatal assessments demonstrate conceptual overlap with measures of temperament,[25] neonatal screening measures may capture some of the early neurobehavioral and physiologic alterations underlying regulation and reactivity in infancy that, in turn, relate to socioemotional development in childhood.

Neonatal Assessment and Infant Temperament

Temperament is the biologically based construct that, with environmental experience, underpins and shapes early personality traits and risks for socioemotional impairments.[26,27] Rudimentary aspects of temperament are observable within the first year of life. From 1 to 12 months old, among the infant's primary developmental tasks is to regulate behavior using basic neurophysiological modulatory mechanisms, such as disengaging from adverse stimuli and engaging in self-soothing behavior, to modulate high levels of arousal and/or distress.[9,22,28] From 9 to 12 months old, sensory-motor regulation steadily improves as motor skills mature, facilitating simple goal-directed behavior as well as the redirection of behavior when needed.[28] Because focused attention and shifting attention skills develop in parallel with sensory-motor regulation skills, infants are increasingly able to regulate reactivity and emotional distress.[28,29]

Temperament in infancy and childhood has been broadly categorized into easy and difficult dimensions defined by positive or negative affect, intensity of reactions, approach and withdrawal behaviors, and the predictability of behavior across situations.[30,31] Conceptually, models of temperament show considerable overlap with constructs included in neonatal screening measures, both often assessing state-organization or arousal, self-regulation, and attention or orientation. Concurrent relationships between neonatal assessments and maternal-report of infant temperament have been reported up to 1 month of age. In 100 mother-infant dyads, principal component analysis (PCA) was performed using the NNNS, the Early Infant Temperament Questionnaire (EITQ), and the Infant Sensory Profile (ISP).[25] Results of the PCA yielded a 3-factor model comprising sensory-affective reactivity, engagement, and state-regulation motor competence. Specific findings showed that the NNNS Regulation and Stress scales loaded onto all 3 factors, and NNNS Arousal scale loaded onto both the Sensory-Affective Reactivity and state-regulation motor competence factors. In addition, EITQ Distractibility, Activity Level, Threshold, Persistence; and ISP Low Threshold also mapped onto sensory-affective reactivity and engagement constructs. Although correlations were strongest between parent reports of infant temperament and sensory processing, the PCA results suggested a common latent structure between the NNNS, temperament, and sensory processing in early infancy.

In addition to concurrent relationships in the first month of life, neonatal screening measures also show longitudinal associations with temperament in later infancy. In a study by Tirosh and colleugues,[32] a small group of healthy neonates ($n = 40$) was assessed with the NBAS 48 to 72 hours after birth. NBAS clusters of interest included Physiologic Regulation, Motor and State Control, and Orientation and Habituation to Stimuli. The state-regulation behaviors, comprising Cuddliness and Consolability items, and the Defense subscale from the NBAS Motor cluster were strong predictors

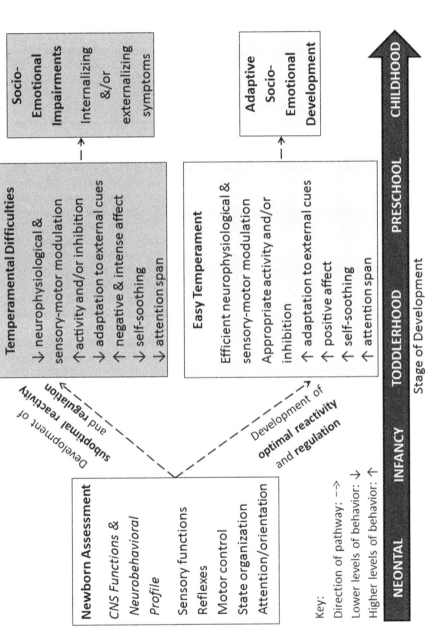

Fig. 1. A conceptual framework linking newborn assessment of CNS functions and the neurobehavioral profile to temperamental difficulties and socio-emotional impairments in childhood.

of temperament at age 4 months, explaining 57% of variance in total Infant Character-istics Questionnaire scores. As well as being an antecedent of infant temperament, neonatal neurobehavior has been found to moderate the relationship between prena-tal exposure to maternal glucocorticoids and emotion-regulation at age 6 months. Bol-ten and colleagues[33] used the NNNS to assess neonatal reactivity to stimulation at 10 to 14 days corrected age and found that high levels of reactivity moderated the asso-ciation between heightened the maternal hypothalamus-pituitary-adrenal axis activity during pregnancy and fewer infant self-soothing activities observed at age 6 months. When taken together, these studies suggest that neonatal neurobehavior relates to temperament within the first year of life and that emerging aspects of temperament may be observable within the neonatal period.

Extending findings from late infancy, neonatal screening measures have also been linked to temperament in early childhood. For example, Costa and Figueiredo[34] assessed 94 infants (80% normal and born at term) with the NBAS at 8 weeks old. Measures of social withdrawal and neuroendocrine reactivity to inoculation were also collected between 8 and 12 weeks old. Cluster analysis was used on the neuro-behavioral, social, and neuroendocrine reactivity measures, which produced 3 psy-chophysiological groups defined as Withdrawn, Extroverted, and Underaroused. Costa and Figueiredo[34] then compared these 3 groups across the maternal-report In-fant Behavior Questionnaire (IBQ) at 1-year follow-up. Findings showed that the With-drawn group had significantly lower activity level ratings on the IBQ than the Extroverted group, and the Underaroused group had lower perceptual sensitivity ratings on the IBQ compared to the Withdrawn group. Findings highlight that maternal perceptions of infant temperament varied as a function of neonatal psycho-physiological profile, suggesting that the NBAS may capture some of the early neuro-behavioral and physiologic alterations related to differences in temperament.

Also using the NBAS, Canals and colleagues[35] examined prospective associations between the NBAS administered at 3 and 30 days old in a sample of healthy infants ($n = 72$), and temperament outcomes to age 6 years. Findings showed significant cor-relations between the NBAS and parent-ratings on the Infant Behavior Record at ages 4 and 12 months and the Dimensions of Temperament Survey, Revised, at age 6 years, though some correlations were modest. Interestingly, NBAS Autonomic Nervous Sys-tem (ANS) stability predicted affect at age 4 months and attention at age 12 months, whereas NBAS state-regulation predicted affect at 4 months and general activity at age 6 years. Furthermore, NBAS Endurance scores related to general activity and persistence or attention at age 6 years. When taken together, the findings of Costa and Figueiredo[34] and Canals and colleagues[35] indicate that the NBAS demonstrates relationships with temperament up to age 6 years. In particular, ANS stability and state-regulation may be relatively stable markers of temperament, highlighting devel-opmental continuity within these constructs.

Neonatal Assessment and Socioemotional Impairments in Childhood

As previously outlined, follow-up studies have reported associations between neonatal neurobehavioral development and temperament in childhood.[35,36] Temper-ament is, in turn, a good marker of the regulatory and affective problems that underlie socioemotional problems in childhood.[27,37–40] Thus, neonatal neurobehavioral screening may help identify infants at-risk of socioemotional impairments in child-hood.[39,41] Socioemotional impairments, including internalizing and externalizing prob-lems, are commonly assessed using dimensional screening tools such as the Child Behavior Checklist (CBCL) and the Strengths and Difficulties Questionnaire (SDQ).[42] For example, a large cohort of infants ($n = 1248$) was assessed with the NNNS at

1 month of age as part of a longitudinal study by Liu and colleagues.[43] Results of latent class analysis indicated that 5.8% of study infants were characterized by an extremely negative NNNS profile. These infants obtained the poorest NNNS scores for attention with handling, self-regulation, hypotonicity, nonoptimal and asymmetric reflexes, quality of movement, and stress abstinence signs. Infants in the extremely negative NNNS profile group had significantly higher odds ratios for externalizing (2.05), internalizing (2.72), and total problems (2.37) on the CBCL relative to the other NNNS profile groups at age 3 years, after adjusting for gestational age and socioeconomic status. In a sample of cocaine-exposed infants ($n = 360$), structural equation modeling similarly showed sequential relationships between the NNNS administered at 1 month of age and temperament at age 4 months, which was, in turn, predictive of CBCL Externalizing, Internalizing, and Total Problem scores at age 3 years.[39]

Like the NNNS, the NBAS demonstrates significant associations with the CBCL[44,45] and the SDQ[46] at follow-up. Canals, Esparó, and Fernández-Ballart[44] examined the extent to which clusters of the NBAS, administered at ages 3 days and 4 weeks old in healthy infants ($n = 80$), predicted CBCL Internalizing and Externalizing Problem scores at age 6 years. Findings showed that lower Orientation and higher Motor and Habituation cluster scores on day 3 of life predicted externalizing outcomes, whereas lower Habituation cluster scores at age 4 weeks predicted internalizing outcomes. Results were adjusted for mother's employment status and mental health and infant birthweight and sex. Another study found that the NBAS administered at 40 and 44 weeks postmenstrual age was able to correctly identify around 75% and 95% of clinical versus normal ratings on the Total Difficulties scale of the SDQ at age 7 to 8 years, respectively.[46]

In contrast, a more recent longitudinal study[45] of preterm infants born 25 to 35 weeks gestational age without perinatal complications or high-grade brain injury, reported that an NBAS composite score comprising the State and Regulation of State clusters did not significantly relate to CBCL Total Problem scores at age 10 years. Feldman[45] instead found that the NBAS composite score was correlated with children's levels of cognitive and emotional empathy, assessed via direct observation and self-ratings of emotional responses. Differences in methodological approaches might account for the discrepancy in results. Whereas Canals, Esparó, and Fernández-Ballart[44] examined individual associations between each of the NBAS clusters and scales of the CBCL, Feldman[45] examined an NBAS composite cluster score in relation to Total Problems on the CBCL. Thus, the extent to which the NBAS predicts internalizing, externalizing, or combined adjustment problems in childhood remains unclear.

Summary

When taken together, findings of existing studies suggest that neonatal neurobehavioral assessments may be useful for early identification of infants at-risk for socioemotional impairments in early childhood. Consistent links were found between less optimal performance on neonatal screening measures and poorer temperament outcomes.[32,34,35,39] In addition to temperamental difficulties increasing risks of socioemotional problems,[27,28,30,39,40] there was evidence for direct associations between newborn NBAS and NNNS assessments and externalizing[46] and internalizing[43,44] outcomes in childhood. Although a study[45] did not find a longitudinal relationship with combined externalizing and internalizing outcomes, they did report an association with emotional empathy, which is a component of socioemotional development.[47] Therefore, although newborn assessments have traditionally been developed from the disciplines of medicine, behavioral pediatrics, and occupational therapy,[25] the inclusion of mental health perspectives is also needed to address the increased risk of socioemotional problems among highly reactive and dysregulated infants.

Conceptually, the findings of the reviewed studies support existing models of temperament and developmental continuity. Several study findings were consistent with Rothbart's model of temperament,[29] which highlights reactivity and regulation as the central tenants underlying individual differences in activity or impulsivity, effortful-control, and attention. For example, neonates with lower levels of ANS stability and state-regulation were more likely to be perceived as fussy, poorly regulated, and/or highly reactive toddlers; and, in turn, be rated more highly on measures of socioemotional problems in childhood.[32,35,45] Similarly, neonates who had poorer state-regulation and motor activity, were viewed as unpredictable and highly active in early childhood and subsequently rated at risk of externalizing problems.[44,46] The apparent developmental continuity between neonatal behavior, temperament, and socioemotional problems indicates that aspects of neonatal neurobehavioral and socioemotional development may be longitudinally expressed components of the same phenotype, and thus stable, within early childhood.[26,48]

In addition to developmental continuity, patterns of heterotypic continuity were found in some studies.[32,35,44] These studies found that a specific component of neonatal neurobehavior was related to a range of socioemotional outcomes in early childhood. For example, a study found NBAS ANS stability predicted both affective and attention outcomes within the first year of life[35] and another study found that NBAS Habituation scores predicted internalizing and externalizing problems at age 6 years.[44] Heterotypic continuity between early neonatal behavior and various socioemotional outcomes occurs when an innate characteristic (eg, the capacity for regulation) underlies a set of conceptually related outcomes (eg, emotional regulation, inhibitory control).[35,48] As such, specific aspects of neonatal behavior may be useful markers for a diverse range of socioemotional problems in childhood.

Although neonatal screening demonstrates developmental continuity with socioemotional outcomes, several issues remain. First, many of the reported associations between neonatal and socioemotional development were established using correlation[35,45] or linear regression methods.[32,39] Although this provides insight on the nature of relations between neonatal and socioemotional measures, it is difficult to determine the extent of agreement between these measures in terms of caseness. To the knowledge of the authors, only 2 studies reported classification agreement between neonatal assessment and socioemotional measures using estimated coefficients from logistic regression.[44,46] Specificity or sensitivity approaches seem to be more common in studies evaluating the validity of neonatal assessment for later motor and cognitive impairments.[4,13,15] As such, there may be some benefit in applying sensitivity or specificity approaches to similarly evaluate the prognostic accuracy of neonatal screening for socioemotional outcomes. Second, methodological differences between studies may explain mixed findings. Regarding the NBAS and NNNS, some studies examined the utility of cluster scores,[32,35,43,44] composite or latent summary scores,[39,45] or study-specific total item summary scores.[34,46] Differences were also noted in terms of the use of individual CBCL Externalizing and Internalizing Problem scales[43,44] or the overall Total Problem scales[45] as outcome measures. Additional research is needed to elucidate specific relationships between neonatal neurobehavioral and socioemotional subscales to determine if neonatal makers are more sensitive to particular socioemotional domains. Future research should also consider evaluating the utility of neonatal assessments besides the NBAS and NNNS, and link findings beyond CBCL and SDQ symptom screening measures to clinical evaluations of child psychopathology.

CLINICAL APPLICATIONS

Despite methodological differences across studies, neonatal neurobehavioral measures seem to capture emerging indicators of reactivity and regulation problems that lead to socioemotional difficulties as early as the newborn period. Based on neonatal screening results, at-risk infants and their families may benefit from embedded child mental health surveillance and intervention provided as part of long-term follow-up after nursery discharge.[49] Strategies to monitor and support early socioemotional outcomes among at-risk infants include the promotion of infant capabilities within the context of the mother–child dyad.

Family-centered neonatal interventions, such as the NBO and NIDCAP, help parents transition to the caregiving role and promote parenting efficacy. Short-term preliminary findings show that the NBO supports the transition to motherhood,[50] reduces postpartum depression symptoms,[51] and promotes quality caregiving among mothers of high-risk infants.[52] Importantly, these interventions help parents recognize and interpret infant behavioral cues and respond to the infant's needs in a timely and sensitive manner.[21,22] Interventions that enhance caregiving-sensitivity and attachment-based parenting have been shown to promote behavioral and cognitive resiliency in at-risk infants and children.[53,54] Although a recent meta-analysis did not find any evidence to suggest that the NIDCAP protocol improves long-term neurosensory, motor, and cognitive outcomes in preterm infants,[14] socioemotional outcomes were not assessed. Thus, NIDCAP may still improve the goodness-of-fit in parent–infant dyads and, in turn, support the development of infant temperament and emotion regulation.[24,55] Of note, a systematic Cochrane review evaluating the NBO and NBAS as interventions that improve a wide range of caregiver and infant outcomes is currently underway.[56]

SUMMARY

Neonatal neurobehavioral screening measures assess CNS functions in conjunction with the neurobehavioral profile of the newborn. Almost all newborn assessments evaluate sensory behavior, reflexes, motor control, state-organization, and attention or interactive capabilities. In high-risk neonates, neonatal neurobehavioral assessments demonstrate clinical utility for the identification of neurosensory, cognitive, and motor impairments in childhood. When used in the same fashion, neonatal screening measures also seem to capture some of the early physiologic and neurobehavioral markers related to longer-term differences in temperament and socioemotional development, due to the (1) conceptual overlap between neonatal and socioemotional outcome measures and (2) developmental continuity in reactivity and regulatory behaviors. Therefore, assessment of the newborn's neurobehavior can inform preventative interventions that target high-risk mother–infant dyads to better support infant socioemotional development and alter trajectories to prevent childhood psychiatric disorders.

REFERENCES

1. Lester BM, Tronick E. Behavioral assessment scales: the NICU Network Neurobehavioral Scale, the Neonatal Behavioral Assessment Scale, and the Assessment Of The Preterm Infant's Behavior. In: Singer LT, Zeskind PS, editors. Biobehavioral assessment of the infant; 2001. New York: Guilford Press; 2001. p. 363–80.
2. Brown N, Spittle A. Neurobehavioral evaluation in the preterm and term infant. Curr Pediatr Rev 2014;10:65–72.

3. Morgan AM, Koch V, Lee V, et al. Neonatal neurobehavioral examination. Phys Ther 1988;68:1352–8.

4. El-Dib M, Massaro AN, Glass P, et al. Neurodevelopmental Assessment of the Newborn: an opportunity for prediction of outcome. Brain Dev 2011;33:95–105.

5. Gardner JM, Karmel BZ, Freedland RL, et al. Arousal, attention, and neurobehavioral assessment in the neonatal period: implications for intervention and policy. J Policy Pract Intellect Disabil 2006;3:22–32.

6. Majnemer A, Mazer B. Neurologic evaluation of the newborn infant: definition and psychometric properties. Dev Med Child Neurol 1998;40:708–15.

7. Hammock EA, Levitt P. The Discipline of Neurobehavioral Development: the emerging interface of processes that build circuits and skills. Hum Dev 2006; 49:294–309.

8. Majnemer A, Snider L. A comparison of developmental assessments of the newborn and young infant. Ment Retard Dev Disabil Res Rev 2005;11:68–73.

9. Vandenberg KA. Individualized developmental care for high risk newborns in the NICU: a practice guideline. Early Hum Dev 2007;83:433–42.

10. Berenbaum SA. Neuropsychological follow-up in neonatal screening: issues, methods and findings. Acta Paediatr Suppl 1999;88:83–7.

11. Calciolari G, Montirosso R. Neonatal neurobehavioral assessment in healthy and at-risk infants. Early Hum Dev 2013;89:S58–9.

12. El-Dib M, Massaro AN, Glass P, et al. Neurobehavioral assessment as a predictor of neurodevelopmental outcome in preterm infants. J Perinatol 2012;32:299–303.

13. Harijan P, Beer C, Glazebrook C, et al. Predicting developmental outcomes in very preterm infants: validity of a neonatal neurobehavioral assessment. Acta Paediatr 2012;101:e275–81.

14. Ohlsson A, Jacobs SE. NIDCAP: a systematic review and meta-analyses of randomized controlled trials. Pediatrics 2013;131:e881–93.

15. Craciunoiu O, Holsti L. A systematic review of the predictive validity of neurobehavioral assessments during the preterm period. Phys Occup Ther Pediatr 2016; 00:1–16.

16. Noble Y, Boyd R. Neonatal assessments for the preterm infant up to 4 Months corrected age: a systematic review. Dev Med Child Neurol 2012;54:129–39.

17. Nugent KJ, Keefer CH, Minear S, et al. Understanding newborn behavior and early relationships: the Newborn Behavioral Observations (NBO) system handbook. Baltimore (MD): Brookes; 2007.

18. Als H, Butler S, Kosta S, et al. The Assessment of Preterm Infants' Behavior (APIB): furthering the understanding and measurement of neurodevelopmental competence in preterm and full-term infants. Ment Retard Dev Disabil Res Rev 2005;11:94–102.

19. Korner AF, Thom VA. Neurobehavioral Assessment of the Preterm Infant (NAPI). San Antonio (TX): The Psychological Corporation; 1990.

20. Brazelton TB, Nugent JK. Neonatal Behavioral Assessment Scale. Cambridge (MA): Cambridge University Press; 1995.

21. Westrup B. Newborn Individualized Developmental Care and Assessment Program (NIDCAP): family-centered developmentally supportive care. Early Hum Dev 2007;83:443–9.

22. Nugent KJ. The Newborn Behavioural Observation (NBO) system as a form of intervention. Zero Three 2015;36:2–10.

23. Als H. Toward a Synactive Theory of Development: promise for the assessment and support of infant individuality. Infant Ment Health 1982;3:229–43.

24. Keenan K. Emotion dysregulation as a risk factor for child psychopathology. Clin Psychol Sci Pract 2000;7:418–34.
25. DeSantis A, Harkins D, Tronick E, et al. Exploring an Integrative Model of Infant Behavior: what is the relationship among temperament, sensory processing, and neurobehavioral measures? Infant Behav Dev 2011;34:280–92.
26. Bornstein MH, Putnick DL, Gartstein MA, et al. Infant Temperament: stability by age, gender, birth order, term status, and socioeconomic status. Child Dev 2015;86:844–63.
27. Derauf C, LaGasse L, Smith L, et al. Infant temperament and high risk environment relate to behavior problems and language in toddlers. J Dev Behav Pediatr 2011;32:125–35.
28. Berger A, Kofman O, Livneh U, et al. Multidisciplinary perspectives on attention and the development of self-regulation. Prog Neurobiol 2007;82:256–86.
29. Rothbart MK, Posner MI, Kieras J. Temperament, attention, and the development of self-regulation. In: McCartney K, Phillips D, editors. Handbook of early childhood development. Malden (MA): Blackwell Publishing; 2006. p. 338–57.
30. Wasserman RC, DiBlasio CM, Bond LA, et al. Infant temperament and school age behavior: 6-year longitudinal study in a pediatric practice. Pediatrics 1990;85:801–7.
31. Rothbart MK, Chew KH, Gartstein MA. Assessment of temperament in early development. In: Singer LT, Zeskind PS, editors. Biobehavioural assessment of the infant. New York: Guilford Press; 2001. p. 190–208.
32. Tirosh E, Harel J, Abadi J, et al. Relationship between neonatal behavior and subsequent temperament. Acta Paediatr 1992;81:829–31.
33. Bolten M, Nast I, Skrundz M, et al. Prenatal Programming of Emotion Regulation: neonatal reactivity as a differential susceptibility factor moderating the outcome of prenatal cortisol levels. J Psychosom Res 2013;75:351–7.
34. Costa R, Figueiredo B. Infant's psychophysiological profile and temperament at 3 and 12 months. Infant Behav Dev 2011;34:270–9.
35. Canals J, Hernández-Martínez C, Fernández-Ballart JD. Relationships between early behavioural characteristics and temperament at 6 years. Infant Behav Dev 2011;34:152–60.
36. Rueda MR, Rothbart MK. The influence of temperament on the development of coping: the role of maturation and experience. New Dir Child Adolesc Dev 2009;124:19–31.
37. Sentse M, Veenstra R, Lindenberg S, et al. Buffers and risks in temperament and family for early adolescent dsychopathology: generic, conditional, or domain-specific effects? The trails study. Dev Psychol 2009;45:419–30.
38. Zentner MR. Temperament, Psychological Development and Psychopathology. Correlations, explanatory models and forms of intervention. Z Klin Psychol Psychopathol Psychother 1993;41:43–68.
39. Lester BM, Bagner DM, Liu J, et al. Infant neurobehavioral dysregulation related to behavior problems in children with prenatal substance exposure. Pediatrics 2009;124:1355–62.
40. Eisenberg N, Cumberland A, Spinrad T, et al. The relations of regulation and emotionality to Children's externalizing and internalizing problem behavior. Child Dev 2001;72:1112–34.
41. Eiden RD, Coles CD, Schuetze P, et al. Externalizing behavior problems among polydrug cocaine-exposed children: indirect pathways via maternal harshness and self-regulation in early childhood. Psychol Addict Behav 2014;28:139–53.

42. Warnick EM, Bracken MB, Kasl S. Screening efficiency of the Child Behavior Checklist and Strengths and Difficulties Questionnaire: a systematic review. Child Adolesc Ment Health 2008;13:140–7.
43. Liu J, Bann C, Lester B, et al. Neonatal neurobehavior predicts medical and behavioral outcome. Pediatrics 2010;125:e90–8.
44. Canals J, Esparó G, Fernández-Ballart JD. Neonatal behaviour characteristics and psychological problems at 6 years. Acta Paediatr 2006;95:1412–7.
45. Feldman R. Mutual influences between child emotion regulation and parent–child reciprocity support development across the first 10 years of life: implications for developmental psychopathology. Dev Psychopathol 2015;27:1007–23.
46. Ohgi S, Takahashi T, Nugent JK, et al. Neonatal behavioral characteristics and later behavioral problems. Clin Pediatr 2003;42:679–86.
47. Thompson RA. Empathy and emotional understanding: the early development of empathy. In: Eisenberg N, Strayer J, editors. Empathy and it's development. New York: Cambridge University Press; 1987. p. 119–45.
48. Caspi A, Roberts BW. Personality development across the life course: the argument for change and continuity. Psychol Inq 2001;12:49–66.
49. Cooper LG, Gooding JS, Gallagher J, et al. Impact of family-centered care initiative on NICU care, staff, and families. J Perinatol 2007;27:S32–7.
50. Cheetham NB, Hanssen TA. The Neonatal Behavioral Observation System: a tool to enhance the transition to motherhood. Nord J Nurs Res 2014;34:48–52.
51. Nugent JK, Bartlett JD, Valim C. Effects of an infant-focused relationship-based hospital and home visiting intervention on reducing symptoms of postpartum maternal depression: a pilot study. Infants Young Child 2014;27:292–304.
52. McManus BM, Nugent JA. A neurobehavioral intervention incorporated into a state early intervention Program is associated with higher perceived quality of care among parents of high-risk newborns. J Behav Health Serv Res 2014;41:381–9.
53. Bakermans-Kranenburg MJ, van IJzendoorn MH, Juffer F. Less is More: meta-analyses of sensitivity and attachment interventions in early childhood. Psychol Bull 2003;129:195–215.
54. Jaffee SR. Sensitive, stimulating caregiving predicts cognitive and behavioral resilience in neurodevelopmentally at-risk infants. Dev Psychopathol 2007;19:631–47.
55. van den Akker AL, Deković M, Prinzie P, et al. Toddlers' Temperament Profiles: stability and relations to negative and positive parenting. J Abnorm Child Psychol 2010;38:485–95.
56. Bartram SC, Barlow J, Wolke D. The Neonatal Behavioral Assessment Scale (NBAS) and Newborn Behavioral Observations system (NBO) for supporting caregivers and improving outcomes in caregivers and their infants. Cochrane Database Syst Rev 2015;6:1–14.

Clinical Assessment of Young Children

Melissa Middleton, PhD, Anna Kelley, PsyD, Mary Margaret Gleason, MD*

KEYWORDS

- Assessment • Early childhood • Diagnosis • Observation • Evaluation

KEY POINTS

- Assessment of young children requires a developmentally specific approach that includes explicit evaluation of qualities of the parent-child relationship.
- Evaluation process should include structured and informal observations that allow for a range of interactions and situations.
- Paper and pencil measures can offer information from multiple providers.

INTRODUCTION

Mental health assessment of young children provides valuable information to shape a formulation and guide treatment. Early childhood mental health assessment can occur in an increasing number of settings beyond traditional mental health practices, including childcare settings, primary care settings, and other innovative settings where children and family are seen.[1] Although many of the components of an early childhood mental health assessment are included in the assessment of older children, assessment of very young children requires some specific developmental adjustments and additional considerations.

Contexts of Early Childhood Mental Health Assessment

In early childhood mental health, the parent-child relationship is the central context of development and clinical status. The relational focus in early childhood mental health is explicit and a formulation invariably includes attention to caregiving as a factor contributing to risk or promoting resilience. This caregiving relationship predicts a diverse set of outcomes, including emotional regulation, peer relationships, cognitive development, disruptive behaviors, as well as physical outcomes such as obesity.[2–4] Attention to this relationship is therefore critical in understanding children's clinical presentation and developing effective treatment plans.

Department of Psychiatry and Behavioral Sciences, Tulane University School of Medicine, 1430 Tulane Avenue, #8055, New Orleans, LA 70115, USA
* Corresponding author.
E-mail address: mgleason@tulane.edu

Child Adolesc Psychiatric Clin N Am 26 (2017) 441–454
http://dx.doi.org/10.1016/j.chc.2017.02.003
childpsych.theclinics.com

The broader context of each child's experience, especially as defined by the presence of supportive structures or early adversity, also has the potential to shape the child's development and is assessed. Children's individual adverse experiences, including exposure to domestic violence, maltreatment, and inconsistent parenting, predict psychiatric diagnoses and other adverse mental health outcomes.[5] Factors that influence the family system, including parental psychiatric disorders and substance use, incarceration, and physical illnesses, can affect parents' emotional and physical availability and can influence health outcomes.[6] Beyond the family, quality of out-of-home childcare, neighborhood experience, and community isolation also play a role in children's development and can be associated mental health problems.[7] It is important to emphasize that exposure to healthy caregivers and caregiving environments can increase the likelihood of positive outcomes.[8]

The caregiving contexts likely influence children's experience directly and indirectly through complex interactions with biological factors that may differ based on genes and epigenetic processes.[9]

Diagnostic Systems

Despite efforts to increase the developmental sensitivity in the Diagnostic and Statistical Manual of Mental Disorders, Fifth Edition (DSM-V), neither the DSM nor the International Classification of Diseases (ICD) systems offer a full diagnostic approach to children less than 5 years old.[10,11] These nosologies intentionally focus on the individual without opportunities to define disorders in relationships or context, as reflected in the elimination of axis IV in DSM-V. DSM-V attempted to incorporate more developmentally specific criteria, such as those for posttraumatic stress disorder, reactive attachment disorder, and disinhibited social engagement disorder, but clinical presentations in infants and preschoolers still must be extrapolated for most disorders. The DC:0–5 (Diagnostic Classification of Mental Health and Developmental Disorders of Infancy and Early Childhood) system includes empirically derived diagnostic criteria for infants, toddlers, and preschoolers, derived from empirical literature and extensive international clinical experience.[12] Crosswalks between this system and billable nosologies are available as part of the nosology.

Developmentally Specific Context

The developmental capacities of very young children require developmentally specific assessment approaches beyond the usual history and observation used in typical child and adolescent psychiatric evaluations. Toddlers and preschoolers express themselves through a combination of language, play, and creative activities, giving observations an important role. In addition, the assessment depends substantially on information from adults. Adults necessarily report through the lens of their own perceptions, which are influenced by past relationships, psychiatric disorders, and other factors.[13,14] Thus, assessment includes direct interview as well as indirect means of assessment that elicit information about internal working models. Because children have distinctly different relationships with different adults, it is imperative to consider perspectives from multiple caregivers.[15] Because of the complexity of the data necessary for a comprehensive early childhood mental health assessment, multiple professional perspectives can also be valuable. Because culture shapes parenting, clinicians should be aware of their own cultural lenses throughout the assessment as well as the patient's cultural practices.

THE ASSESSMENT PROCESS
Planning for the Appointment

Assessments should include time with parents and children together with opportunities to observe the parent-child interactions, and time alone with the adult, allowing sensitive history taking about the pregnancy, parental relationships, and trauma experiences without exposing the child to negative content or extremes of parental affect. Because most children and parents are not sure what to expect at an early childhood mental health assessment, it is useful to orient them to the structure of the appointments. It is true in all settings, but particularly in early childhood mental health, that open-ended questions and strength-based reflections can promote a supportive environment during the assessment.

Taking the History

As with older children, the chief complaint should be elicited from both the parent and the child of about 36 months or more. This process gives insight into the child's experience and allows clarification about common misconceptions, such as concern about needles, and to reframe negative attributions, such as that the child was brought because the child is bad.

The structure of the history of present illness in an early childhood mental health assessment is similar to that in older children. The assessment should explore the precipitants to the symptom development, symptom duration, intensity, parental/other adults' responses, factors that exacerbate the symptoms, and how they resolve. Throughout the history, it is important to consider the symptoms in the developmental context of the particular child. Impairment is an important characteristic that allows clinicians to differentiate between clinical disorders and normative behaviors. Impairment can occur within the child, such as inability to participate in developmentally typical activities, and in the family. For example, a child's separation anxiety can cause impairment by resulting in a mother not being able to keep a job she loves in order to avoid separations. The child may not appear to be impaired, but the significant accommodations should be considered impairing.

All symptoms should be assessed for relationship or context specificity compared with generalized presentation across multiple relationships or contexts of life. In young children, patterns of behavior that occur within a single relationship may be better characterized as relationship-specific problems, as they are in DC:0–5, than as disorders within the child.[15]

Review of systems

Because so many disorders may present with similar chief complaints (commonly dysregulated emotions or behaviors), it is critical to include most domains of problems in the review of systems, including fears and anxiety, mood regulation, social reciprocity, response to sensory inputs, developmental level (especially communication), sleep, and feeding. Compliance with rules and authority, activity level, attentional capacity, stereotyped behavior patterns, compulsions, and attachment behaviors are part of the psychiatric review of systems. Physical review of systems should include growth trajectory as well as central nervous system signs or symptoms in all children. Specific physical signs and symptoms should be explored to the extent they correlate with the clinical presentation. For example, pain or sleep apnea should be considered in children with unexplained irritability or dysregulation and limited verbal communication.

Medical history

A medical history in a mental health evaluation begins preconception, and includes the pregnancy and details of the delivery to yield information about biological risks from medical complications and teratogens, experiences shaping parent perceptions of the child, and the family's environmental risk factors. Perinatal events all contribute to the understanding of the child's medical status and the parent's narrative about the child. Beyond delivery, common medical problems, including reflux, reactive airways disease or asthma, injuries resulting in fractures or lacerations, lead exposure, and central nervous system injuries or disorders all warrant attention. Such conditions may influence development through direct effects on the brain or body; effects of medications; indirect effects of the disorder, such as social isolation for immunologic suppression or inability to participate with other children in normative activities; or through impacts on parents' emotions or employment status. In addition, these illnesses influence the parental perception of the child, potentially resulting in increased resilience or increased risk through disengagement or overprotection.

Developmental history

An assessment addresses development across multiple domains, including language, fine and gross motor, social communication, self-help, and preschool readiness skills to understand the distribution of developmental levels as well as global level.

Family history

As with older children, family history contributes to children's development directly through genetics in early childhood and through the caregiving environment. A substantial literature highlights the influence of maternal depression on children's development, beginning with neonatal outcomes and through the lifespan, and paternal depression can also be influential.[16,17] Clinicians consider how caregivers' symptoms may influence parenting. Parental physical conditions may also influence caregiving patterns or emotional availability through pain, medication effects, or anxiety/distress. A multigeneration history allows for further exploration of the parents' own caregiving histories, including family interpersonal violence and caregiving separations.

Social history

The social history for a young child includes attention to each level of the child's caregiving environment: the primary caregiving environment, the extended family and out-of-home caregiving environment, as well as the neighborhood context. Attention to factors described earlier that promote resilience as well as those that may influence risk can be helpful in developing the formulation. A history can begin with stressors identified in the Adverse Childhood Experiences Study, but history also includes a broader definition of both supportive factors and resilience factors.[6]

UNSTRUCTURED OBSERVATIONS

A wealth of information can be gained through observation of the young child, including, but not limited to, observation of the child and the child's behavior, observation of the interactions between the child and caregiver, and observation of the child's behavior toward the clinician. The duration of contact with the young child and the caregiver is an opportunity to gather relevant clinical data through observation. Informal observation begins on first contact with the child, often in the waiting room, where it can be helpful to observe physical proximity, parent-child interactions, and child interactions with others.[18]

The initial introduction to the clinician offers a valuable opportunity to observe the child with an unfamiliar adult. This event should activate the attachment system and trigger referencing or seeking proximity to a caregiver, shown by eye contact, verbalizations, and physical approach. Red flags might include lack of social referencing or indiscriminate behavior (eg, embracing or seeking comfort from the clinician). Observations begin walking from the waiting room, including the child's gait, activity level, and ability to follow directions. The waiting room greeting represents just the first step in the assessment and all observations should be further assessed.

Throughout the assessment, context-specific factors, including anxiety related to being in an unknown environment, the child's sleep status, the child's nap time with respect to the time of day, and any medications the child is taking, may influence interpretation. Differences in responsiveness to the caregiver or clinician should be noted, because they may reflect qualities of the parent-child relationship and the degree to which the symptoms generalize.

Mental Status Examination

Appearance
Any signs of dysmorphology should be noted, including specific features related to prenatal exposure to substances, such as fetal alcohol syndrome, as well as possible genetic syndromes.[19] Size for age should be noted as a marker of potential genetic or endocrine conditions, or of nutritional sufficiency, insufficiency, or excessive caloric intake. Clothing in young children often represents a parent's judgment, attention to caregiving, or resources. Scars or bruises may indicate past or present injuries, including possible maltreatment.

Behavior
Stereotypical movements (eg, hand flapping) may represent signs of an autism spectrum disorder or sensory deficit. Tics, including motor and vocal patterns, should be observed. Eye contact, between the child and caregiver as well as the child and the clinician, provides information about the parent-child relationship, the child's social skills, and possible signs of an autism spectrum disorder. The child's level of exploration should be noted, as should affective reactions to any transitions and novelty, including excitement and curiosity, or with fear, avoidance, or indifference as indices of flexibility. In addition, frustration tolerance can be observed through naturally frustrating experiences or limit setting. Activity level, impulse control, and attention span can be observed throughout the observation, with careful consideration of the child's age and developmental level and the context of the assessment. Behavioral observations may not be representative of a child's patterns in other contexts.

Speech
Noting vocalizations and speech throughout the interview process is an additional component of a mental status examination with young children, and includes prosody, volume, and comprehensibility, as well as repetitive verbalizations. This process provides clinicians with information regarding the child's developmental level, cognitive functioning, and any possible speech delays, anxiety patterns, or autism spectrum disorder.

Mood and affect
Throughout the initial meeting, the clinician attends to the young child's stated mood and range of affect. In typically developing children around 3 years of age, children may be able to identify some emotions, often with the help of feeling charts, drawings, or puppets. How the child expresses emotions (including verbalizations, facial

expressions, and body language) and the level of intensity and range of the emotional expression should be observed. Fear responses and their triggers inform clinicians' understanding of anxiety. Observed anhedonia is of particular note because it is unusual in this age group.

Thought content

Play can offer valuable insight into children's thought content, as well as thought process, and cognitive development. Beginning at 24 months, children may express relevant thematic content through their play, offering a window into the children's life experiences or preoccupations. Nonfunctional repetitive play may reflect autism spectrum disorder, whereas repetitive functional play characterized by an urgent quality and a lack of enjoyment may provide valuable information by reflecting traumatic experiences and triggers.

Thought process

The quality of children's play may range from organized and coherent to scattered and disorganized, providing further information about thought processes, again in a developmentally specific manner.

Development

Asking the child to draw a picture can provide information regarding cognitive functioning and developmental level. Information from the entire mental status examination should be used to inform the understanding of the child's cognitive functioning. Helpful information on milestones can be found at http://www.cdc.gov/ncbddd/actearly/milestones/.

Observation of Caregiver-Child Interaction

Early childhood experts suggest observing caregiver-child interactions in terms of the sequence of behaviors that occur between the caregiver and child in certain domains.[20,21]

Reciprocity

Reciprocity refers to the pattern of back and forth communication or mutual attunement between the child and caregiver. It can be helpful to think of this in terms of a dance between the child and caregiver. Noting whether the caregiver and child respond to each other's cues and whether there is a general smoothness in the interactions provides information about each partner's awareness of the other and their comfort in interactions. Low reciprocity can be seen in dyads with limited familiarity or attunement difficulties reflecting possible relationship patterns, depression, or autism spectrum disorder.

Mutual enjoyment and shared affective experiences

Clinicians note the affective quality of the interactions between the dyad, specifically with regard to dyadic delight in each other's presence. An example of mutual enjoyment might include a father smiling at an infant, who in turn smiles back. Minimal or complete lack of mutual enjoyment is noteworthy as a sign of relationship difficulties, context-specific pattern, or mood disturbance in child or parent.

Emotional availability and emotion regulation

The clinician should note whether the caregiver anticipates the child's emotional needs, including frustration or anger, and the ability to help the child recover when distressed. Additional observations include how the child expresses emotion, especially frustration, fear, or anger, in the caregiver's presence and how the caregiver reacts to the child expressing these emotions. For example, how does the caregiver engage with the child if frustrated or is it the caregiver who becomes disengaged or activated?

Comfort seeking and distress responses
Young children depend on caregivers for comfort. How the child signals distress reflects the child's effectiveness in expressing a need for help to the caregiver as well as the caregiver responsiveness. Clinicians consider responsiveness to children's signals and ways they offer support. Does the caregiver interpret the child's need for comfort as developmentally appropriate and does the caregiver validate the child's need through a sensitive response, or are the child's signals dismissed or belittled?

Play
Valuable information can be gathered by observing children and caregivers at play. Areas of observation include the ability of the child and caregiver to engage in play together, the ability of the caregiver to follow the child's lead, shared attention, the quality of the play (ie, is there a forced quality to the play or does it appear to flow naturally), and any themes that arise in the play.

Limit setting and cooperation
There are likely to be several natural opportunities for caregivers to set and enforce limits in assessments. Clinicians note the threshold for limit setting, the clarity of the limits set, as well as the child's reaction to limit setting and interest in and demonstration of following directions given by the caregiver. Provocative interactions also provide a valuable window into the relationship patterns. Observations about the caregiver's relative focus on compliance or negative behaviors, intensity of affect related to limits, and inadvertent reinforcement of negative behaviors.

Separation and reunion response
In children more than 7 to 9 months' developmental age, creating an opportunity for a brief period of separation and a reunion between the child and caregiver provides valuable clinical information about how the child uses the parent to reduce distress. This procedure can be incorporated into the assessment when separating to review sensitive history with parents and on reentry, intentionally allowing the parent to enter first. Whether and how the caregiver prepares the child for the separation and how the child signals distress and uses the parent at reunion offers valuable information about everyday separations and the attachment system (see Boris NW and Renk K's article, "Beyond Reactive Attachment Disorder: How Might Attachment Research Inform Child Psychiatry Practice?," in this issue).[21] In a healthy relationship, a parent acknowledges the upcoming separation and the child seeks proximity or visually references the parent on reunion, with resolution of distress.

Throughout, it is especially important to note any differences in the child's interactions with the caregiver versus the clinician.

Additional Informal Observations

Because of the context sensitivity of young children, appointments at multiple times of days and observations in multiple contexts, including childcare or home, can provide valuable information to the clinician about the child's experiences.

STRUCTURED ASSESSMENT TOOLS

Several structured tools allow formal assessment of the parent-child relationship, including the Crowell parent-child relationship assessment[22] and the Working Model of the Child Interview (WMCI),[23] which provide a comprehensive evaluation of the child-parent relationship. Other measures offer structured review of diagnostic criteria and symptom report.

Crowell Parent-child Interaction Procedure

The Crowell parent-child interaction procedure is designed for children aged 6 months to 6 years. The parent and child are observed in a series of 9 activities: free play, cleanup, bubbles, 4 structured tasks, as well as a separation and reunion. The Crowell provides a method of assessing several aspects of the child-parent relationship, including shared emotions, comforting behavior and comfort seeking, teaching and learning, play, limit setting and response to limits, and self-regulation.[21,22]

The free-play episode allows assessment of the dyad's comfort with one another, the affection they share, and their style of play. In cleanup, the clinician observes the dyad's cooperation, how the parent sets limits, and the child's response. The bubbles interaction offers the potential to observe shared positive affect as well as turn taking. In teaching tasks, the clinician observes the child's use of the parent in structured and potentially challenging activities, cooperation, self-regulation skills, and whether the dyad can have fun despite needing to complete tasks. The separation and reunion provides information about an activated attachment system as described earlier.

Working Model of the Child Interview

The WMCI focuses on the caregiver's internal representation of the child and of their relationship.[23,24] When used in clinical settings, clinicians attend to the affective tones of the interview as well as the narrative themes. The interview begins with a developmental history of the infant, beginning preconception, and includes questions about the child's personality and of whom the child reminds the parent. Parents are also asked about their relationships with their child and what they would change if they could, as well as hopes and fears regarding their child's future. Although the content of these responses is valuable, the clinician learns about the parent's internal representation by attending to the content of the caregiver's narrative qualities. Specifically, the richness of details, flexibility of the sense of the child, narrative coherence and consistency, intensity of emotional involvement, acceptance of the children as they are, sensitivity to the child's unique needs, perceived difficulty of the child, and fears of loss.

WMCI can be characterized through formal coding as:

1. Balanced, in which the parent provides a detailed sense of the child as a unique individual while showing an empathic appreciation for the infant
2. Disengaged, in which the parent shows an emotionally distant narrative and uses generic terms to describe the child
3. Distorted, in which the parent shows confusion, inconsistencies, or an unrealistic representation of the child

These narrative classifications differentiate between clinical and nonclinical groups.[24,25] Notably, prenatal WMCI at 28 weeks predicts the infant's attachment behaviors at 12 months.[26] Anecdotally, the process of the WMCI can be therapeutic for parents, allowing them to consider their children through a new perspective.

Structured Diagnostic Interviews

In addition to parent-child relationship assessments, diagnostic interviews provide a systematic approach to assess parental report of child symptoms, level of impairment, and family functioning. The independent report of the parents should be used in conjunction with a more comprehensive assessment.

Preschool Age Psychiatric Assessment

The Preschool Age Psychiatric Assessment (PAPA) was the first interviewer-based psychiatric diagnostic specifically for young children.[27] The PAPA reviews assessment of Diagnostic and Statisical Manual (DSM)-IV, Research Diagnostic Criteria:Preschool Age (RDC:PA), Diagnostic Criteria:0-3R, and International Classification of Diseases-10 criteria in children between the ages of 2 and 5 years. Because of the training and time required, this tool is primarily used in research.

This interview yields symptom counts, level of functional impairment, and specific diagnoses. The test-retest reliability of the PAPA is comparable with that of the structured psychiatric interviews used to assess older children and adults, and outcomes correlate with the Child Behavior Checklist results.[28] Recently, a Web-based version of the PAPA, the ePAPA, was created to aid in clinical use.

Diagnostic Infant Preschool Assessment

The Diagnostic Infant Preschool Assessment (DIPA) is a structured interview designed to administer to caregivers of children 18 to 60 months of age.[29] The interview of 30 to 60 minutes covers 16 disorders and yields diagnoses derived from the RDC:PA and is updated for the DSM-V. The initial testing of the DIPA showed concurrent criterion validity with the Child Behavior Checklist and test-retest reliabilities.[29]

Parent-report Measures

In addition to diagnostic interviews and parent-child relationship assessments, validated parent-report checklists of young children can be useful in identifying specific child behaviors and symptoms compared with symptom levels of a larger population. Parent-report checklists should be considered within the context of a more comprehensive assessment because parental report has been shown to be influenced by a myriad of factors, including parental depression.[30] The Edinburgh Postnatal Depression Scale[31] and the Patient Health Questionnaire[32] are nonproprietary tools that can be helpful to assess for parental depression. **Table 1** presents selected measures for young children.

Laboratory Evaluation

There are few indications for an extensive medical work-up for young children presenting with mental health problems. The history of the presenting problem, medical history, social history (especially living environment), family history, and observations of the child should guide a specific medical work-up. Children who do not have an active relationship with a medical home should be referred to a medical home for a full physical examination and preventive care. Commonly considered work-ups in early childhood mental health evaluations are lead levels, genetics evaluations, and referrals to neurology. Genetics testing or referrals may be considered for children whose clinical presentation is suggestive of a specific disorder, such as fragile X or trisomy 21, or those with a developmental delay in multiple developmental domains of otherwise unknown cause. In keeping with the American Academy of Pediatrics' 2014 recommendations, chromosomal microarray is the preferred test when a specific disorder is not suspected and fluorescence in situ hybridization may be used for specific disorders.[33] Referral to genetics or other local specialists may be helpful in cases of suspected fetal alcohol spectrum disorders for specialized advocacy and family counseling. A complete blood count and lead level should be considered for all

Table 1
Selected parent-report measures for young children

Measure	Age (mo)	Scales	Validity/Reliability	Cost?	Scoring Information and Additional Information
ASQ-3[35]	1–66	Gross motor, fine motor, problem solving, personal-social	TRT: 0.92 IRR: 0.93 Specificity: 77.9%–92.1% Sensitivity: 82.5%–89.2%	Yes	Typical development, need for monitoring, or needs further assessment for each domain
ASQ:SE-2[36]	1–72	Self-regulation, compliance, communication, adaptive functioning, autonomy, affect, and interaction with people	TRT: 0.89 Validity: 0.83 Specificity: 0.83 Sensitivity: 0.81	Yes	Typical development, need for monitoring, or needs further assessment for total score
BITSEA[37]	12–36 mo	Internalizing, externalizing, dysregulation, and competence	TRT (problem scale): 0.85 TRT (competency scales): 0.87		Positive if above cutoff on problem scale and below the cutoff on competence scale Companion measure to ITSEA
CBCL[38]	18–60	Broadband: internalizing, externalizing, and total problems	TRT (parent): 0.85 TRT (teacher): 0.81 Higher scores in clinically referred children than in non-clinically referred children (effect size = 0.3)		Symptom domain typical, borderline, or clinical scores for broadband, narrowband, and DSM-IV Includes companion validated teacher rating form
ECSA[39]	18–60	Child mental health problems, parent distress	S test-retest reliability: 0.81 Sensitivity (predicting DIPA): 0.86 Specificity: 0.83 Significant correlations with CBCL and BITSEA		Child score ≥18 is positive Parent score on PHQ 2>0 positive Includes validated parent depression items and distress items and opportunity to indicate concern about individual items

ITSEA[40]	12–36	Internalizing, externalizing, dysregulation, and competence	TRT (competency scale) = 0.76 T TRT (dysregulation scale): 0.91 C correlation with CBCL total problem scores: 0.47 (internalizing problems) and 0.67 (externalizing problems)	Companion to BITSEA
ECBI[41]	24 mo–16 y	Externalizing	TRT (intensity scale): 0.86 TRT (problem scale): 0.88 Interparent reliability (intensity scale): 0.69 Interparent reliability (problem scale): 0.61 Internal consistency: 0.95 (IS) and 0.93 (PS)	Clinical cutoff 131 for IS and 15 for PS
Preschool Feelings Checklist[42]	36–66	Internalizing symptoms	Sensitivity: 0.92 Specificity: 0.84 Internal consistency: 0.77	Score of 3 or more cutoff for clinically relevant depressive symptoms
MCHAT-R	16–30	ASD symptoms	Internal consistency = 0.63 Sensitivity >0.9 Specificity >0.9	0–2, low risk; 3–7, medium risk; 8–20, high risk Medium risk requires follow-up interview

Abbreviations: ASD, autism spectrum disorder; ASQ, Ages and Stages Questionnaire; ASQ:SE, Ages and Stages Questionnaire: Social-Emotional; BITSEA, Brief Infant-Toddler Social-Emotional Assessment; CBCL, Child Behavior Checklist; DIPA, Diagnostic Infant Preschool Assessment; ECBI, Eyberg Child Behavior Inventory; ECSA, Early Childhood Screening Assessment; IRR, interrater reliability; IS, intensity scale; ITSEA, Infant-Toddler Social and Emotional Assessment; MCHAT-R, Modified Checklist for Autism in Toddlers; PS, problem scale; TRT, test-retest reliability.

children with known exposure risks, those with pica, and/or children with hyperactivity who did not complete recommended testing.[34] Brain imaging should only be considered in children with microcephaly or macrocephaly, or those with observable neurologic symptoms or developmental regression in conjunction with a referral to neurology.[33] Children with suspected neurologic issues, like absence seizures, or possible metabolic storage diseases should be referred to specialists for further work-up. In general, a high level of suspicion is warranted for other organ involvement in young children presenting with comorbid emotional, behavioral, and developmental symptoms.

FORMULATION: PUTTING IT ALL TOGETHER

The formulation requires the consolidation of all interview, observational, procedural, and written information obtained through the assessment. Although diagnosis offers a systematic, categorical description of the child's patterns, the formulation provides the links among the biological, psychological, and environmental factors that may confer risk of the presenting problems and those that have protected against worsening morbidity. The formulation may also identify the entry points that may offer the highest likelihood of change in the family system. The entry point into the family system may be through the parent, the child, or the parent-child relationship, and the formulation may guide the clinician in recognizing the part of the family system that will be most amenable to intervention. For example, treatment of parental depression before direct treatment of preschool attention-deficit/hyperactivity disorder may increase the effectiveness of the indicated parent management training. In all cases, it should be noted that assessment is not a single event but an ongoing process of using existing information to guide formulation, hypothesis development, treatment planning, and continuous reassessment throughout the treatment process.

REFERENCES

1. Zeanah PD, Bailey LO, Berry S. Infant mental health and the "real world"-opportunities for interface and impact. Child Adolesc Psychiatr Clin N Am 2009;18(3): 773–87.
2. Halfon N, Larson K, Slusser W. Associations between obesity and comorbid mental health, developmental, and physical health conditions in a nationally representative sample of US children aged 10 to 17. Acad Pediatr 2013;13(1): 6–13.
3. Barlow J, van der Voort A, Juffer F, et al. Sensitive parenting is the foundation for secure attachment relationships and positive social-emotional development of children. J Child Serv 2014;9(2):165–76.
4. Drake K, Belsky J, Fearon R. From early attachment to engagement with learning in school: the role of self-regulation and persistence. Dev Psychol 2014;50(5): 1350.
5. Shonkoff JP, Garner AS, Committee on Psychosocial Aspects of Child and Family Health, Committee on Early Childhood, Adoption, and Dependent Care, Section on Developmental and Behavioral Pediatrics. The lifelong effects of early childhood adversity and toxic stress (technical report). Pediatrics 2012;129: e232–46.
6. Felitti VJ, Anda RF, Nordenberg D, et al. Relationship of childhood abuse and household dysfunction to many of the leading causes of death in adults: the Adverse Childhood Experiences (ACE) study. Am J Prev Med 1998;14:245.

7. Yoshikawa H, Aber JL, Beardslee WR. The effects of poverty on the mental, emotional, and behavioral health of children and youth: implications for prevention. Am Psychol 2012;67(4):272.

8. Panter-Brick C, Leckman JF. Editorial commentary: resilience in child development–interconnected pathways to wellbeing. J Child Psychol Psychiatry 2013; 54(4):333–6.

9. Drury SS, Gleason MM, Theall KP, et al. Genetic sensitivity to the caregiving context: the influence of 5httlpr and BDNF val66met on indiscriminate social behavior. Physiol Behav 2012;106(5):728–35.

10. APA. Diagnostic and statistical manual of mental disorders 5. Washington, DC: American Psychiatric Press; 2013.

11. WHO. The IDC-10 classification of mental and behavioral disorders: clinical descriptions and diagnostic guidelines. 10th edition. Geneva (Switzerland): World Health Organization; 1992.

12. Zero to Three. Diagnostic classification of mental health and developmental disorders of infancy and early childhood. Washinton, DC: Zero to Three; 2016.

13. Dozier M, Stovall KC, Albus K, et al. Attachment for infants in foster care: the role of the caregiver state of mind. Child Development 2001;72(5):1467–77.

14. Biederman J, Mick E, Faraone SV. Biased maternal reporting of child psychopathology? J Am Acad Child Adolesc Psychiatry 1998;37(1):10.

15. Zeanah CH, Lieberman A. Defining relational pathology in early childhood: the diagnostic classification of mental health and developmental disorders of infancy and early childhood DC:0-5 approach. Infant Ment Health J 2016;37(5):509–20.

16. Apter-Levy Y, Feldman M, Vakart A, et al. Impact of maternal depression across the first 6 years of life on the child's mental health, social engagement, and empathy: the moderating role of oxytocin. Am J Psychiatry 2013;170(10):1161–8.

17. Gutierrez-Galve L, Stein A, Hanington L, et al. Paternal depression in the postnatal period and child development: mediators and moderators. Pediatrics 2015;135(2):e339–47.

18. Gleason MM. Relationship assessment in clinical practice. Child Adolesc Psychiatr Clin N Am 2009;18(3):581.

19. Moldavsky M, Lev D, Lerman-Sagie T. Behavioral phenotypes of genetic syndromes: a reference guide for psychiatrists. J Am Acad Child Adolesc Psychiatry 2001;40(7):749–61.

20. Powell B, Cooper G, Hoffman K, et al. The circle of security intervention: enhancing attachment in early parent-child relationships. New York: Guilford Publications; 2013.

21. Zeanah CH, Larrieu JA, Valliere J, et al. Infant-parent relationship assessment. In: Zeanah CH, editor. Handbook of infant mental health. New York: Guilford; 2000. p. 222–35.

22. Crowell JA. Assessment of attachment security in a clinical setting: observations of parents and children. J Dev Behav Pediatr 2003;24(3):199–204.

23. Zeanah CH, Benoit D. Clinical applications of a parent perception interview in infant mental health. Child Adolesc Psychiatr Clin N Am 1995;4(3):539–54.

24. Zeanah CH, Benoit D, Hirschberg L, et al. Mothers' representations of their infants are concordant with infant attachment classifications. Developmental Issues Psychiatry Psychol 1994;1:9–18.

25. Main M, Goldwyn R, Hesse E. Adult attachment scoring and classification system. Berkeley (CA): University of California at Berkeley; 1998.

26. Benoit D, Zeanah CH, Parker KC, et al. "Working model of the child interview": infant clinical status related to maternal perceptions. Infant Ment Health J 1997; 18(1):107–21.
27. Egger HL, Erkanli A, Keeler G, et al. Test-retest reliability of the Preschool Age Psychiatric Assessment (PAPA). J Am Acad Child Adolesc Psychiatry 2006; 45(5):538–49.
28. Achenbach T, Roscorla L. Manual for the ASEBA preschool form. Burlington (VT): University of Vermont; 2000.
29. Scheeringa MS, Haslett N. The reliability and criterion validity of the diagnostic infant and preschool assessment: a new diagnostic instrument for young children. Child Psychiatry Hum Dev 2010;41(3):299–312.
30. Dawson G, Ashman SB, Panagiotides H, et al. Preschool outcomes of children of depressed mothers: role of maternal behavior, contextual risk, and children's brain activity. Child Dev 2003;74(4):1158–75.
31. Cox JL, Holden JM, Sagovsky R. Detection of postnatal depression: development of the 10-item Edinburgh postnatal depression scale. Br J Psychiatry 1987;150: 782–6.
32. Kroenke K, Spitzer R, Williams J. The patient health questionnaire-2: validity of a two-item depression screener. Med Care 2003;41(11):1284–92.
33. Moeschler JB, Shevell M, Moeschler JB, et al. Comprehensive evaluation of the child with intellectual disability or global developmental delays. Pediatrics 2014;134(3):e903–18.
34. Lanphear BP, Lowry JA, Ahdoot S, et al. Prevention of childhood lead toxicity. Pediatrics 2016;138(1).
35. Squires J, Bricker D. Ages & stages questionnaires. 3rd edition (ASQ-3). Baltimore (MD): Brookes Publishing; 2009.
36. Squires J, Bricker D, Twombly E. Ages & stages questionnaires: social-emotional. Baltimore (MD): Paul H Brookes Publishing; 2002.
37. Briggs-Gowan M, Carter AS. Brief Infant Toddler Social Emotional Assessment (BITSEA) manual version 2.0. New Haven (CT): Yale University; 2002.
38. Achenbach TM, Rescorla LA. Manual for the ASEBA preschool forms & profiles: an integrated system of multi-informant assessment; child behavior checklist for ages 1 1/2-5; language development survey; caregiver-teacher report form. Burlington (VT): University of Vermont; 2000.
39. Gleason MM, Zeanah CH, Dickstein S. Recognizing young children in need of mental health assessment: development and preliminary validity of the early childhood screening assessment. Infant Ment Health J 2010;31(3):335–57.
40. Briggs-Gowan M. Preliminary acceptability and psychometrics of the Infant-Toddler Social and Emotional Assessment (ITSEA): a new adult-report questionnaire. Infant Ment Health J 1998;19(4):422–45.
41. Eyberg SM, Pincus D. Eyberg child behavior inventory & Sutter-Eyberg student behavior inventory. Odessa (FL): Psychological Assessment Resources; 1999.
42. Luby JL, Heffelfinger A, Koenig-McNaught AL, et al. The preschool feelings checklist: a brief and sensitive screening measure for depression in young children. J Am Acad Child Adolesc Psychiatry 2004;43(6):708–16.

Psychopathology and Intervention

Beyond Reactive Attachment Disorder
How Might Attachment Research Inform Child Psychiatry Practice?

Neil W. Boris, MD[a],*, Kimberly Renk, PhD[b]

KEYWORDS

- Attachment • Therapy • Reactive attachment disorder
- Disinhibited social disengagement disorder

KEY POINTS

- Attachment in early childhood shapes early regulatory and brain function, making an understanding of caregiver-child attachment important for any practitioner working with young children.
- Child psychiatrists who are not expert in assessing attachment but who see a significant number of young children who have experienced early disruption in caregiving need to work in care coordination teams with infant mental health specialists. Such specialists should be familiar with assessments that include elements of standardized observations of caregiver-child interactions as well as interviews that capture caregivers' states of mind regarding attachment and caregivers' capacity to mentalize.
- Compared with children who have experienced early maltreatment leading to disorganized attachment, reactive attachment disorder and disinhibited social engagement disorder are rare conditions, although assessment and intervention approaches for both disorganization and disorder are similar.
- Evidence-based, attachment-focused interventions do not focus on changing child behavior directly. Instead, such interventions focus on fostering caregivers' mentalization capacities and shaping caregivers' responses to their children's attachment behaviors.

 Video content accompanies this article at www.childpsych.theclinics.com.

In a recent article, Allen[1] argued that reactive attachment disorder should be removed from the Diagnostic and Statistical Manual of Mental Disorders (DSM) Fifth Revision. Allen[1] focused on 2 serious challenges in the application of research on

Disclosure: Dr N.W. Boris is a paid consultant to and trainer for Circle of Security International.
[a] Center for Prevention and Early Intervention Policy, Florida State University, 1339 East Lafayette Street, Tallahassee, FL 32301, USA; [b] Department of Psychology, University of Central Florida, 4111 Pictor Lane, Psychology Building (99), Room 353, Orlando, FL 32816, USA
* Corresponding author.
E-mail address: nboris212@gmail.com

Child Adolesc Psychiatric Clin N Am 26 (2017) 455–476
http://dx.doi.org/10.1016/j.chc.2017.03.003
childpsych.theclinics.com

attachment and attachment disorders. First, he noted that mental health practitioners diagnose children with reactive attachment disorder not based on the criteria from the DSM or International Classification Of Diseases systems, but simply because these children have histories of early disruption in caregiving along with current, and often severe, behavioral issues, such as aggression, defiance, and impulsivity.[2,3] Second, he highlighted that, although most of these children do not meet published criteria for an attachment disorder,[3] the association of long-standing behavior problems in the historical context of inadequate attachment has spawned interventions to treat these attachment problems (so-called attachment therapies). Some of these attachment therapies are clearly not evidence based, and there have been at least 6 documented child deaths in the United States associated with therapy for attachment disorders.[4]

In the same article, Allen[1] reviewed recent research on the natural history of attachment disorders in institutionalized children and how these data have informed changes in diagnostic criteria while also informing interventions needed to improve the functioning of institutionalized children.[5] Were reactive attachment disorder to somehow be removed from the DSM-5 or other diagnostic systems, growing the thin research base on disorders of attachment would become more difficult.

What Allen's[1] article underscores are 2 known and interrelated challenges. First, the care of children with mental health problems, particularly the youngest children, suffers because of significant gaps in the translation of research into practice.[6,7] One clear research-to-practice gap has to do with the construct of attachment. With tens of thousands of studies in the last 50 years, research on attachment has been called "one of the broadest, most profound and most creative lines of research in 20th century (and now 21st century) psychology."[8(pxi)] Although attachment research includes studies across the lifespan, many of the clinical applications are focused on young children and their caregivers. At the same time, few communities have enough early childhood practitioners to meet demand,[9] and it is not clear how many child psychiatry training programs even offer an early childhood or attachment focus.

The second issue underscored by Allen's[1] article is that child mental health service systems in the United States (and elsewhere) are not developed enough to allow evidence-based practice to take root.[10] There is much complexity in child mental health systems, and many factors likely affect the degree to which evidence-based practice is adopted.[11] Given that knowledge transfer is poor and systems of care are lacking, the fact that inadequate or even dangerous care of children occurs is cause for alarm. However, it is by no means clear that removing reactive attachment disorder from the nosology will change the care that young children receive.

This article does not focus on reactive attachment disorder or disinhibited social engagement disorder in spite of the controversy regarding these diagnoses. There are recent comprehensive reviews on attachment disorders, including Allen's[1] own review, which are available to practicing child psychiatrists.[5] Furthermore, a 2016 practice parameter published by the American Academy of Child and Adolescent Psychiatry presents a series of recommendations on assessment and intervention for disorders of attachment.[12] As the practice parameter and associated reviews detail, disorders of attachment are rare when criteria are appropriately applied.[1,12] Beyond reactive attachment disorder, all children have some form of attachment to a select group of caregivers, and so both assessment and intervention in early childhood should be informed by the broader research on attachment. The primary focus of this article, therefore, is to provide an updated review of attachment theory and research for child psychiatrists.

This article presupposes that most child psychiatrists will not become expert in assessing early relationships and attachment. Even so, treatment planning for young children requires that child psychiatrists be expert in case formulation,[13] and understanding how attachment informs comprehensive evaluation in early childhood is critical.[14] As Allen's[1] provocative recent article underscores, the stakes are high. Poor case formulation has led to diagnostic imprecision, untested psychotherapies, and child harm.

This article begins with a review of attachment as a developmental process, followed by a review of individual differences in attachment. Individual differences in attachment are about patterns of attachment in relationships and the caregiving context influencing these relationship patterns. It then turns to a review of attachment and psychological function, focusing on key findings that have influenced intervention research. Next, the extreme cases of early deprivation that sometimes lead to diagnosis of an attachment disorder are considered, and a brief overview of how recent data have informed diagnostic classification is provided.

The remaining focus of this article is on assessment and intervention. Given that most practicing child psychiatrists do not specialize in attachment assessment or intervention, working with young children who have histories of early maltreatment and/or disruption in caregiving requires being part of a care coordination team.[6,15] With regard to assessment, this article focuses on how to identify a specialist who uses research-based tools for assessing early childhood development and attachment.[16] Rather than reviewing these tools fully, this article provides examples of how the tools are used and the types of clinical data that can be derived from a comprehensive attachment-focused intervention. The article reviews both interactional assessment and parental interviews and links these instruments to the developmental research reviewed earlier.

In addition, intervention is discussed. Although there are discredited therapies used for so-called attachment problems (eg, the harrowing example of rebirthing therapy[17]), there are also recently developed psychotherapy approaches directly derived from attachment theory and research that have a growing evidence base. Child psychiatrists should be aware of these emerging intervention approaches, how they are different from traditional behaviorally oriented parent management training, and their growing evidence base.[18] In addition, this article closes with consideration of the role of pharmacotherapy in the care of young children for whom there are attachment concerns.

ATTACHMENT AND DEVELOPMENTAL PROCESS

In the current era, child development is viewed as a transactional process involving the interplay of genes and environment. Even if various domains of human function unfold along a fairly specific timeline, gene-environment transactions driving change continually shape developing children.[19] For example, language development unfolds across childhood with the most rapid changes evident in the preschool years. Expressive language lags behind receptive language development in infancy. As toddlers begin to talk, their vocabulary quickly increases. By the preschool period, children's capacities, from articulation to letter recognition, follow along a fairly predictable timeline. At the same time, environmental input significantly affects language development. For example, vocabulary acquisition at 2 years of age is strongly associated with maternal speech, and maternal speech is associated with socioeconomic status.[20] Children who meet criteria for language disorders can be recognized in the preschool period. These children's developmental progression is atypical, and impairment associated with language disorders can be long lasting and can influence other domains of functioning.[21]

Like language development, the development of attachment is a transactional process that unfolds over a predictable timeline. The idea that human infants are biologically predisposed to attach to caregivers arose from decades of animal studies, and Bowlby[22] came to believe that the process of attachment was rooted in evolution.[23,24] The goals of language development, including why the forces of evolution might conserve expressive language, seem clear. Such communication allows the transfer of knowledge between individuals and groups, although how language evolved in humans remains mysterious.[25] The goals of attachment are likewise clear. Infants depend on caregivers, with social bonds serving a protective function.[23] Furthermore, animal studies reveal that caregiver-infant interactions serve a regulatory function for offspring, and recent progress in studying neurobiology at the molecular level clearly shows that early interactions shape brain development and can have long-lasting effects in offspring.[26] Studying the neurobiology of attachment in humans also underscores that attachment plays an important regulatory function and, in so doing, shapes the developing brain (Video 1).[27,28]

As with language development, optimal functioning of the attachment system can be observed, and significant deviations in optimal functioning are associated with later impairment.[29,30] For child psychiatrists, understanding what an optimal attachment relationship looks like relative to one in which there is dysfunction, or even clinical disorder, is important. The key word here is relationship. Although language development is influenced by environmental input, attachment is truly an interpersonal or relational process. Evaluating attachment therefore requires assessing the child and caregivers as a unit. Furthermore, because disturbances in child attachment are mostly driven by the caregiving context, expert assessors use tools to understand how given caregivers' psychological models of relationships influence them in their relationship with their offspring. The development of attachment is addressed next, and concepts of security, insecurity, disorganization, and disorder are introduced.

THE DEVELOPMENT OF ATTACHMENT

Infants are highly responsive social creatures, and there is evidence that, even before birth, the fetus's regulatory systems are influenced by environmental input. It is clear as well that caregivers begin to psychologically connect with their infants in the prenatal period,[31] suggesting that the process of attachment starts even before children are born. Furthermore, there is increasing evidence that the prenatal environment can be influenced by the caregiver's psychological state. For example, longitudinal research has made it clear that prenatal exposure to maternal anxiety is associated with children's behavioral functioning years after birth.[32] More broadly, a remarkable area of research, known as the developmental origins of health and disease, is focusing on fetal and/or early postnatal exposure to allostatic loads and how early exposure affects later emotional, behavioral, and physiologic functioning. A review of the study of causal mechanisms regarding how the regulatory systems of developing young children are programmed to respond to stimuli and how that programming affects psychosocial and health outcomes later in life[33] is beyond the scope of this article. It is enough to say that the long-term developmental impact of environmental perturbations in the prenatal and early postnatal period has important implications for public health interventions and for health care in general.[34]

Throughout the first 2 months of life, infants show little observable preference for particular caregivers. Nevertheless, even in the first days of life, infants are able to discriminate their mothers from other caregivers. For example, newborns just days old work (through nonnutritive sucking) to produce a recording of their mother's voice compared with the voice of another woman.[35] A qualitative shift in infant capacities at about 2 to 3 months of age ushers in a host of new social abilities for human infants.[36] The advent of the social smile is accompanied by infants gazing in more sustained ways at caregivers, crying less, cooing, and engaging in sophisticated social "conversations" with their caregivers.[37]

Although infants tend to interact differently with fathers, mothers, and strangers, they do not express strong preference for any caregiver in the first 6 months of life. However, careful analysis shows that the degree to which interactions between the infant and the closest caregiver are characterized by synchrony and mutual responsiveness is predictive of later attachment security with that caregiver.[38] There is an evolving body of research on how caregiver-infant synchrony is influenced by the neuroendocrine system and how these factors, in turn, predict later attachment.[39] However, few providers have access to laboratory analysis of key neuroendocrine factors or have the capacity to study caregiver-infant interactions using microanalysis of video. Instead, specialists in attachment assessment must wait until the infant is about 7 to 9 months of age, when infants seem to "fall in love" with a small number of preferred attachment figures, to assess the quality of attachment observationally in real time.

In the months before the first birthday, infants behave in ways that show their formation of discriminated attachments. They seek comfort, support, and nurturance from a few (ie, typically <4) caregivers. In the presence of unfamiliar adults, 8-month-olds show what has been termed stranger anxiety, marked by wariness, anxiety, and even distress. Around the same age, separation protest begins, peaking between 9 and 18 months of age cross-culturally.

As infants begin to walk, their natural interest in exploring the physical world leads to a new "dance" between caregiver and child, a dance that is shown in **Fig. 1**.

Toddlers use their attachment figures as secure bases from whom they go out and explore the world and as safe havens to whom they return (ie, come in) for protection,

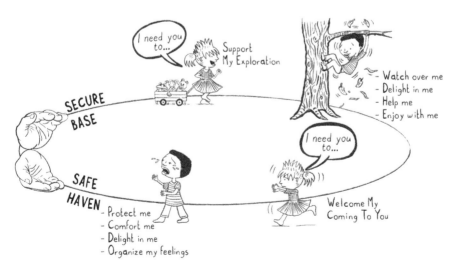

Fig. 1. Circle of Security: Parent attending to the child's needs. (*From* Circle of Security International. Early Intervention Program for Parents & Children. Available at: http://circleofsecurityinternational.com/handouts. Accessed March 6, 2017; with permission.)

comfort, delight, or to have their feelings organized. Each day, repeated trips around the circle occur, with toddlers going out and coming in. At times when toddlers' exploration leads them further away from their attachment figures than is comfortable or when some frightening or confusing event occurs, they feel the urge to return to the caregiver. Attachment patterns evolve through experience, and these patterns reflect the dance that begins in the first months as a cry and a cuddle and that transitions to exploring and returning in toddlerhood and on through adolescence. As most providers are aware, the degree to which an individual caregiver is able to provide a secure base or safe haven for a given child varies widely. One of the most remarkable strands of attachment research has been the study of individual differences in attachment and the implications of those differences for a child's social and emotional functioning across time.[40]

INDIVIDUAL DIFFERENCES IN ATTACHMENT: SECURE, INSECURE, AND DISORGANIZED

The study of individual differences in attachment began with the strange situation procedure (SSP), which was created in the 1970s.[41] The name strange situation is based on the fact that novel situations, especially when combined with separation from the caregiver, activate young children's attachment systems. The SSP begins with a free play period, followed by the introduction and approach of an adult whom the infant or young child has never met (the stranger). The infant or young child experiences 2 separations from, and 2 reunions with, the caregiver over the course of the approximately 25-minute SSP. These separations, including one in which the child remains alone in the room, maximally activate the attachment system. The pattern of the child's response on reunion with the caregiver is used to classify the child into 1 of 4 groups.

Secure children signal clearly to their caregivers when they are distressed. They seek comfort and are welcomed in (see **Fig. 1**) in a warm and efficient manner, such that they are able to return to exploration. Although secure infants may be very distressed by separation, they signal their distress clearly, and their feelings are organized by their responsive caregivers quickly. Insecure-ambivalent children also signal their caregivers when distressed. The difference is that they cannot be calmed quickly or efficiently. Instead, the dance between caregiver and child is characterized by strain, with the return to exploration coming slowly and only as distress moderates over time. Children labeled insecure-avoidant resist directly signaling their caregivers. At reunion, avoidant children turn, whether distressed or not, to the toys that are provided as part of the SSP, outwardly appearing to calm themselves rather than signaling to the caregiver that they need to be comforted. In addition, disorganized attachment is characterized by the lack of a coherent strategy for managing the distress of separation at the time of reunion. Disorganized young children appear fearful or confused when distressed and in the presence of their caregivers. They may seek comfort but then veer away from their caregivers, for example, and their reunion responses leave the impression that they are uncertain about the responses that they will receive from their caregivers. These 4 patterns of attachment can be reliably coded by clinicians who are trained to recognize them and have been studied intensively, including in longitudinal studies.[40]

ATTACHMENT AND PSYCHOLOGICAL FUNCTION

Bowlby[42] argued, in expounding the theory of attachment, that caregivers' repeated response patterns to their children's bids for proximity seeking or exploration (eg, repeated trips around the circle depicted in **Fig. 1**) would influence the child's thoughts, feelings, and expectations about relationships. Bowlby[42] used the term internal working model to reflect the psychological representations about relationships that arise through experience.[42,43] For example, a toddler whose reunion response shows uncertainty, fear, and confusion (ie, a response that fits best with a disorganized attachment pattern) becomes a preschooler whose internal working model of relationships is marked by the same uncertainty, fear, and confusion. Children's early experiences can be shown to influence how they talk about close relationships, through play or verbally even before they reach school age.[43] Thus, a child whose state of mind about relationships has been influenced by disorganized attachment with a primary caregiver will reflect some degree of uncertainty, fear, or confusion in how to perceive relationships. In turn, this state of mind affects the child's behavior with others.[44]

There are now several instruments used to capture an individual's state of mind with regard to close relationships. One method used in the preschool period through middle childhood is Story Stems, during which the child is asked to play out and narrate a story line for which the examiner has provided a standardized beginning, or stem.[45] For adolescents and adults, coding interview responses regarding how the individual talks about experiences with caregivers likewise gets at an individual's state of mind. This article returns to further discussion of instruments that assess state of mind or working models regarding attachment later, but it is also important to note that recent attachment research has studied not just how experience encodes internal working models of attachment but how the process of thinking about others' internal states might be related to early attachment.

Recent research has made it clear that there are important links between the capacity to reflect on others' mental states, a phenomenon called mentalization, and attachment security in childhood.[46] There are compelling data that what comes with attachment security is both a better capacity to regulate emotions[47] and a better capacity to recognize emotions in others and to appreciate how those emotions might influence another individual's behavior.[46,48] In contrast, attachment insecurity or disorganization is associated with challenges in emotion regulation, which are also reflected in the expectable corollary of executive function deficits[49] as well as difficulty with mentalizing.[50]

The issue of mentalization is not simply academic. Experienced clinician recognize that central to many forms of psychotherapy is the capacity of the therapist to recognize and respond to the internal states of the patient. What makes a therapeutic alliance therapeutic is the therapist's capacity to mentalize about the patient's experience and empathize with that experience. Given that difficulties in this process of reflecting on another's mental states are associated with attachment insecurity and/ or disorganization, therapy approaches that assist caregivers in mentalizing about their infants or young children's experiences have been developed and represent the vanguard of attachment-based interventions.[51] Mentalization-based therapies are reviewed in more detail later.

There is much that clinicians do not yet know about how insecure or disorganized attachment in early childhood is related to social outcomes across time.[47] Even if there is complex interplay between genetic and environmental factors that influence attachment specifically[52] and development more generally, there is strong evidence that early disorganization is linked in longitudinal studies to later mental disorder.[48,49] Disorganized attachment is associated with social risk. The kinds of challenges that leave caregivers struggling to even engage their toddlers' needs as those toddlers travel the Circle of Security include issues like substance abuse, mental illness, and a history of trauma or loss. Such factors predict disorganized attachment.[53] The most extreme early deprivation has long been recognized to affect young children's development profoundly, and research on maltreated or institutionalized young children led to the development and refinement of criteria for attachment disorders.[12,54]

ATTACHMENT DISORDERS

Since first appearing in the DSM-III in 1980, the criteria for attachment disorders have evolved considerably.[16,55] In DSM-5, there are 2 separate disorders listed: reactive attachment disorder and disinhibited social engagement disorder. These two separate disorders parallel the 2 reactive attachment disorder subtypes (an inhibited subtype and a disinhibited subtype) that were included in each of the earlier versions of the DSM since the DSM-III. Research has borne out that reactive attachment disorder and disinhibited social engagement disorder seem to have different courses.[5] However, it is noteworthy that most of this research has been done with children who have been institutionalized and, therefore, exposed to highly atypical caregiving environments.

In DSM-5, both disorders are included in the section for disorders associated with traumatic stress, reflecting the extreme early deprivation that has always been associated with attachment disorders.[54] It has been argued that it is perhaps better to conceptualize these disorders as disorders of nonattachment.[54,55] For example, children with reactive attachment disorder do not seek out a safe haven. Instead of returning to their caregivers when distressed, these children seem helpless or disengaged. In contrast, those with disinhibited social engagement disorder seek out contact with any number of individuals who might become potential caregivers. It is their lack of selectivity in social engagement that is most remarkable. Children who have consistent caregivers, even if those caregivers are sometimes hostile or emotionally unavailable, are unlikely to develop either disorder, although the limits of caregiving deficiency associated with each disorder are hard to establish. In any case, each of the attachment disorders seems to be rare.[1,12]

As noted in the recently published practice parameter,[12] child psychiatrists should screen for each attachment disorder in children who have been in foster care or have been raised in institutional settings. Simply inquiring about reticence with strangers and comfort seeking behaviors is a first step in this assessment process, and any question about young children's patterns of social engagement should lead to a more intensive assessment, including observation of each child's interactions with the primary caregiver. Assessment of potential comorbid diagnoses, including developmental delays but also attention-deficit/hyperactivity disorder or an autism spectrum disorder, is likewise important. The safety of the child's current placement is a paramount concern. Comprehensive assessment is time intensive, and many child psychiatrists find that working with a specialist in attachment assessment is necessary both for diagnostic purposes and to create a multifocal and safe intervention plan.

ASSESSMENT OF ATTACHMENT

A general key principle of psychiatric assessment of young children is that clinical history needs to be bolstered by observational data from caregiver-child interactions. The American Academy of Child and Adolescent Psychiatry's practice parameters on assessment in infancy and early childhood and on assessment and intervention for attachment disorders give helpful overviews of recommended practice for comprehensive assessment of young children.[12,56] From an attachment perspective, observing how the infant or young child goes out to explore on the top half of the circle and how the caregiver's capacity to watch over, enjoy with, and delight in the child is most relevant (see **Fig. 1**). In order to assess interactions on the bottom half of the circle, it is important to activate the attachment system by placing some stress on the caregiver-child dyad. By asking the child to learn a challenging new task or to separate from a caregiver, the natural tendency to come in to the caregiver and express bottom-half needs is likely to occur. Caregivers then have the opportunity to show their capacity to be safe havens for the children, and their capacity to comfort the children and organize their feelings is important to track.

Table 1 summarizes the kind of interactive assessment that allows for observations that will help sort out the quality of children's attachment to their caregivers and/or signs

Table 1
Recommended clinical observation of attachment assessment

Episode	Duration (min)	Action	Observation
1	5	Clinician observes parent-child free play	Note especially familiarity, comfort, and warmth in child as the child interacts with attachment figure
2	3	Clinician talks with, then approaches, then attempts to engage child in play	Most young children show some reticence, especially initially, about engaging with an unfamiliar adult
3	3	Clinician picks up child and shows child a picture on the wall or looks out window with child	This increases the stress for the child. Again, note the child's comfort and familiarity with this stranger
4	3	Caregiver picks up child and shows child a picture on the wall or looks out window with child	In contrast with stranger pick-up, child should feel obviously more comfortable during this activity
4a[a]	1	Child is placed between caregiver and stranger and remote control novel (eg, scary/exciting) toy is introduced	Child should seek comfort preferentially from parent. If interested rather than frightened, child should share positive affect with parent
5	3	Clinician leaves the room	This separation should not elicit much of a reaction in the child, because the clinician is a stranger
6	1	Clinician returns	Similarly, the child should not be much affected by the stranger's return
7	3	Caregiver leaves the room	Child should take notice of caregiver's departure, although not necessarily show obvious distress. If the child is distressed, the clinician should be of little comfort to the child
8	1	Caregiver returns	Child's reunion behavior with caregiver should be congruent with separation behavior. That is, distressed children should seek comfort, and nondistressed children should reengage positively with caregiver, by introducing caregiver to the toy or activity or talking with caregiver about what occurred during the separation

[a] Optional episode.
From Zeanah CH, Chesher T, Boris NW, the American Academy of Child and Adolescent Psychiatry (AACAP) Committee on Quality Issues (CQI). Practice parameter for the assessment and treatment of children and adolescents with reactive attachment disorder and disinhibited social engagement disorder. J Am Acad Child Adolesc Psychiatry 2016;55(11):998; with permission.

of reactive attachment disorder or disinhibited social engagement disorder. The observation column of **Table 1** also highlights some key behaviors that are important to identify. **Table 2** focuses on caregiver behavior, caregiver state of mind, and child behavior, with each column highlighting what clinically concerning caregiver-toddler dyadic interactions would look like on the top and the bottom of the circle (see **Fig. 1**). For example, on the top of the circle when children go out to explore the world, caregivers may have difficulty with supporting children's exploration, missing children's cues indicating that help is needed, becoming overly intrusive in their efforts to help, and/or failing to delight in children's achievements. Repeated lack of delight, lack of help, or intrusion when the child needs the caregiver to simply watch over the child's exploration leads the child to miscue the parents by choosing not to seek out the caregiver's assistance (even though it might be needed), hiding the child is feeling, and even becoming watchful or fearful of the caregiver. On the bottom of the circle, when children come in for connection, interactions of concern include caregivers being mean (eg, rejecting children's attempts for connection, being harsh), weak (eg, pleading with children, acting overwhelmed by children's behavior), or gone (eg, being emotionally or even physically unavailable when children need connection). Over time, as children learn that caregivers consistently are not able to provide needed connection, children's responses may include withdrawal from their caregivers, seeking out comfort from others indiscriminately, or showing extreme behavior (eg, tantrums, aggression) in an effort to communicate that their attachment needs have not been met.

It is expected that only some child psychiatrists have either the expertise or the latitude in their clinical practices to conduct like the assessment laid out in **Table 1**. Consequently, working with a community expert in assessing attachment may be essential, particularly if the child psychiatrist sees a significant number of young children who, for example, are in foster care because of concerns about their parents' capacity to care for them. Standardized interaction procedures are what most specialists in attachment assessment use, and **Table 3** lists what would distinguish a provider who is a generalist from one who would be considered a specialist. For infants less than 12 months of age, specialists use something like the Still Face Paradigm[37] to assess dyadic synchrony. In contrast, for toddlers and preschool-aged children, a procedure like the one summarized in **Table 1**, which combines elements of the SSP[41] and the Caregiver Child Structured Play Interaction (also called the Crowell Procedure after one of its creators),[57] would be ideal. Most of these assessments require toys, a playroom with a one-way window, and an observation room with a video camera.

Specialists in attachment or infant mental health also know about assessing the caregiver's state of mind and capacity for mentalization (see **Table 3**). For example, narrative interviews require caregivers to reflect on key relationships. Specialists are familiar with interviews like the Adult Attachment Interview (George C, Kaplan N, Main M, unpublished data, University of California, Berkeley; 1985)[58] and the Working Model of the Child Interview (Zeanah CH, Benoit D, Barton ML, et al, unpublished data, Louisiana State University School of Medicine; 1996), both of which have a strong research base but are also valuable as clinical tools. Column 1 in **Table 2** summarizes the kinds of clinical data that specialist are concerned about when listening to caregivers talk about their relationships with their children. Overall, such interviews push caregivers to mentalize about key relationships, giving information both about their states of mind about attachment and their capacity for mentalization. As noted, caregivers who struggle to talk about their children's internal states are particularly concerning given the link between mentalization and attachment security. Often, caregivers with histories of interpersonal trauma struggle to connect with their children because their traumatic experiences lead them to view their children's behavior as manipulative or purposefully negative.[59] Furthermore, there is evidence that care-givers' unresolved trauma limits their capacity to mentalize, such that intergenera-tional transmission of insecure or disorganized attachment ensues.[59,60]

For children who may be showing signs of reactive attachment disorder or disinhi-bited social engagement disorder, assessing the caregiving context is no less impor-tant. The first consideration for such children is the provision of an emotionally available caregiver.[12] Longitudinal studies, like the Bucharest Early Intervention Proj-ect, show that the caregiving context predicts symptom expression and develop-mental outcomes across time in institutionalized children. However, the older children are when they are adopted, the more likely it is that lasting cognitive and/or socioemotional deficits will be evident across time.[54,61] Nevertheless, the appropriate target for intervention is the family context, whether the work is with a family who has adopted an institutionalized child or one in which there are concerns about attachment disorganization and social risk. However, there is emerging evidence that a variety of therapeutic interventions can help promote attachment security in young children.

EVIDENCE-BASED THERAPEUTIC INTERVENTIONS TO FOSTER ATTACHMENT

Evidence-based attachment-focused interventions focus on the caregiver and on addressing the caregiver's state of mind and capacity to mentalize. Although child behavior is obviously important, the primary goal is to help caregivers understand that their children's behavior reflects unmet attachment needs. The attachment rela-tionship becomes the focus of intervention and the caregiver's mentalization becomes the process through which change occurs.[48] Practitioners should be wary of any attachment therapy that focuses on trying to address proxies of children's attachment behaviors (eg, by forcing eye contact, holding, some kind of rebirthing).[2,62] Such ther-apies are risky and have caused significant harm.[4]

Most child psychiatrists are aware of parent management training approaches that are often used for disorders like attention-deficit/hyperactivity disorder and opposi-tional defiant disorder. These parenting approaches, with parent-child interaction therapy being a well-researched example,[63] focus on rewarding positive behavior and ignoring or actively intervening with negative behavior. Although there are no head-to-head trials of such approaches versus attachment-based approaches in young children, both types of approaches have garnered support.[64] Nonetheless, ex-perts in behaviorally based interventions agree that, when behaviorally based ap-proaches fail, untreated attachment issues may be the issue. As Scott and Dadds[65] argue, attachment-based interventions acknowledge "the emotional importance of having a trustable, secure figure who can be relied upon to be responsive to [chil-dren's] needs, especially around times of distress"[65(p1443)] and that behavioral ap-proaches may fail when such a secure figure is not established. If behavioral approaches prove ineffective, seeking out a specialist in attachment and attachment-based interventions is clearly indicated.

One example of an explicitly mentalization-focused intervention is the Mothers and Toddlers Program (MTP).[66] Designed for substance-involved mothers with children who are 12 to 36 months of age, MTP is based on the psychosocial and neurobiolog-ical mechanisms of attachment and addiction. Therapists use a developmental pro-gression to foster change in mothers. As part of this progression, therapists begin by fostering a strong therapeutic alliance so that mothers are willing to honestly examine how their substance misuse has affected their parenting and their children's attachment. Therapists also ensure that mothers develop the tools and engage the supports necessary to tolerate and regulate the strong affect that they experience

Table 2
Clinical aspects of significantly disturbed attachment using the Circle of Security framework

The caregiver is unable to provide a secure base and cannot consistently provide a safe haven. Relationships in this range are marked by serious concerns in all areas such that immediate intervention is warranted. For many dyads in this range, involvement of child protective services or use of intensive in-home services should be considered. Not only are the caregiver's representations of the child concerning but the caregiver's behavior toward the child is grossly insensitive. Moments of positive interactions are not sustained. The child, in turn, shows concerning behavior on 1 or both sides of the circle. Although the caregiver may voice concerns about the relationship with the child, the capacity to recognize the child's needs around the circle is lacking. Family stressors are likely to be high, and the child's safety and developmental trajectory are of great concern

Caregiver Representation	Caregiver Behavior	Child Behavior
Attributions about the child are: • Negative to the degree of derogation: direct expression of anger about the child's needs breaks through • Marked by distortion, such that the child's needs are characterized as hurtful, frightening, or overwhelming; in some cases, the child is seen as primarily responsible for the caregiver's distress or the picture of the child is lost in the caregiver's own issues or in marked tangential responses that are not about the relationship • Generically positive (eg, loving or caring) but the story of the relationship is characterized by extreme disengagement such that the caregiver struggles to find language to talk about the child's needs and seems disinterested The tone of the interview: • May be marked by indifference or disappointment • May be shaped by moments of anger or hostility • May be colored by guilt or shame	On the top half of the circle, the caregiver: • Reads cues poorly and therefore: 1. Has difficulty watching over the child; either takes charge by intruding or withdrawing, or does both unpredictably 2. Misses help-me moments • Restricts the child's exploration through intrusion, pressuring to achieve, or teasing • Rarely delights in or enjoys being with the child On the bottom half of the circle, the caregiver: • May respond to cues for comfort or protection by: 1. Simply avoiding or rejecting the cue 2. Showing harsh or mocking affect or tone of voice • Responds to cues that the child needs his or her feelings organized, by: 1. Ignoring or rejecting the child's cue 2. Behaving as if the child's need is overwhelming or irritating 3. Begging or pleading with the child rather than being calming	On the top half of the circle, the child: • Shows little delight and may miscue that they are disinterested in the caregiver • Seems tentative about affect sharing or avoids it altogether; exploration is rudimentary and play muted • May be hypervigilant, such that tracking the caregiver supplants exploration On the bottom half of the circle, the child: • Seeks proximity by approaching strangers or simply withdraws from caregiver, showing fear, confusion, or even dissociation • Organize-my-feelings moments may look extreme, such as showing self-endangering behavior or periods of defiance • Attempts to miscue through organize-my-feelings moments break down into tantrums that are difficult to extinguish • The child may be overbright or solicitous, as if trying to set the emotional tone of the interaction, particularly at reunion

The caregiver's capacity to have insight into the child's experience:

- Is limited such that the caregiver shows little capacity to imagine what the child is feeling
- Stage salient issues like negotiating separation or starting toilet training are likely to be experienced as burdensome or overwhelming or even uninteresting; challenges with independence are blamed, at least in part, on the child

The caregiver's memories about the child:

- Are few
- Lack detail, positive emotion, and richness; no autonoetic awareness
- Are contradictory, such that, for example, specific memories of the child described as loving focus instead on the child being manipulative or difficult

Other features of the interview:

- Moments of confusion or even dissociation may be evident
- Previous experience of loss or trauma may be talked about even if not clearly related to the interview question

The caregiver's hands are characterized by:

- Being only bigger and stronger (without being kind) or being weak and withdrawing in fear or helplessness

Courtesy of N.W. Boris, MD, Orlando, FL; and C.H. Zeanah, MD, New Orleans, LA; and M.M. Gleason, MD, New Orleans, LA.

Table 3
Differentiating providers and their level of experience and training

Generalist	Specialist
Early intervention training and familiarity with attachment theory	Advanced training in infant mental health
Works with families at moderate risk; consults to early intervention programs	Works with highest-risk families (eg, those with internationally adopted children or those in the child welfare system)
Familiar with attachment patterns from secure to disorganized but no formal training	Trained in classifying attachment patterns (infant, preschool, or both systems)
Uses general clinical interview rather than narrative interviews	Trained in the use of narrative interviews like the Working Model of the Child Interview or the Adult Attachment Interview
Supportive treatment provider with limited training in dyadic therapy	Experienced dyadic therapist

From Boris NW, Chesher T, Wajda-Johnston V. Assessment of attachment. In: Carmen-Wiggins RD, Carter A, editors. Oxford handbook of infant and early childhood mental health. New York: Oxford University Press, in press; with permission.

during group sessions. With these tools and supports in place, therapists then work to enhance mothers' capacities to reflect on themselves and their children, attempting to move mothers from distorted, harsh, incoherent, and insensitive states of mind to a coherent and integrated understanding of themselves and their children.

In sum, the theory of change with MTP is that parent–young child interactions are promoted by fostering mothers' sensitivity and responsiveness to their young children's emotional cues via a focus on the mothers' states of mind regarding attachment and their reflective capacities. Mentalization is the main target of this intervention, with parent behavior and psychological symptoms being secondary effects.[67] Follow-up studies show that substance-involved mothers who participate in MTP have better mentalization capacity and attachment-based caregiving behaviors immediately after the intervention[67] and in 6 weeks of follow-up.[68]

Other interventions use video feedback as a tool both for increasing parents' sensitivity to the quality of their interactions with their children and for getting parents to mentalize regarding their children's needs. Video provides parents with the unique experience of observing their own interaction with their children as a means of spurring mentalization as well as enhancing identification with their children.[69] For some parents seeing the child (or another parent's child) helps to underscore the child's experience. Video is also an effective tool to provide information about attachment as a developmental process.[59]

Attachment and Biobehavioral Catch-Up (ABC) is a home-based intensive parenting intervention that is designed to enhance parents' nurturance and to increase synchronous interactions between high-risk parents and their young children through the use of videotaped dyadic interaction and video review.[70,71] This model of intervention includes direct coaching of parents, with a focus on attachment needs. Coaches help caregivers guess at children's attachment needs even when children might be acting in ways that suggest that they do not need to be nurtured. Thus, caregivers are encouraged to override their natural tendency to respond to their children's miscues by moving away from their children when the children may really need the opportunity to come in for nurturing. ABC has been shown to foster a more secure state of mind for caregivers.[72] Further, coaches help caregivers to provide predictable and controllable interpersonal interactions as a means of fostering the regulatory capabilities of children who experience dysregulation at the biobehavioral level in conjunction with their attachment difficulties.[73] Mothers participating in ABC while receiving treatment in a residential substance treatment program show more sensitive and supportive parenting of their infants.[74]

The Circle of Security intervention was developed to harness group process (much like MTP) and video review (like ABC) to get parents to reflect on their children's attachment needs.[59] The Circle of Security begins with video-based psychoeducation about attachment using video clips of the caregivers in the group interacting with their children. In effect, caregivers get a review of key attachment concepts enhanced by graphic aides (see **Fig. 1** for an example) while also learning to observe children's behavior as an attachment coder would. As the intervention builds, the therapist selects clips from a preintervention SSP conducted with the caregiver and the child. The first set of individualized tape reviews allows the therapist to spur a given caregiver to reflect on the specific pattern of interactions with the child. A second set of tape reviews asks the caregiver to think about the struggles in meeting the child's specific attachment needs and often spurs reflection on intergenerational issues from the caregiver's own childhood. Through group process, the therapist works to foster caregivers' resilience, nurturing, and capacity for empathic understanding, whereas video review enhances caregivers' capacity to mentalize about their own attachment needs and those of their children.[59,75]

Circle of Security has been shown to shift attachment classification when delivered to groups of high-risk caregivers.[76,77] Changes in child internalizing and externalizing behavior problems following intervention have also been documented, as have shifts in caregivers' states of mind regarding attachment and caregivers' capacity to mentalize.[77,78] Circle of Security groups for incarcerated women with infants have been shown to promote secure attachment through improving caregiver sensitivity.[79] The model has also been adapted for home visiting[80] and is used individually and with couples.[59]

Recently, an 8-week version of the intervention has been developed (Cooper G, Hoffman K, Powell B. COS-P facilitator DVD manual 5.0, unpublished data. Circle of Security International; 2009). Video review is still incorporated as a means of enhancing parents' understanding of attachment-focused concepts, but stock video footage of parent–young child interactions (rather than individualized video footage) is used. The limited research on this less intensive intervention has documented a decrease in caregiver unsupportive responses to their children's distress matched by improvements in children's inhibitory control after 10 weeks.[81] Furthermore, improvements in self-reported parental locus of control, parenting attributions, discipline practices, and emotion regulation have been documented.[82,83]

Mom Power, a 13-session multifamily intervention meant to address the mental health and parenting competence of high-risk mothers who have experienced trauma and who are experiencing psychological symptoms, such as posttraumatic stress disorder or depression, is another promising intervention.[84] This family group intervention focuses on attachment and mentalization but incorporates specific intervention components to address caregivers' histories of trauma and psychological symptoms. As part of the Mom Power program, mothers participate in 3 individual sessions and 10 weekly 3-hour group sessions. Parenting skills that promote secure attachment are introduced alongside self-care skills that help caregivers cope with their own trauma and emotional distress. Participants have been shown to experience decreases in depressive and posttraumatic stress symptoms and report less caregiving helplessness, and improvements in parenting have been documented.[84] A similar intervention focused on caregivers in military families has also been developed and is promising.[85]

There are many recently developed attachment-focused interventions, and special-ists in attachment or infant mental health may be trained in one such intervention. At the same time, young children referred with aggression, behavioral disruption, and difficulties with emotion regulation in the context of early maltreatment, foster care, and/or institutionalization are frequently referred for evaluation regarding pharmacotherapy.

PHARMACOTHERAPY AND ATTACHMENT

As the practice parameter on attachment disorders from the American Academy of Child and Adolescent Psychiatry notes, psychopharmacologic interventions are not indicated for the core features of reactive attachment disorder or disinhibited social engagement disorder.[12] Some children with reactive attachment disorder or disinhi-bited social engagement disorder and some children with disturbances of attachment (but who do not meet criteria for an attachment disorder) have comorbid conditions (eg, anxiety, attention-deficit/hyperactivity disorder), and pharmacologic intervention may be indicated for that select group of children. The challenge for practitioners who are qualified to prescribe is that children with early disruption in attachment and/or early traumatic experiences can present with multiple internalizing and externalizing symp-toms. If assessment is incomplete and case formulation and care coordination are inad-equate, ineffective interventions may ensue. It seems likely that recent data on the abrupt increase in polypharmacy for young children in the child welfare system[86] reflect the pressure that prescribers feel to manage symptoms (eg, aggression in young chil-dren) with pharmacotherapy. With few, if any, longitudinal studies of pharmacotherapy in early childhood, which is a time when neural networks are in rapid development, the potential harm of pharmacotherapy is a concern.[87] If child psychiatrists are to serve symptomatic young children well, family-based care should be a first consideration, with pharmacotherapy playing an adjunctive role, and polypharmacy being avoided if possible.[88] If the prescriber feels that attachment-based psychotherapeutic interven-tions have not been tried and there is increasing pressure for pharmacotherapy trials, reviewing the case with a local specialist (see **Table 3**) would be prudent. The authors agree with Reebye and Elbe,[89] who noted that: "Regulation difficulties in preschoolers and young children have to be resolved through a multifaceted, responsible approach. Of these approaches, psychopharmacological intervention is an important avenue that should not be ignored even if it is only helpful to a select subset of this popula-tion."[89(p156)] However, when a child's dysregulation is associated with attachment disruption, disorganization, or disorder, pharmacotherapy alone is not likely to be sufficient.

One interesting development in attachment research has been the identification of key neurohormones that are linked to social bonding.[28,39] In the last 5 years, interven-tion trials of oxytocin, a neuropeptide at the center of this area of research, have been conducted with caregivers of young children, yielding variable results.[90] It is too soon to tell whether oxytocin will prove to be clinically useful in, for example, boosting care-givers' response to attachment-based therapies, although recent investigations of its use more broadly in psychiatry suggest that prescribing practitioners will be hearing more about this line of research.[91]

SUMMARY

Attachment is a key developmental process in childhood. Although child psychiatrists may have occasion to consider diagnosis of reactive attachment disorder or disinhi-bited social engagement disorder, they are more likely to see young children with early maltreatment or family disruption who have significant behavioral challenges but do not fit criteria for an attachment disorder. Understanding key principles of attachment assessment and intervention allows proper care coordination. For those psychiatrists not themselves expert in attachment assessment and intervention, accessing a local specialist to join a care coordination team may be important. However, standardized attachment assessments are informing clinical evaluation and several attachment-based interventions have recently been developed. Selecting the appropriate intervention may mean avoiding untested therapies that cause harm. Judicious use of pharmacotherapy can be helpful for young children with early disrupted attachment, although targeting behavior with medication alone is unlikely to be effective. In the end, coordinated care involving providers with sufficient expertise holds promise for helping the most vulnerable young children to thrive.

SUPPLEMENTARY DATA

Supplementary data related to this article can be found online at http://dx.doi.org/10.1016/j.chc.2017.03.003.

REFERENCES

1. Allen A. RADical idea: a call to eliminate "attachment disorder" and "attachment therapy" from the clinical lexicon. Evid Based Pract Child Adolesc Ment Health 2016;1:60–71.
2. Boris NW. Attachment, aggression and holding: a cautionary tale. Attach Hum Dev 2003;5:245–7.
3. Woolgar M, Baldock E. Attachment disorders versus more common problems in looked after and adopted children: comparing community and expert assessments. Child and Adolescent Mental Health 2015;20(1):34–40.
4. Mercer J. Attachment therapy. In: Lilienfeld SO, Lynn SJ, Lohr JM, editors. Science and pseudoscience in clinical psychology. 2nd edition. New York: The Guilford Press; 2015. p. 466–99.
5. Zeanah CH, Gleason MM. Annual research review: attachment disorders in early childhood–clinical presentation, causes, correlates, and treatment. J Child Psychol Psychiatry 2015;56:207–22.
6. American Academy of Child and Adolescent Psychiatry, Workgroup on Systems of Care. Best principles for early childhood systems of care. 2002. Available at: https://www.aacap.org/App_ Themes/AACAP/docs/clinical_practice_center/systems_of_care/B est_Principles_for_Early_Childhood_SOC.pdf. Accessed October 14, 2016.
7. McLennan JD, Wathen CN, MacMillan HL, et al. Research–practice gaps in child mental health. J Am Acad Child Adolesc Psychiatry 2006;45:658–65.
8. Cassidy J, Shaver PR. Preface. In: Cassidy J, Shaver PR, editors. Handbook of attachment: theory, research and clinical applications. 2nd edition. New York: Guilford Publications; 2008. p. xi–xvi.
9. Brauner CB, Stephens CB. Estimating the prevalence of early childhood serious emotional/behavioral disorders: challenges and recommendations. Public Health Rep 2006;121:303–10.
10. Hoagwood K, Burns BJ, Kiser L, et al. Evidence-based practice in child and adolescent mental health services. Psychiatr Serv 2001;52:1179–89.
11. Aarons GA. Measuring provider attitudes toward evidence-based practice: consideration of organizational context and individual differences. Child Adolesc Psychiatr Clin N Am 2005;14:255–8.

12. Zeanah CH, Chesher T, Boris NW, the AACAP Committee on Quality Issues. Practice parameter for the assessment and treatment of children and adolescents with reactive attachment disorder and disinhibited social engagement disorder. J Am Acad Child Adolesc Psychiatry 2016;55:990–1003.

13. Henderson SW, Martin A. Case formulation and integration of information in child and adolescent mental health. In: Rey JM, editor. IACAPAP e–Textbook of child and adolescent mental health. Geneva (Switzerland): International Association for Child and Adolescent Psychiatry and Allied Professions; 2014.

14. Boris NW, Fueyo M, Zeanah CH. The clinical assessment of attachment in children less than five. J Am Acad Child Adolesc Psychiatry 1997;36:291–3.

15. Winters NC, Pumariga A, Work Group on Community Child and Adolescent Psychiatry; Work Group on Quality Issues. Practice parameter on child and adolescent mental health care in community systems of care. J Am Acad Child Adolesc Psychiatry 2007;46:284–99.

16. Boris NW, Chesher TL, Wajda-Johnston V. Assessment of attachment in infancy and early childhood. In: DelCarmen R, Carter A, editors. Handbook of infant, toddler, and preschool mental health assessment. 2nd edition. Oxford University Press, in press.

17. Mercer J, Sarner L, Rosa L. Attachment therapy on trial: the torture and death of Candace Newmaker. Westport (CT): Praeger; 2003.

18. Zeanah CH, Berlin LJ, Boris NW. Practitioner review: clinical applications of attachment theory and research for infants and young children. J Child Psychol Psychiatry 2011;52:819–33.

19. Sameroff AA. A unified theory of development: a dialectic integration of nature and nurture. Child Dev 2010;81:6–22.

20. Hoff E. The specificity of environmental influence: socioeconomic status affects early vocabulary development via maternal speech. Child Dev 2003;74:1368–78.

21. Lewis BA, Patton E, Freebairn L, et al. Psychosocial co-morbidities in adolescents and adults with histories of communication disorders. J Commun Disord 2016;61: 60–70.

22. Bowlby J. By ethology out of psycho-analysis: an experiment in interbreeding. Anim Behav 1980;28:649–56.

23. Cassidy J. The nature of the child's ties. In: Cassidy J, Shaver PR, editors. Handbook of attachment: theory, research and clinical applications. 2nd edition. New York: Guilford Publications; 2008. p. 3–22.

24. Suomi SJ. Attachment in rhesus monkeys. In: Cassidy J, Shaver PR, editors. Handbook of attachment. New York: Guilford Press; 2008. p. 173–91.

25. Hauser MD, Yang C, Berwick RC, et al. The mystery of language evolution. Front Psychol 2014;5:40.

26. Landers MS, Sullivan RM. The development and neurobiology of infant attachment and fear. Dev Neurosci 2012;34:101–14.

27. Drury SS, Sánchez MM, Gonzalez A. When mothering goes awry: challenges and opportunities for utilizing evidence across rodent, nonhuman primate and human studies to better define the biological consequences of negative early caregiving. Horm Behav 2016;77:182–92.

28. Strathearn L. Maternal neglect: oxytocin, dopamine and the neurobiology of attachment. J Neuroendocrinol 2011;23:1054–65.

29. Carlson EA. A prospective longitudinal study of attachment disorganization/disorientation. Child Dev 1998;69:1107–28.

30. Sroufe LA, Egeland B, Carlson E, et al. The development of the person: the Minnesota Study of Risk and Adaptation from birth to adulthood. New York: Guilford Press; 2015.

31. Brandon AR, Pitts S, Denton WH, et al. A history of the theory of prenatal attachment. J Prenat Perinat Psychol Health 2009;23:201–22.

32. O'Connor TG, Heron J, Golding J, et al. Maternal antenatal anxiety and behavioural/emotional problems in children: a test of a programming hypothesis. J Child Psychol Psychiatry 2003;44:1025–36.

33. Gage SH, Munafò MR, Davey Smith G. Causal inference in developmental origins of health and disease (DOHaD) research. Annu Rev Psychol 2016;67:567–85.

34. Wallack L, Thornburg K. Developmental origins, epigenetics, and equity: moving upstream. Matern Child Health J 2016;20:935–40.

35. Decasper AJ, Spence MJ. Prenatal maternal speech influences newborns' perception of speech sound. Infant Behav Dev 1986;9:133–50.

36. Zeanah CH, Boris NW, Scheeringa MS. Infant development: the first three years of life. In: Tasman A, Kay J, Lieberman JA, editors. Psychiatry. New York: WB Saunders; 1996. p. 75–100.

37. Tronick E, Als H, Adamson L, et al. Infants response to entrapment between contradictory messages in face-to-face interaction. J Am Acad Child Adolesc Psychiatry 1978;17:1–13.

38. Beebe B, Jaffe J, Markese S, et al. The origins of 12-month attachment: a microanalysis of 4-month mother-infant interaction. Attach Hum Dev 2010;12:3–141.

39. Feldman R, Weller A, Zagoory-Sharon O, et al. Evidence for a neuroendocrinological foundation of human affiliation: plasma oxytocin levels across pregnancy and the postpartum period predict mother-infant bonding. Psychol Sci 2007;18: 965–70.

40. Weinfield NS, Sroufe LA, Egeland B, et al. Individual differences in infant-caregiver attachment. In: Cassidy J, Shaver PR, editors. Handbook of attachment: theory, research and clinical applications. 2nd edition. New York: Guilford Publications; 2009. p. 78–101.

41. Ainsworth MDS, Blehar MC, Waters E, et al. A psychological study of the strange situation. Hillsdale (NJ): Earlbaum; 1978.

42. Bowlby J. A secure base. New York: Basic Books; 1988.

43. Bretherton I, Munholland KA. Internal working models in attachment relationships. In: Cassidy J, Shaver PR, editors. Handbook of attachment: theory, research and clinical applications. 2nd edition. New York: Guilford Publications; 2009. p. 102–27.

44. Berlin LJ, Cassidy J, Appleyard K. The influence of early attachments on other relationships. In: Cassidy J, Shaver PR, editors. Handbook of attachment: theory, research and clinical applications. 2nd edition. New York: Guilford Publications; 2009. p. 333–47.

45. Page TF, Boris NW, Heller SS, et al. Narrative story-stems with high risk six year-olds: differential associations with mother- and teacher-reported psycho-social adjustment. Attach Hum Dev 2011;13:359–80.

46. Fonagy P, Gergely G, Target M. Psychoanalytic constructs and attachment theory and research. In: Cassidy J, Shaver PR, editors. Handbook of attachment: theory, research and clinical applications. 2nd edition. New York: Guilford; 2009. p. 783–810.

47. Thompson R. Early attachment and later development: familiar questions, new answers. In: Cassidy J, Shaver PR, editors. Handbook of attachment: theory,

research and clinical applications. 2nd edition. New York: Guilford; 2009. p. 348–65.

48. Fonagy P, Bateman AW. Mechanisms of change in mentalization-based treatment of BPD. J Clin Psychol 2006;62:411–30.

49. Lyons-Ruth K, Jacobvitz D. Attachment disorganization: genetic factors, parenting contexts, and developmental transformation from infancy to adulthood. In: Cassidy J, Shaver PR, editors. Handbook of attachment: theory, research and clinical applications. 2nd edition. New York: Guilford; 2009. p. 666–97.

50. Dykas MJ, Cassidy J. Attachment and the processing of social information across the life span: theory and evidence. Psychol Bull 2011;137:19–46.

51. Suchman NE, Mayes L, Conti J, et al. Rethinking parenting interventions for drug dependent mothers: fostering maternal responsiveness to children's emotional needs. J Subst Abuse Treat 2004;27:179–85.

52. Gervai J. Environmental and genetic influences on early attachment. Child Adolesc Psychiatry Ment Health 2009;3:25–37.

53. Cyr C, Euser EM, Bakermans-Kranenburg MJ, et al. Attachment security and disorganization in maltreating and high-risk families: a series of meta-analyses. Dev Psychopathol 2010;22:87–108.

54. Nelson CA, Fox NA, Zeanah CH. The effects of early psychosocial deprivation on brain and behavioral function: findings from the Bucharest Early Intervention Project. In: Cicchetti D, editor. Developmental psychopathology: risk, resilience and intervention. New York: Wiley; 2016. p. 934–70.

55. Zeanah CH, Boris NW. Disturbances and disorders of attachment in early childhood. In: Zeanah CH, editor. Handbook of mental health. 2nd edition. New York: Guilford Press; 2000. p. 353–68.

56. American Academy of Child and Adolescent Psychiatry. Practice parameters for the assessment of infants and toddlers (0–36 months). J Am Acad Child Adolesc Psychiatry 2007;44:1206–19.

57. Aoki Y, Zeanah CH, Heller SS, et al. Parent-Infant Relationship Global Assessment Scale: a study of its predictive validity. Psychiatry Clin Neurosci 2002;56: 493–7.

58. Steele H, Steele M. 10 clinical uses of the adult attachment interview. In: Steele H, Steele M, editors. Clinical applications of the adult attachment interview. New York: Guilford Press; 2008. p. 3–30.

59. Powell B, Cooper G, Hoffman K, et al. The Circle of Security intervention: enhancing attachment in early parent-child relationships. New York: Guilford Press; 2014.

60. Berthelot N, Ensink K, Bernazzani O, et al. Intergenerational transmission of attachment in abused and neglected mothers: the role of trauma-specific reflective functioning. Infant Ment Health J 2015;36:200–12.

61. Beckett C, Maughan B, Rutter M, et al. Do the effects of early severe deprivation on cognition persist into early adolescence? Findings from the English and Romanian adoptees study. Child Dev 2006;77:696–711.

62. Chaffin M, Hanson R, Saunders BE, et al. Report of the APSAC task force on attachment therapy, reactive attachment disorder, and attachment problems. Child Maltreat 2006;11:76–89.

63. Hembree-Kigin TL, McNeil CB. Parent-child interaction therapy. New York: Plenum Press; 1995.

64. Renk K, Boris NW, Kolomeyer E, et al. The state of evidence-based parenting interventions for parents who are substance-involved. Pediatr Res 2016;79:177–83.

65. Scott S, Dadds MR. Practitioner review: when parent training doesn't work: theory-driven clinical strategies. J Child Psychol Psychiatry 2009;50:1441–50.

66. Suchman NE, DeCoste C, Castiglioni N, et al. The mothers and toddlers program: preliminary findings from an attachment-based parenting intervention for substance-abusing mothers. Psychoanal Psychol 2008;25:499–517.

67. Suchman NE, DeCoste C, Castiglioni N, et al. The Mothers and Toddlers Program, an attachment-based parenting intervention for substance using women: post-treatment results from a randomized clinical pilot. Attach Hum Dev 2010; 12:483–504.

68. Suchman NE, DeCoste C, McMahon TJ, et al. The Mothers and Toddlers Program, an attachment-based parenting intervention for substance-using women: results at 6-week follow-up in a randomized clinical pilot. Infant Ment Health J 2011;32:427–49.

69. Rusconi-Serpa S, Sancho Rossignol A, McDonough SC. Video feedback in parent-infant treatments. Child Adolesc Psychiatr Clin N Am 2009;18:735–51.

70. Bernard K, Meade EB, Dozier M. Parental synchrony and nurturance as targets in an attachment based intervention: building upon Mary Ainsworth's insights about mother-infant interaction. Attach Hum Dev 2013;15:507–23.

71. Bick J, Bernard K, Dozier M. Attachment and biobehavioral catch-up: an attachment-based intervention for substance using mothers and their infants. In: Suchman NE, Pajulo M, Mayes LC, editors. Parenting and substance abuse: developmental approaches to intervention. New York: Oxford University Press; 2013. p. 303–20.

72. Dozier M, Peloso E, Lindhiem O, et al. Developing evidence-based interventions for foster children: an example of a randomized clinical trial with infants and toddlers. J Social Issues 2006;62:767–85.

73. Dozier M. Attachment-based treatment for vulnerable children. Attach Hum Dev 2003;5:253–7.

74. Berlin LJ, Shanahan M, Appleyard Carmody K. Promoting supportive parenting in new mothers with substance-use problems: a pilot randomized trial of residential treatment plus an attachment-based parenting program. Infant Ment Health J 2014;35:81–5.

75. Marvin R, Cooper G, Hoffman K, et al. The Circle of Security project: attachment-based intervention with caregiver-preschool child dyads. Attach Hum Dev 2002; 4:107–24.

76. Hoffman K, Marvin R, Cooper G, et al. Changing toddlers' and preschoolers' attachment classifications: the Circle of Security intervention. J Consult Clin Psychol 2006;74:1017–26.

77. Huber A, McMahon C, Sweller N. Efficacy of the 20-week Circle of Security intervention: changes in caregiver reflective functioning, representations, and child attachment in an Australian clinical sample. Infant Ment Health J 2015;36:556–74.

78. Huber A, McMahon C, Sweller N. Improved child behavioural and emotional functioning after Circle of Security 20-week intervention. Attach Hum Dev 2015;17: 547–69.

79. Cassidy J, Ziv Y, Stupica B, et al. Enhancing attachment security in the infants of women in a jail-diversion program. Attach Hum Dev 2010;12:333–53.

80. Cassidy J, Woodhouse S, Sherman L, et al. Enhancing infant attachment security: an examination of treatment efficacy and differential susceptibility. Dev Psychopathol 2011;23:131–48.

81. Cassidy J, Brett BE, Gross JT, et al. Circle of Security-parenting: a randomized controlled trial in Head Start. Dev Psychopathology, in press.

82. Horton E, Murray C. A quantitative exploratory evaluation of the Circle of Security-parenting program with mothers in residential substance-abuse treatment. Infant Ment Health J 2015;36:320–36.

83. Renk K, Boris NW. Creating a circle of security for substance-involved mothers and their parenting. Poster presented at the Biannual Convention of the Society for Research in Child Development. Philadelphia, Pennsylvania, March 19–21, 2015.

84. Muzik M, Rosenblum K, Alfafara EA, et al. Mom power: preliminary outcomes of a group intervention to improve mental health and parenting among high-risk mothers. Arch Womens Ment Health 2015;18:507–21.

85. Rosenblum KL, Muzik M. STRoNG intervention for military families with young children. Psychiatr Serv 2014;65:399–408.

86. Olfson M, King M, Schoenbaum M. Treatment of young people with antipsychotic medications in the United States. JAMA Psychiatry 2015;72:867–74.

87. Vitiello B. Principles in using psychotropic medication in children and adolescents. In: Rey JM, editor. IACAPAP e-textbook of child and adolescent mental health. Geneva (Switzerland): International Association for Child and Adolescent Psychiatry and Allied Professions; 2012. Available at: http://iacapap.org/wp-content/uploads/TABLE-OF-CONTENTS-2015.pdf. Accessed April 4, 2017.

88. Gleason MM, Egger HL, Emslie GJ, et al. Psychopharmacological treatment for very young children: contexts and guidelines. J Am Acad Child Adolesc Psychiatry 2007;46:1532–72.

89. Reebye PN, Elbe D. The role of pharmacotherapy in the management of self-regulation difficulties in young children. J Can Acad Child Adolesc Psychiatry 2009;18:150–9.

90. Bhandari R, van der Veen R, Parsons CE, et al. Effects of intranasal oxytocin administration on memory for infant cues: moderation by childhood emotional maltreatment. Soc Neurosci 2014;9:536–47.

91. Romano A, Tempesta B, Micioni Di Bonaventura MV, et al. From autism to eating disorders and more: the role of oxytocin in neuropsychiatric disorders. Front Neurosci 2016;12:497–516.

Trauma and Very Young Children

Melissa Jonson-Reid, MSW, PhD*, Ellie Wideman, MSW

KEYWORDS

- Trauma • Early childhood • Best practices • Therapeutic interventions • Screening

KEY POINTS

- Trauma experiences in early childhood are not as rare as once thought and pose significant challenges to healthy development and clinical intervention.
- Evidenced-based screening and treatment practices are emerging for this age range but remain limited, particularly for children younger than the age of 4 years.
- Currently, parent-involved treatments have the most evidence for effectiveness for this population.

It is easier to build strong children than to repair broken adults.

—*F. Douglas*

INTRODUCTION

Although research on the impact of trauma on children is not new, the attention to the effects of trauma for the very young child was renewed and strengthened by the work of Dr. Jack Shonkoff. Broadly focused on the intersection of early brain and the environment, his work also popularized the use of the words toxic stress in relation to early childhood development.[1,2] What do we mean by the word trauma?

- Trauma is defined in various ways across studies but typically includes exposure to events or conditions such as child abuse and neglect, domestic violence, community violence, war, and so forth. It may also include natural disasters or accidents.
- Trauma can occur as a discrete event, can be repeated, or can be a cumulative experience across multiple forms of violence or negative events.

How Common Is Trauma Exposure?

Children, particularly those living in poverty, have high rates of exposure to trauma. Child maltreatment is among the most common, with neglect being the most common

George Warren Brown School of Social Work, Washington University, Campus Box 1196, 1 Brookings Drive, St Louis, MO 63130, USA
* Corresponding author.
E-mail address: jonsonrd@wustl.edu

Child Adolesc Psychiatric Clin N Am 26 (2017) 477–490
http://dx.doi.org/10.1016/j.chc.2017.02.004
1056-4993/17/© 2017 Elsevier Inc. All rights reserved.

form of maltreatment. Nearly 69 out of 1000 infants and about 50 out of 1000 children ages 1 through 5 are investigated or assessed for report of abuse or neglect annually; children younger than the age of 3 years make up 71% of child maltreatment fatalities.[3] Although the exact rate of young children who are also exposed to intimate partner violence (IPV) is less clear, the overlap between these conditions is estimated to be between 30% and 60%.[4,5] Of course, children are also exposed to other forms of violence. Using the parent self-report for the Juvenile Victimization Questionnaire, Finkelhor[6] found rates of victimization for young children ranged from a low of about 50 per 1000 for indirect, to nearly 200 per 1000 for maltreatment, and more than 400 per 1000 for assault. Two-thirds of surveyed parents of children participating in Head Start (ages 3–5) reported that their child or children had witnessed or were victimized by community violence.[7]

How Does Trauma Affect Development?

Both retrospective surveys of cumulative adverse experiences[8] and prospective studies of maltreatment and IPV exposure[9–13] find that children who experience trauma are at risk of poor outcomes across a range of developmental and health domains. This risk accrues both because of direct harm through serious injury,[14] insults to attachment (See Boris NW, Renk K: Beyond Reactive Attachment Disorder: How Might Attachment Research Inform Child Psychiatry Practice?, in this issue), deficits in positive stimulation and modeling critical to early brain development, and repeated taxing of the neurobiological response system related to stress.[2] Being mindful of the direct and indirect nature of the influence of trauma that occurs within the first 2 years of life, before lasting memories of specific events can be formed,[15,16] is particularly important. Just because a child may be too young to recall traumatic events does not mean those experiences are without consequence.

Very young children lack a clear conception of time and cause and effect, they are susceptible to believing that their wishes, fears, and thoughts can become real or make things happen. The development of logical understanding and the ability to see different points of view are only just emerging by kindergarten.[17,18] The normal egocentrism, lack of understanding cause, and magical thinking can result in blaming themselves when trauma occurs. These normative developmental issues also make it impossible to anticipate danger or attempt to secure their personal safety, which leads to an increased vulnerability for physical harm. All of these factors combined may compound the negative effects of trauma on a child's development.[19]

Trauma, particularly persistent trauma, can result in the development of dysfunctional fear-related neurophysiologic patterns affecting emotional, behavioral, cognitive, and social functioning.[20] For example, increased and/or near constant activation of the stress response system (or hypothalamic-pituitary-adrenal [HPA] axis) leads to inappropriate levels of adrenaline and cortisol circulating through the body. Research indicates that this overactivation may lead to physical changes in the structure of the brain, such as in the hippocampus.[21,22] This overactivated stress response may also increase vulnerability to later mental health problems, particularly depression.[22] Interestingly many of these studies indicate that emotional neglect has a similarly powerful affect as other forms of maltreatment. A clear understanding of these effects on the developing brain and potential interaction with genetics is still emerging.[22]

Many readers may have heard about the Adverse Childhood Experiences (ACES) study. As noted in the brief discussion of prevalence and illustrated in **Fig. 1**, there are other contextual risks, such as poverty or having a parent with a mental health disorder, that may co-occur with, or enhance the risk of, experiencing trauma. The

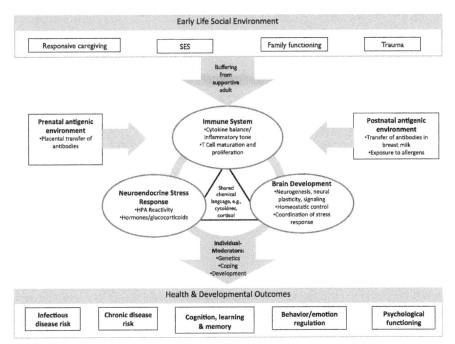

Fig. 1. Mediating role of the neuroendocrine-immune (NEI) network in linking early life experiences to individual differences in health and functioning. SES, socioeconomic status. (*From* Johnson SB, Riley AW, Granger DA, et al. The science of early life toxic stress for pediatric practice and advocacy. Pediatrics 2013;131(2):322; with permission.)

ACES study of longer term health and mental health consequences among adults recalling childhood experiences measured a mixture of what the authors would consider trauma and contextual risks.[8] Some of these contextual risks, such as early prolonged exposure to poverty, may have their own independent impact on developmental harm.[22,23]

Before reviewing some of the clinically relevant consequences of trauma, however, it is important to remember that early childhood development is a result of a complex interaction of risk, protective, and buffering factors. **Fig. 1** illustrates the number of neurobiological structures involved in a child's response to stress, and the various other positive and negative factors that influence this response.[24] A risk of negative outcome is not the same as certainty that a child so exposed will develop behavioral or emotional difficulties.

CLINICAL CONSEQUENCES AMONG YOUNG CHILDREN

As previously referenced, there are a variety of harms that can accrue following trauma. Clinical consequences of the traumatic event experience may affect a 12-month-old differently than a 6-year-old because of the varying stage of neural development, as well as individual characteristics.[25,26] This can make assessment challenging. Research on very young children suggests that it is important for clinicians not to rely on *Diagnostic and Statistical Manual of Mental Disorders, 4th Edition, Text Revision* or the *Diagnostic Classification of Mental Health and Developmental*

Disorders of Infancy and Early Childhood: Revised Edition, 0–3 (DC: 0–3R) exclusively but to also assess developmental symptoms as a consequence of trauma exposure that may be particularly relevant to an infant or toddler[11,27]:

- Some children (estimates vary depending on criteria used and the age range included in the study from <25% to 69%) who experience trauma will develop posttraumatic stress disorder, which can manifest in problems sleeping, hyperarousal, and difficulty concentrating.[11]
- Overactivation of the HPA may lead to greater vulnerability to later depression.[22]
- Young children may regress to earlier milestones (eg, bedwetting), be very clingy, and so forth[28]
- Impacts on early development may manifest in problems regulating emotion[29] and/or insecure attachment,[30] which can lead to enduring difficulties in relationships with others.
- Children may become hypervigilant even to very mild perceived threats (attention bias), which may lead to anxiety disorder symptoms.[31]

PROTECTIVE FACTORS AND RESILIENCE

Not all young children exposed to trauma will develop serious or chronic symptoms that lead to lasting impairment. Resilience is an individual's ability to survive through adverse life events, move forward with life tasks, and sustain their quality of life despite the negative circumstances. The proportion of children who are resilient following trauma varies widely between studies and measurement criteria used.[32,33] It is generally conceptualized as a balance of factors from pre-existing individual characteristics (eg, intelligence, genetic factors, coping strategies) and environmental factors in the home and community.[34,35] Family factors that may buffer or offset risk include things like responsive caregiving and secure attachment to an adult, whereas community factors include things such as social cohesion and available resources.[36,37] Although some protective factors may be difficult for a clinician to affect, others are less so.

Recent research suggests that even neurochemical changes associated with trauma may be affected by intervention.[38] The timing of a positive intervention along with the developmental stage of the child may have a tremendous impact on how the therapeutic intervention will influence the brain. Early interventions may more quickly and effectively or efficiently shape the development of attachment and optimal neuropathways versus later remediation.[25,26]

ASSESSMENT AND INTERVENTION

When young children experience a traumatic stressor, their first response is typically to look for support from the adults who care for them. In addition to treatment, mental health practitioners can offer tips for caregivers to help reestablish safety and constancy for young children who have experienced a trauma, including

- Answering children's questions in language at their level of current understanding
- Developing family safety plans
- Engaging in age-appropriate activities
- Finding ways to have fun and relax together
- Helping children increase their feelings vocabulary
- Honoring family traditions that bring them close to the people they love
- Noting changes in behaviors to discuss with clinicians
- Helping children to get back to their routines before the event

- Establishing and following routines and schedules
- Setting boundaries and limits with consistency and patience
- Showing love and affection.[19,26]

Assessment of Trauma Symptoms

Assessment of trauma in young children must focus on the presenting problem in the context of the child's overall development. Clinical assessment should include broad analysis of the traumatic experiences including

- Reactions of the child and parents or caregivers
- Changes in the child's behavior
- Available resources in the environment to stabilize the child and family
- Quality of the child's primary attachment relationships
- Ability of parents or caregivers to facilitate the child's healthy socioemotional, psychological, and cognitive development.[25,26]

A helpful age-appropriate checklist is available online from the National Child Traumatic Stress Network[39] and included in **Table 1** to guide clinicians' thinking about behavioral signs that may indicate a problematic reaction to trauma.

Only a handful of formal trauma assessment instruments exist for this age range. There is considerable debate regarding the relative utility of various approaches to assessing trauma symptoms for this population.[11,27,40] It is beyond the scope of this article to attempt to review the relative strengths and weaknesses of each tool. **Table 2** contains links to training or purchase for scales that include a lower age range of 3 years or younger.[41–47] Two caveats should be noted. First, although the Child Behavior Checklist (CBCL) for children ages 1.5 to 5 years is sometimes used to assess trauma symptoms, it was not designed for that purpose and some practitioners question its use.[40] Second, the DC: 0–3R is not a scale but rather a system for diagnoses of mental health and development disorders in very young children.[41] Clinicians should review the properties of the measures along with the characteristics of their client in determining which approach to assessment is most useful in case planning.

Intervention

Interventions for young children who have experienced trauma range from adopting a trauma-informed care or systems approach to specific treatment modalities. In many cases, the ideas for appropriate care as yet far exceed the available data to judge their effectiveness.

Trauma-informed systems

Providers operating in a trauma-informed system are able to understand the influence of trauma and use the best available evidenced-based practices to address a child or family's needs. Common elements of these systems include

- Routinely screening for trauma exposure and related symptoms
- Using culturally appropriate evidence-based assessment and treatment of trauma symptoms
- Making resources available to children, families, and providers on trauma exposure, its impact, and treatment
- Engaging in efforts to strengthen the resilience and protective factors of children and families affected by and vulnerable to trauma
- Addressing parent and caregiver trauma and its impact on the family system

Table 1
Assessment checklist provided by the National Child Trauma Stress Network, 2003

	Ages 0–2 y	Ages 3–6 y
Cognitive		
Poor verbal skills	✔	—
Memory issues	✔	—
Focus in school	—	✔
Development of a disability	—	✔
Poor skill development	—	✔
Behavioral		
Excessive temper	✔	✔
Demanding of attention: positive and negative	✔	✔
Regression in Behaviors	✔	✔
Aggression in behaviors	✔	✔
Acting out in social situations	—	✔
Imitate the trauma event in play and so forth	—	✔
Verbally abusive	—	✔
Screams or cries more easily	✔	—
Startles easily	✔	✔
Unable to trust others or make friends easily	—	✔
Believes to be the blame for trauma event	—	✔
Fears adults who remind them of trauma event	✔	✔
Fear of separation for adult parents or caregiver	✔	✔
Anxious, fearful, avoidant	—	✔
Increase in feelings of anxiety, sadness, irritability	✔	✔
Noticeably withdrawn	✔	✔
Lowered self-confidence	—	✔
Physical		
Poor appetite, weight changes (loss or gain), digestion issues	✔	—
Stomachaches, headaches	—	✔
Sleep changes (insomnia)	✔	✔
Nightmares or night terrors	✔	✔
Regression (bedwetting after milestone was reached and achieved)	—	✔

Adapted from The National Child Trauma Stress Network. Symptoms and behaviors associated with exposure to trauma. Available at: http://www.nctsn.org/trauma-types/early-childhood-trauma/Symptoms-and-Behaviors-Associated-with-Exposure-to-Trauma. Accessed February 7, 2017; with permission.

- Emphasizing continuity of care and collaboration across child-service systems
- Maintaining an environment of care for staff that addresses, minimizes, and treats secondary traumatic stress, and that increases staff resilience.[48]

As yet, although there are numerous calls to implement this approach from preschool settings to juvenile courts, there is little research on what influence these systems have on child outcomes.[48–53]

Table 2
Instruments and tools for assessing traumatic stress in young children

Assessment Tool	Authors	Age Range (y)
Child Behavior Checklist (CBCL), not designed spec	Achenbach & Rescorla,[41] 2001 http://www.aseba.org/preschool.html	1.5–5
The DC: 0–3R Multi-Axial System	Zero to Three,[42] 2005 https://www.zerotothree.org/resources/services/dc-0-3r	0–3
Posttraumatic Stress Disorder Semi-Structured Interview and Observation Record	Scheeringa & Zeanah,[45] 1994 http://www.nctsn.org/content/posttraumatic-stress-disorder-semi-structured-interview-and-observational-record	0–4
Preschool-Age Psychiatric Assessment (PAPA)	Egger et al,[44] 1999; Egger et al,[43] 2006 http://devepi.duhs.duke.edu/papa.html	2–5
Posttraumatic Stress Disorder symptoms in Preschool-Aged Children (PTSD-PAC)	Levendosky et al,[46] 2002 http://www.nctsnet.org/content/ptsd-preschool-aged-children	3–5
Trauma Symptom Checklist for Young Children	Briere et al,[47] 2001 http://www4.parinc.com/Products/Product.aspx?ProductID=TSCYC&tp=tscyc	3–12

Data from Refs.[41–47]

Trauma interventions

Age-appropriate trauma treatment interventions have been increasingly developed and tested as the awareness of the prevalence and influence of trauma on very young children has grown. These approaches share many of the same core components. They are generally relationship-based, focus on healing and supporting the child-parent relationship, and promote the use of positive parenting skills.[49,54] A brief overview is provided of the few available evidence-based treatments for this age range that were either specifically designed to work with trauma or have been found effective with a population exposed to trauma (eg, child welfare). It is unclear to what extent trauma treatments, compared with parenting programs that are focused on attachment and positive parenting, are most useful for this population.[55,56]

Table 3 summarizes the intended population, outcomes assessed, effect sizes (if possible), and means of accessing training for interventions with the highest ratings from the California Evidence-Based Clearinghouse (CEBC). The exception to this is Attachment, Self-Regulation, and Competency, which is not yet rated by CEBC but is listed as an evidence-based program by the National Child Traumatic Stress Network for addressing complex trauma. **Table 3** is followed by a brief description of the content and approach of each intervention.

Attachment and biobehavioral catch-up

- For young children who have experienced early traumatic disruptions in care and/or maltreatment to focus on attachment reconstruction.
- This intervention targets 3 areas: (1) nurturance, (2) a child's dysregulation at the behavioral and biological levels, and (3) parenting practices to alleviate child's

Table 3
Recommended evidence-based practice interventions: ratings and effectiveness

Intervention or Treatment & Training Information	Child Age (y)	Outcomes Tested	Population Characteristics	Effects	CEBC Rating[a]
Attachment, Regulation, and Competency (ARC) http://www.nctsn.org/sites/default/files/assets/pdfs/arc_general.pdf	0–21	Parent-child aggression, conduct problems, shame	Children with chronic and complex traumas	None available specific to this age range	NR
Attachment and Biobehavioral Catch-Up (ABC) http://www.nctsn.org/sites/default/files/assets/pdfs/abc_general.pdf	0–2	Attachment & cortisol	Infants and toddlers with known trauma and traumatic break with primary caregiver	$d = 1.06$	1
Child-Parent Psychotherapy http://www.nctsn.org/sites/default/files/assets/pdfs/cpp_general.pdf	0–5	Attachment, self-representation, maternal sensitivity	Trials were done with child welfare involved families	$h = 0.64-1.39$	2
Incredible Years http://incredibleyears.com/workshop-info/training-descriptions/	4–8 0–3[b]	Increasing prosocial behaviors	Parents of children with behavior problems and also with child welfare-involved families	$d = 0.27$	1
Parent-Child Interaction Therapy (PCIT) http://www.nctsn.org/sites/default/files/assets/pdfs/pcit_general.pdf	2–7	Disruptive behaviors in children with trauma	Children with behavior and parent-child relationship issues	Fathers ($d = 1.88$), mothers $d = 1.99$	1
Trauma-Focused Cognitive Behavior Therapy (TF-CBT) http://www.nctsn.org/sites/default/files/assets/pdfs/tfcbt_general.pdf	3–18	Reduction of trauma symptoms	Children with known trauma history	$d = 0.40-.70$	1

d, Cohen's d and is a measure of effect size; h, Cohen's measure of effect size with Arcsin transformation.
[a] 1, well-supported; 2, supported by research evidence; NR, not rated.
[b] An infant toddler version is available but effects from the randomized clinical trial are not yet known.

behavioral concerns.[57–59] Attachment and biobehavioral catch-up (ABC) includes 10 1-hour sessions, usually in the home with the caregiver and child together.

Attachment, regulation, and competency
- Attachment, regulation, and competency (ARC) is a structure for treatment designed for youth from early childhood to adolescence and their parents or caregivers or caregiving systems.[60,61]
- ARC was developed to address complex trauma and can be used within a wide range of systems. ARC addresses 3 core domains: (1) attachment, (2) self-regulation, and (3) developmental competency. ARC as a structure is not a 1-size-fits-all model, meaning the treatment duration will vary.

Child-parent psychotherapy
- This dyadic psychotherapy is focused on the caregiver-child attachment relationship and can be done in the home or clinic.
- The focus is on (1) safety, (2) affect regulation, (3) reciprocity in relationships, and (4) parent understanding of trauma and adaptive behavior. This is a long-term intervention with 50 1-hour sessions with the child and caregiver together.[55,62,63]

The incredible years
- The incredible years (IY) was designed as a parenting program not a trauma treatment and promotes emotional and social competence to prevent and reduce behavior and emotional problems in young children.
- There are treatment versions of the program, as well as prevention versions for high-risk populations. The program has been adapted for and implemented with child welfare–involved and homeless populations.[56,64–66] The number of sessions vary by the age of the child and are conducted in group format.

Parent-child interaction therapy
- Parent-child interaction therapy (PCIT) is also a parent training intervention that focuses on improving the parent or caregiver-child relationship and on increasing children's positive behaviors. It has been adapted for children who have experienced trauma.
- Parents or caregivers are coached by a therapist while engaging in specific play and discipline skills with their child. PCIT is a short-term, mastery-based treatment that is provided for an average of 14 weeks.[67–69]

Trauma-focused cognitive behavioral therapy
- Trauma-Focused Cognitive Behavioral Therapy (TF-CBT) is a cognitive behavioral intervention adapted for children who have experienced trauma. Although not originally designed for very young children, at least 1 randomized clinical trial indicates feasibility and benefit for preschool children.
- Treatment, on average, consists of 12 sessions. The approach helps children and their nonabusing family members practice emotional identification and appropriate reaction to thoughts, feelings, and behaviors that are associated with past traumas. They practice these techniques during graduated exposure to abuse-constructed trauma. Several joint parent or caregiver and child sessions are included to enhance family communication.[55,70–72]

These interventions have the strongest research supporting use with this population. Treatments involving the child alone (eg, day treatment or play therapy) were excluded because, thus far, studies have not been of sufficient rigor, and/or the evidence is poor for effectiveness, and/or there is no indication that they can be used with traumatized children in this age range.[73–75] On the other hand, at least 28 different interventions are currently being explored as promising practices on various Web-based collections for evidence-based practices. Clinicians are encouraged to check these Web sites for updated assessment and treatment information:

- http://www.cebc4cw.org/ud
- http://www.nctsn.org/
- http://www.samhsa.gov/ebp-web-guide/mental-health-treatment.

SUMMARY

The relatively common occurrence of trauma in the lives of young children in the United States and around the world creates a sense of urgency for improving knowledge in this area. Many questions remain regarding adequate assessment and triage for further intervention, as well as the relative impact of specific treatment packages across varying populations, degrees of trauma, and family characteristics. Clinicians can help move the field forward by partnering with researchers (eg, practice-based research networks) to build knowledge of the adoption of and outcomes noted for evidence-based and promising programs across varying populations. Assessment and treatment work also needs to be coordinated with neuroscience, genetic, and epigenetic studies. Improved understanding of the therapeutic effect of interventions at the neurobiological level for populations with varying degrees of vulnerability[22,25,38] may lead to more effective targeting of preventive approaches while supporting efforts to increase access to effective treatment.[2,24] Although the prevalent nature and significant harm associated with trauma should inspire clinicians to action, research also indicates significant hope for children who receive early and effective intervention.

REFERENCES

1. National Research Council and Institute of Medicine. From neurons to neighborhoods: the science of early childhood development. Committee on integrating the science of early childhood development. In: Shonkoff JP, Phillips DA, editors. Board on children, youth, and families, commission on behavioral and social sciences and education. Washington, DC: National Academy Press; 2000. p. 182–217.
2. Shonkoff JP, Garner AS, Siegel BS, et al. The lifelong effects of early childhood adversity and toxic stress. Pediatrics 2012;129:e232–46.
3. US DHHS, Children's Bureau. Child maltreatment 2014. Washington, DC: Author; 2016. Available at: http://www.acf.hhs.gov/programs/cb/resource/child-maltreatment-2014. Accessed September 1, 2016.
4. Kelleher K, Gardner W, Coben J, et al. Co-occurring intimate partner violence and child maltreatment: local policies/practices and relationships to child placement, family services and residence. Final Report (Doc No 213503). 2006. Available at: https://www.ncjrs.gov/pdffiles1/nij/grants/213503.pdf. Accessed August 15, 2016.
5. Millett LS, Seay KD, Kohl PL. A national study of intimate partner violence risk among female caregivers involved in the child welfare system: the role of nativity, acculturation, and legal status. Child Youth Serv Rev 2015;48:60–9.
6. Finkelhor D. Childhood victimization: violence, crime, and abuse in the lives of young people. New York: Oxford University Press; 2008.

7. Shahinfar A, Fox NA, Leavitt LA. Preschool children's exposure to violence: relation of behavior problems to parent and child reports. Am J Orthop 2000;70:115–25.

8. Felitti VJ, Anda RF, Nordenberg D, et al. Relationship of childhood abuse and household dysfunction to many of the leading causes of death in adults: the Adverse Childhood Experiences (ACE) study. Am J Prev Med 1998;14:245–58.

9. Graham-Bermann SA, Perkins S. Effects of early exposure and lifetime exposure to intimate partner violence (IPV) on child adjustment. Violence Vict 2010;25(4): 427–39.

10. Lanier P, Jonson-Reid M, Stahlschmidt M, et al. Child maltreatment and pediatric health outcomes: a longitudinal study of low-income children. J Pediatr Psychol 2009;35(5):511–22.

11. Levendosky AA, Bogat GA, Martinez-Torteya C. PTSD symptoms in young children exposed to intimate partner violence. Violence Against Women 2013;19: 187–201.

12. Jonson-Reid M, Drake B, Kohl P. Is the overrepresentation of the poor in child welfare caseloads due to bias or need? Child Youth Serv Rev 2009;31:422–7.

13. Jonson-Reid M, Kohl P, Drake B. Child and adult outcomes of chronic child maltreatment. Pediatrics 2012;129(5):839–45.

14. Leventhal JM, Gaither JR. Incidence of serious injuries due to physical abuse in the United States: 1997 to 2009. Pediatrics 2012;130(5):e847–52.

15. Bauer PJ, Leventon JS. Memory for one-time experiences in the second year of life: implications for the status of episodic memory. Infancy 2013;18(5):755–81.

16. Howe ML. Memory development: implications for adults recalling childhood experiences in the courtroom. Nat Rev Neurosci 2013;14(12):869–76.

17. Piaget J. The language and thought of the child, vol. 5. New York: Psychology Press; 1959.

18. Erikson EH. Childhood and society. New York: WW Norton & Company; 1993.

19. National Child Trauma Stress Network. Complex trauma. 2003. Available at: http://www.nctsnet.org/nctsn_assets/pdfs/edu_materials/ComplexTrauma_All.pdf. Accessed August 15, 2016.

20. Perry BD, Pollard R. Homeostasis, stress, trauma, and adaptation: a neurodevelopmental view of childhood trauma. Child Adolesc Psychiatr Clin N Am 1998;7:33–51.

21. National Scientific Council on the Developing Child. Excessive stress disrupts the architecture of the developing brain: working paper 3. Updated edition. 2014. Available at: http://www.developingchild.harvard.edu. Accessed August 15, 2016.

22. Frodl T, O'Keane V. How does the brain deal with cumulative stress? A review with focus on developmental stress, HPA axis function and hippocampal structure in humans. Neurobiol Dis 2013;52:24–37.

23. Luby JL. Poverty's most insidious damage: the developing brain. JAMA Pediatr 2015;169(9):810–1.

24. Johnson SB, Riley AW, Granger DA, et al. The science of early life toxic stress for pediatric practice and advocacy. Pediatrics 2013;131(2):319–27.

25. Perry BD. Examining child maltreatment through a neurodevelopmental lens: clinical applications of the neurosequential model of therapeutics. J Loss Trauma 2009;14(4):240–55.

26. Child Welfare Information Gateway. Understanding the effects of maltreatment on brain development. Washington, DC: U.S. Dept of Health and Human Services, Children's Bureau; 2015. Available at: https://www.childwelfare.gov/pubPDFs/brain_development.pdf. Accessed September 1, 2016.

27. Scheeringa MS, Zeanah CH, Myers L, et al. New findings on alternative criteria for PTSD in preschool children. J Am Acad Child Adolesc Psychiatry 2003;42:561–70.

28. Malarbi S, Muscara F, Stargatt R. Cognitive deficits and posttraumatic stress disorder in children: a diagnostic dilemma illustrated through a case study. J Trauma Dissociation 2016;17(2):199–206.
29. Dvir Y, Ford JD, Hill M, et al. Childhood maltreatment, emotional dysregulation, and psychiatric comorbidities. Harv Rev Psychiatry 2014;22(3):149–61.
30. Howell KH, Barnes SE, Miller LE, et al. Developmental variations in the impact of intimate partner violence exposure during childhood. J Inj Violence Res 2016; 8(1):43–57.
31. Briggs-Gowan MJ, Pollak SD, Grasso D, et al. Attention bias and anxiety in young children exposed to family violence. J Child Psychol Psychiatry 2015;56(11): 1194–201.
32. Cicchetti D. Annual research review: resilient functioning in maltreated children–past, present, and future perspectives. J Child Psychol Psychiatry 2013;54(4):402–22.
33. Klika JB, Herrenkohl TI. A review of developmental research on resilience in maltreated children. Trauma Violence Abuse 2013;14(3):222–34.
34. Enlow MB, Blood E, Egeland B. Sociodemographic risk, developmental competence, and PTSD symptoms in young children exposed to interpersonal trauma in early life. J Trauma Stress 2013;26(6):686–94.
35. Feldman R, Vengrober A, Eidelman-Rothman M, et al. Stress reactivity in war-exposed young children with and without posttraumatic stress disorder: relations to maternal stress hormones, parenting, and child emotionality and regulation. Dev Psychopathol 2013;25(4 pt 1):943–55.
36. Coatsworth JD, Duncan L. Fostering resilience. A strengths-based approach to mental health. A CASSP discussion paper. Harrisburgh (PA): Pennsylvania CASSP Training and Technical Assistance Institute; 2003.
37. Zolkoski SM, Bullock LM. Resilience in children and youth: a review. Child Youth Serv Rev 2012;34(12):2295–303.
38. McCrory E, De Brito SA, Viding E, et al. Research review: the neurobiology and genetics of maltreatment and adversity. J Child Psychol Psychiatry 2010; 51(10):1079–95.
39. National Child Trauma Stress Network. Possible reactions of children 0-6 exposed to traumatic stress; ND. Available at: http://www.nctsn.org/trauma-types/early-childhood-trauma/Symptoms-and-Behaviors-Associated-with-Exposure-to-Trauma. Accessed September 1, 2016.
40. Stover CS, Berkowitz S. Assessing violence exposure and trauma symptoms in young children: a critical review of measures. J Trauma Stress 2005;18(6):707–17.
41. Achenbach TM, Rescorla LA. Manual for ASEBA preschool forms and profiles. Burlington (Canada): University of Vermont; 2001.
42. Zero To Three. Diagnostic classification of mental health and developmental disorders of infancy and early childhood: revised edition (DC: 0–3R). Washington, DC: Zero To Three Press; 2005.
43. Egger HL, Erkanli A, Keeler G, et al. Test–retest reliability of the preschool age psychiatric assessment (PAPA). J Am Acad Child Adolesc Psychiatry 2006;45: 538–49.
44. Egger HL, Ascher BH, Angold A. The preschool age psychiatric assessment: version 1.1. Durham (NC): Center for Developmental Epidemiology, Department of Psychiatry and Behavioral Sciences, Duke University Medical Center; 1999.
45. Scheeringa MS, Zeanah CH. PTSD semi-structured interview and observational record for infants and young children. New Orleans (LA): Department of Psychiatry and Neurology, Tulane University Health Sciences Center; 1994.

46. Levendosky AA, Huth-Bocks AC, Semel MA, et al. Trauma symptoms in preschool-age children exposed to domestic violence. J Interpers Violence 2002;17(2):150–64.

47. Briere J, Johnson K, Bissada A, et al. The trauma symptom checklist for young children (TSCYC): reliability and association with abuse exposure in a multi-site study. Child Abuse Negl 2001;25(8):1001–14.

48. National Child Traumatic Stress Network. Creating trauma-informed systems. ND. Available at: http://www.nctsnet.org/resources/topics/creating-trauma-informed-systems. Accessed September 1, 2016.

49. Holmes C, Levy M, Smith A, et al. A model for creating a supportive trauma-informed culture for children in preschool settings. J Child Fam Stud 2015; 24(6):1650–9.

50. Ko S, Ford J, Kassam-Adams N, et al. Creating trauma-informed systems: child welfare, education, first responders, health care, juvenile justice. Prof Psychol Res Pract 2008;39:396–404.

51. Pilnik L, Kendall J. Identifying polyvictimization and trauma among court involved children and youth: a checklist and resource guide for attorneys and other court-appointed advocates. Bethesda (MD): Safe Start Center, Office of Juvenile Justice and Delinquency Prevention, Office of Justice Programs, US Dept. of Justice; 2012.

52. Taylor S, Steinber A, Wilson C. The child welfare trauma referral tool. San Diego (CA): Chadwick Center for Children and Families, Rady Children's Hospital; 2006.

53. Statman-Weil K. Creating trauma sensitive classrooms. Young Child 2015;72–9. Available at: http://www.naeyc.org/yc/files/yc/file/201505/YC0515_Trauma-Sensitive_Classrooms_Statman-Weil.pdf. Accessed September 1, 2016.

54. Hodas GR. Responding to childhood trauma: the promise and practice of trauma informed care. Pennsylvania: Pennsylvania Office of Mental Health and Substance Abuse Services; 2006.

55. Fraser JG, Lloyd S, Murphy R, et al. A comparative effectiveness review of parenting and trauma-focused interventions for children exposed to maltreatment. J Dev Behav Pediatr 2013;34(5):353–68.

56. Rogers KC, Bobich M, Heppell P. The impact of implementing an "Incredible Years" group within a family living unit in a transitional living shelter: the case of "Cathy". Pragmat Case Stud Psychother 2016;12(2):65–112.

57. Dozier M, Dozier D, Manni M. Recognizing the special needs of infants' and toddlers' foster parents: development of a relational intervention. Zero Three 2002; 22:7–13.

58. Dozier M, Lindhiem O, Lewis E, et al. Effects of a foster parent training program on young children's attachment behaviors: preliminary evidence from a randomized clinical trial. Child Adolesc Social Work J 2009;26(4):321–32.

59. Bernard K, Dozier M, Bick J, et al. Enhancing attachment organization among maltreated children: results of a randomized clinical trial. Child Dev 2012;83(2): 623–36.

60. Blaustein ME, Kinniburgh KM. Treating traumatic stress in children and adolescents: how to foster resilience through attachment, self-regulation, and competency. New York: Guilford Press; 2010.

61. Arvidson J, Kinniburgh K, Howard K, et al. Treatment of complex trauma in young children: developmental and cultural considerations in application of the ARC intervention model. J Child Adolesc Trauma 2011;4(1):34–51.

62. Lieberman AF, Van Horn P, Ippen CG. Toward evidence-based treatment: child-parent psychotherapy with preschoolers exposed to marital violence. J Am Acad Child Adolesc Psychiatry 2005;44(12):1241–8.
63. Toth SL, Maughan A, Manly JT, et al. The relative efficacy of two interventions in altering maltreated preschool children's representational models: implications for attachment theory. Dev Psychopathol 2002;14:877–908.
64. Reid MJ, Webster-Stratton C. The Incredible Years parent, teacher, and child intervention: targeting multiple areas of risk for a young child with pervasive conduct problems using a flexible, manualized, treatment program. Cogn Behav Pract 2001;8:377–86.
65. Hurlburt MS, Nguyen K, Reid J, et al. Efficacy of the Incredible Years group parent program with families in Head Start who self-reported a history of child maltreatment. Child Abuse Negl 2013;37(8):531–43.
66. Webster-Stratton C, Reid M. Adapting the Incredible Years, an evidence-based parenting programme, for families involved in the child welfare system. J Child Serv 2010;5(1):25–42.
67. Abrahamse ME, Junger M, Chavannes EL, et al. Parent–child interaction therapy for preschool children with disruptive behaviour problems in The Netherlands. Child Adolesc Psychiatry Ment Health 2012;6:24–34.
68. Chaffin M, Funderburk B, Bard D, et al. A combined motivation and parent–child interaction therapy package reduces child welfare recidivism in a randomized dismantling field trial. J Consult Clin Psychol 2011;79(1):84–95.
69. Lanier P, Kohl PL, Benz J, et al. Preventing maltreatment with a community-based implementation of parent–child interaction therapy. J Child Fam Stud 2014;23(2):449–60.
70. Deblinger E, Lippmann J, Steer R. Sexually abused children suffering posttraumatic stress symptoms: initial treatment outcome findings. Child Maltreat 1996;1(4):310–21.
71. Bigfoot DS, Schmidt SR. Honoring children, mending the circle: cultural adaptation of trauma-focused cognitive-behavioral therapy for American Indian and Alaska Native children. J Clin Psychol 2010;66(8):847–56.
72. Scheeringa MS, Salloum A, Arnberger RA, et al. Feasibility and effectiveness of cognitive-behavioral therapy for posttraumatic stress disorder in preschool children: two case reports. J Trauma Stress 2007;20(4):631–6.
73. Kanine RM, Tunno AM, Jackson Y, et al. Therapeutic day treatment for young maltreated children: a systematic literature review. J Child Adolesc Trauma 2015;8(3):187–99.
74. Lin YW, Bratton SC. A meta-analytic review of child-centered play therapy approaches. J Couns Dev 2015;93(1):45–58.
75. Shaheen S. How child's play impacts executive function–related behaviors. Appl Neuropsychol Child 2014;3:182–7.

Disruptive Behavior Disorders in Children 0 to 6 Years Old

Mini Tandon, DO, Andrea Giedinghagen, MD*

KEYWORDS

- Preschool children • Disruptive behavior • Oppositional defiant disorder
- Conduct disorder

KEY POINTS

- Disruptive behavior disorders (DBDs) are among the most common reasons preschoolers present for psychiatric care, and frequently presage later psychiatric, legal, and educational issues.
- Exposure to harsh and inconsistent parenting increases preschoolers' risk of DBDs, and partially mediates the adverse effects of economic hardship, neighborhood violence, and parental depression.
- Childhood DBDs are associated with decreased size and activity of bilateral amygdalae and insulae, and with related deficits in fear modulation and empathic emotional processing.
- Preschoolers with DBDs show executive functioning deficits, in part related to attention-deficit/hyperactivity disorder comorbidity. Decreased response inhibition to emotionally salient stimuli is particularly linked to reactive aggression.
- Parent management training programs focused on decreasing coercive parenting techniques and encouraging positive, consistent engagement with children are the gold standard treatments for preschool DBDs.

Disruptive behaviors are among the most common reasons preschool children present for psychiatric care. Disruptive behavior disorders (DBDs), specifically oppositional defiant disorder (ODD) and conduct disorder (CD), are some of the most common diagnoses in preschoolers. Prevalence of ODD in preschoolers is estimated at 4% to 16.6%, with CD incidence at 3.9% to 6.6%. ODD specifically is associated with later mood disorders; childhood-onset CD predicts later educational and legal

Disclosures: Dr M. Tandon has a copyright and receives royalties on a children's book.
Division of Child and Adolescent Psychiatry, Washington University in St. Louis School of Medicine, 660 South Euclid Avenue, Box 8134, St Louis, MO, USA
* Corresponding author. Department of Psychiatry, Washington University in St. Louis School of Medicine, 660 South Euclid Avenue, Box 8134, St Louis, MO 63110.
E-mail address: giedinga@psychiatry.wustl.edu

issues.[1] Preschool-age ODD is a less robust predictor than preschool CD of poor school-age and adolescent outcomes, but still confers the risk of later impairment, likely through progression to CD.[2] These disorders are costly, not only in terms of children and families' suffering but also for society as a whole in terms of mental health (and criminal justice) resources. Solid evidence supports treating DBDs with parent management training and other psychosocial methods, but early intervention offers the best chance for recovery.[3] Thus, identification and treatment of children with early-onset DBDs is vital.

In the last decade, evidence for and acceptance of the existence of DBDs in preschool-aged children has grown. There has been a proliferation of research into DBDs' earliest manifestations, with numerous studies showing it is possible to identify ODD and CD before 6 years of age.[4] In answer to concerns about the reliability and validity of DBD diagnoses in preschoolers, a series of studies by Keenan and Wakschlag[5] compared the incidence of ODD and CD symptoms between clinically referred and nonreferred preschool-aged children.[6–8] The seminal 2004 study compared 2.5-year-olds with 5.5-year-olds at a preschool behavior problems clinic with age-matched, non–psychiatrically referred peers. Of the referred children, 59.5% met criteria for ODD and 41.8% met CD criteria; only 2% of nonreferred children met criteria for either.[6]

Adopting a developmental perspective in DBD diagnosis has also helped to differentiate early mental disorder from normative individuation attempts. Some oppositional behaviors are common to all children (eg, occasional defiance in 2-year-olds). Differences in frequency, intensity, and kind demarcate the onset of disorder.[8] For instance, hitting is common among 3-year-olds, but for a child to use aggression frequently or as an initial interpersonal strategy generally indicates disorder.[6,8] Physical aggression, property destruction, deceitfulness, and theft are markers of preschool CD as well as predictors of CD persistence. In contrast, actions like loss of temper or telling stories not intended for gain are not associated with later CD.[1]

COMORBIDITY

Almost all individuals with CD also carry an ODD diagnosis. ODD frequently progresses to CD, and roughly 10% of children with CD then develop antisocial personality disorder as adults. Attention-deficit/hyperactivity disorder (ADHD) is also frequently comorbid, particularly the hyperactive and combined subtypes.[4] Children with comorbid ADHD have greater executive functioning deficits and increased emotional impulsivity compared with pure CD or ODD.[9] Comorbid ADHD is also associated with earlier DBD onset.[10,11] In one study of children diagnosed with CD before the age of 9 years, more than 70% of patients previously carried an ODD diagnosis. Preschool-onset DBDs are associated with persistent conduct and psychiatric problems.[12]

ENVIRONMENTAL RISK FACTORS

Perhaps the clearest case of an environmental exposure that predisposes to DBDs is exposure to active maternal smoking during pregnancy (MSDP).[13] MSPD has been shown to increase the risk of externalizing behavior in children as young as 18 months.[14–16] It increases the risk of ODD and CD during the preschool years and beyond, independent of ADHD.[17,18] Children exposed to MSDP were more likely to show conduct problems in a recent genetically sensitive analysis as well. Children of mothers who smoked more than 10 cigarettes daily during pregnancy showed the most disruptive behaviors.[19]

Another environmental exposure related to preschool DBD incidence is termed neighborhood effect: children from economically disadvantaged neighborhoods manifest DBDs more often. However, neighborhood disadvantage is also associated with exposure to neighborhood violence, which independently increases DBD risk.[20] One analysis found proximal factors like neighborhood violence, exposure to intrafamilial conflict, and harsh parenting likely account for the increased incidence of DBDs in disadvantaged neighborhoods.[21] Children exposed to chronic violence also have faulty processing of interpersonal cues, with more negative/hostile attributions about others' behavior, leading to increased aggression.[22] Chaos (ie, noise, disorganization, and instability) in the home, which is common in economically disadvantaged neighborhoods, is also associated with childhood conduct issues, with greater chaos associated with more conduct problems.[23,24]

There are indirect associations between family income and children's behavioral problems mediated by maternal depression and parental stress.[25] Exposure to maternal depression during infancy increases preschool children's likelihood of developing DBDs, likely mediated by the effects of disengaged, harsh, or overly permissive parenting.[21,26] Women with depression frequently have parenting issues related to disengagement and withdrawal, and may also show hostile parenting (ie, frequent negative, irritable statements and demands).[27] Parental hostility and depression during early childhood are associated with increased development of DBDs.[28]

Parental stress is a related indicator; parents living in low-income and high-violence neighborhoods are subject to constant psychological stress, which exacerbates parental mental health issues.[29,30] Parental stress predicts both hostile and inconsistent parenting.[29] Harsh and inconsistent parenting practices are then associated with the development of DBDs, irrespective of socioeconomic status (**Fig. 1**).[31] In Patterson's[32] model of coercive family process, worsening of disruptive behavior is in part the result of a cascade of coercive interaction between child and caregiver, who challenge one another until the fatigued parent relents, unintentionally reinforcing the child's coercive behaviors.[32,33] Oppositional and aggressive behaviors by preschoolers elicit more controlling and negative maternal responses, which are then associated with conduct symptom persistence in preschoolers.[34] Mothers of preschoolers with conduct problems also report decreased feelings of parental competence and use fewer assertive problem-solving skills.[35] Parental discipline of

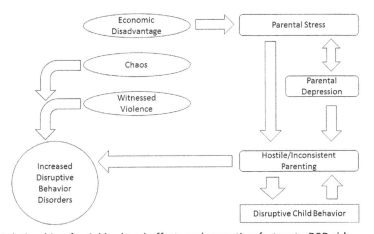

Fig. 1. Relationship of neighborhood effects and parenting factors to DBD risk.

children with DBDs is not only frequently harsh but there is also less positive parenting. Positive parenting techniques include close monitoring of the child, positive reinforcement, and regular engagement. These techniques are associated with decreased DBD risk, and are taught in parent management training programs used for prevention and treatment of preschool ODD and CD. Training in these skills increases parental confidence and competence and improve child behavior.[36]

GENETIC RISK FACTORS

DBDs cluster in families with ADHD, CD, ODD, and depression.[37] The association between maternal depression and the development of preschool DBDs is partially mediated by parenting practices, but there is also a genetic association between the two, and ODD shows heterotypic continuity with depression and anxiety.[38] Substance use disorders in close family also predispose to preschool ODD and CD. This predisposition may be mediated by the effects of substance use on parenting in addition to genetics.[39] Undertreated ADHD and childhood CD also increase the risk of substance use disorders; this may be an additional genetic signal for association with ADHD or CD.[40]

Recent studies have also investigated genetic polymorphisms that may predispose to DBDs through interaction with childhood adversity. Polymorphisms in the 5-hydroxy-tryptamine transporter–linked polymorphic region (5HTTLPR) and monoamine oxidase A (MAOA) gene are the most intensely investigated.[41] The 2 most common variants in 5-HTTLPR are the L (long, high expressing) and S (short, low expressing) alleles. The S allele results in decreased production of serotonin transporters, and thus decreased serotonin clearance from the synaptic cleft.[42] 5HTTLPR and MAOA were originally investigated for modulating the effects of childhood adversity on later affective disorders.[43,44] Early 5HTTLPR studies found that the S allele increases vulnerability to externalizing disorders in the context of childhood adversity, whereas later studies found increased vulnerability among children homozygous for the L allele. Many others found no effect.[41,45] 5-HTTLPR's modulation of mental disorder in the setting of early adversity warrants further study.[46]

The MAOA polymorphism's modulation of the relationship between childhood adversity and DBD development has been well studied. The high-activity allele results in increased monoamine oxidase A transcription, and decreased serotonin and dopamine concentration in the synaptic cleft. This allele seems to convey protection from developing antisocial behavior against a background of childhood maltreatment in boys.[43,44] However, there have been contradictory findings. For instance, the MAOA polymorphism that confers protection from antisocial behavior in boys may have no protective activity in girls. Further research is needed.[41]

NEUROIMAGING

Literature on brain structural and functional abnormalities in preschoolers with DBDs is sparse. However, work on adolescents and young adults exists. Recent meta-analysis of 12 structural MRI and 17 functional MRI studies found that children with ODD and CD have smaller bilateral amygdalae and insulae, as well as decreased brain activity in these areas on functional MRI. There was a particularly strong association between decreased amygdala volume and activity and CD/ODD, even accounting for comorbid ADHD.[47] These areas are associated with so-called hot executive function (decision making driven by emotional stimuli). Decreased volume in the right striatum, left medial and superior frontal gyrus, and left precuneus was also found.

Another meta-analysis of regional gray matter volume differences in youth with and without conduct issues also found gray matter reduction in the bilateral insulae, left amygdala, and medial superior frontal gyrus and left fusiform gyrus in children with DBDs.[48] Childhood-onset conduct disorder was associated with decreased bilateral amygdalar and right insular volume in adolescent boys.[49] A study of children 6 to 9 years old also associated greater aggression with smaller amygdalae.[50] Hyporesponsivity to threat, an expected correlate of diminished amygdalar function, is also seen in children with CD/ODD.[51,52] These children have decreased startle responses when exposed to unpleasant stimuli, understood as aberrant fear modulation.[51] Lack of empathy is also common in children with DBDs, and may be correlated with insular findings: insular activity is related to pain perception, as in empathetically processing another's (emotional) pain and placing it in a social context.[53,54]

NEUROPSYCHOLOGICAL PROFILES AND NEUROPHYSIOLOGIC CORRELATES

Literature on executive functioning in young children with DBDs is mixed, and the executive dysfunction associated with CD and ODD is frequently linked with comorbid ADHD. A 2015 study found significant executive function deficits in preschool children with ADHD and ADHD with comorbid ODD (but not ODD alone).[9] A study of Norwegian preschoolers found that those with comorbid ADHD and ODD, as well as ADHD alone, also scored lower than controls on measures of response inhibition and working memory.[55] Other studies have found significant negative effects on response inhibition among patients with ADHD, DBDs, and both when rewards were immediate and highly emotionally salient (ie, required use of hot executive functioning).[56]

Children with ODD and CD also show more risk-taking behavior in experimental conditions.[57] This behavior is associated with the previously discussed orbitofrontal cortex hyporeactivity to reward in these children,[58] which is the proposed connection to increased sensation seeking in DBDs. Orbitofrontal and cingulate cortex impairment in modulation of inhibitory control also impairs behavioral regulation if there are hot (highly affectively charged) stimuli. This impairment is then associated with decreased control of emotional behavior, leading to increased reactive aggression.[52]

Other studies related to fear response in preschool (and older) patients with aggressive behavior have associated decreased baseline autonomic nervous system arousal with later aggressive behavior. Measuring skin conductance is one method of quantifying sympathetic nervous system activity. Low sympathetic activity during aversive exposures has been interpreted as evidence of fearlessness or punishment insensitivity.[52] For example, low skin conductance in 1-year-old infants, at baseline and during fear challenge, is associated with increased aggression at 3 years.[59] The same pattern of decreased skin conductance is also associated with high levels of aggression in 4-year-olds.[60] Explanations for the relationship between decreased sympathetic activity and later aggression have focused on these children's attenuated responses to aversive stimuli. The hypothesis runs that children with this neurologic phenotype do not respond to punishment with appropriate learning, stalling socialization.[52,61,62]

ASSESSMENT

The Achenbach System of Empirically Based Assessment (ASEBA) is one of the most comprehensive report forms for assessment of DBDs, and there is a version for children 1.5 to 5 years of age. In addition to an ODD Diagnostic and Statistical Manual of Mental Disorders (DSM)–oriented scale and emotionally reactive and aggressive behavior syndrome scales, the ASEBA also screens for comorbid conditions.[63] It does not offer a specific CD scale. The Preschool Aged Psychiatric Assessment, developed by Egger and Angold,[65] is a semistructured interview that includes assessment for conduct problems, validated for use in children aged 2 to 5 years. However, it requires training to administer and is not widely available for clinical use.[64,65]

The Disruptive Behavior Diagnostic Observation Schedule is an observational method of assessing preschool disruptive behavior. Child behavior is assessed during interactions with parents, and with the examiner, both while the examiner is engaged with the child and while the examiner is busy with another task.[66,67] It has moderate sensitivity and specificity for DBDs.[68] It also predicts impairment: children who show disruptive behavior in the child-examiner interaction show greater impairment overall.[69]

TREATMENT

Psychosocial interventions are the first-line treatments for preschool DBDs.[70] Several specific programs are often grouped together under the heading of parent management training, including the Parent Management Training–Oregon Model (PMTO), parent-child interaction therapy (PCIT), and the Incredible Years (IY) program. They focus primarily on providing caregivers with effective communication and disciplinary tools while enhancing positive parental engagement.[7,71] These interventions, as a group, decrease childhood behavioral problems and improve parental mental health and parental competence.[72]

The PMTO focuses on training caregivers rather than focusing on the child directly. In the PMTO model, children's disruptive behaviors result in part from parents' unintentional reinforcement of children's use of coercive methods to obtain what they want.[32] The program involves a concerted effort to reshape parenting techniques, paring down reliance on coercion and focusing instead on positive reinforcement for prosocial behavior. Modules focus on reducing coercive interactions and instead encourage limit-setting, effective communication, and positive caregiver involvement.[73]

PCIT is a dyadic therapy focusing on the ways in which parent-child interactions can improve parents' and children's abilities to regulate strong emotions. Parents learn ways to engage positively with their children via praise and reflection, and how to ignore negative behaviors.[74] After parents learn these skills, therapists observe parent-child interactions through a 1-way mirror, then discuss observed maladaptive interactional styles. In later sessions, therapists coach parents through interactions with their children, delivering instructions via earpiece. In cross-cultural investigations, the effect size of PCIT on preschool disruptive behavior is consistently moderate to large.[75] It has been extensively modified for different populations, with successful adaptations targeting children with autism spectrum disorders and parent-child dyads with a history of maltreatment.[76,77] The use of online platforms for PCIT delivery is currently being investigated.[78]

The IY program is one of the best-studied psychosocial treatments for preschool DBDs. It includes parent, child, and teacher training. Meta-analysis has shown significant, moderate to large effects of IY parent training on childhood disruptive behavior.[70,79] The IY program also improves parental confidence and skill, and satisfaction with the program is characteristically high. Decreases in childhood DBD symptoms after IY intervention are partially mediated by increases in parental skill, most notably decreases in coercive and critical parenting behaviors.[36,80] In a study of young children who received IY interventions for ODD, high levels of maternal criticism at 2-year follow-up predicted persistent conduct problems.[81] Combining IY parent training and teacher training improved child behavior outcomes at 2-year follow-up compared with either intervention alone; including child training also improves outcomes.[81,82]

Numerous adaptations have allowed the implementation of parent management training in diverse venues and in more cost-effective ways. The IY program remains effective at improving parenting competence and confidence in a wide range of delivery settings, whether through daycare centers in impoverished urban areas,[83] among Chinese immigrants to the United States,[84] or among mothers from multicultural backgrounds in Head Start.[85] A study of abbreviated PCIT delivered in part via videotape and telephone call showed that although standard therapy was superior immediately after treatment, differences in effectiveness were minimal 6 months later.[86] Brief interventions delivered in conjunction with pediatric primary care can also reduce preschool behavior problems and improve parental feelings of competence.[87] Parent training programs using Web-based platforms can also improve children's behavioral outcomes.[88]

REFERENCES

1. Hong JS, Tillman R, Luby JL. Disruptive behavior in preschool children: distinguishing normal misbehavior from markers of current and later childhood conduct disorder. J Pediatr 2015;166(3):723–30.
2. Burke JD, Waldman I, Lahey BB. Predictive validity of childhood oppositional defiant disorder and conduct disorder: implications for the DSM-V. J Abnorm Psychol 2010;119(4):739–51.
3. Comer JS, Chow MA, Chan PT, et al. Psychosocial treatment efficacy for disruptive behavior problems in very young children: a meta-analytic examination. J Am Acad Child Adolesc Psychiatry 2013;52(1):26–36.
4. Egger HL, Angold A. Common emotional and behavioral disorders in preschool children: presentation, nosology, and epidemiology. J Child Psychol Psychiatry 2006;47:313–37.
5. Keenan K, Wakschlag LS. Can a valid diagnosis of disruptive behavior disorder be made in preschool children? Am J Psychiatry 2002;159(3):351–8.
6. Keenan K, Wakschlag LS. Are oppositional defiant and conduct disorder symptoms normative behaviors in preschoolers? A comparison of referred and nonreferred children. Am J Psychiatry 2004;161(2):356–8.
7. Keenan K, Wakschlag LS, Danis B, et al. Further evidence of the reliability and validity of DSM-IV ODD and CD in preschool children. J Am Acad Child Adolesc Psychiatry 2007;46(4):457–68.
8. Wakschlag LS, Tolan PH, Leventhal BL. "Ain't misbehavin": towards a developmentally-specified nosology for preschool disruptive behavior. J Child Psychol Psychiatry 2010;51(1):3–22.
9. Ezpeleta L, Granero R. Executive functions in preschoolers with ADHD, ODD and comorbid ADHD-ODD: evidence from ecological and performance-based measures. J Neuropsychol 2014;9(2):258–70.
10. Willcutt EG, Pennington BF, Chhabildas NA, et al. Psychiatric comorbidity associated with DSM-IV ADHD in a nonreferred sample of twins. J Am Acad Child Adolesc Psychiatry 1999;38(11):1355–62.
11. Moffitt TE, Caspi A, Harrington H, et al. Males on the life-course-persistent and adolescence-limited antisocial pathways: follow-up at age 26 years. Dev Psychopathol 2002;14(1):179–207.
12. Brennan LM, Shaw DS, Dishion TY, et al. Longitudinal predictors of school-age academic achievement: unique contributions of toddler-age aggression,

oppositionality, inattention and hyperactivity. J Abnorm Child Psychol 2012;40(8): 1289–300.

13. Wakschlag LS, Pickett KE, Cook E, et al. Maternal smoking during pregnancy and severe antisocial behavior in offspring: a review. Am J Public Health 2002;92(6): 966–74.

14. Wakschlag LS, Leventhal BL, Pine DS, et al. Elucidating early mechanisms of developmental psychopathology: the case of prenatal smoking and disruptive behavior. Child Dev 2006;77(4):893–906.

15. Stene-Larsen K, Borge AI, Vollrath ME. Maternal smoking in pregnancy and externalizing behavior in 18 month old children: results from a population based prospective study. J Am Acad Child Adolesc Psychiatry 2009;48(3):283–9.

16. Dolan CV, Geels L, Vink JM, et al. Testing causal effects of maternal smoking during pregnancy on offspring's externalizing and internalizing behavior. Behav Genet 2016;46(3):378–88.

17. Ellis LC, Berg-Nielsen TS, Lydersen S, et al. Smoking during pregnancy and psychiatric disorders in preschoolers. Eur Child Adolesc Psychiatry 2012;21(11): 635–44.

18. Nigg JT, Breslau N. Prenatal smoking exposure, low birth weight, and disruptive behavior disorders. J Am Acad Child Adolesc Psychiatry 2007;46(3):362–9.

19. Gaysina D, Fergusson M, Leve LD, et al. Maternal smoking during pregnancy and offspring conduct problems: evidence from 3 independent genetically sensitive research designs. JAMA Psychiatry 2013;70(9):956–63.

20. Briggs-Gowan MJ, Carter AS, Ford JD. Parsing the effects of violence exposure in early childhood: modeling developmental pathways. J Pediatr Psychol 2012; 37(1):11–22.

21. Heberle AE, Thomas YM, Wagmiller RL, et al. The impact of neighborhood, family and individual risk factors on toddler's disruptive behavior. Child Dev 2014;85(5): 2046–61.

22. Ziv Y. Exposure to violence, social information processing, and problem behavior in preschool children. Aggress Behav 2012;38(6):429–41.

23. Coldwell J, Pike A, Dunn J. Household chaos–links with parenting and child behaviour. J Child Psychol Psychiatry 2006;47(11):1116–22.

24. Deater-Deckard K, Mullineaux PY, Beekman C, et al. Conduct problems, IQ, and household chaos: a longitudinal multi-informant study. J Child Psychol Psychiatry 2009;50(10):1301–8.

25. Shelleby EC, Votruba-Drzal E, Shaw DS, et al. Income and children's behavioral functioning: a sequential mediation analysis. J Fam Psychol 2014;28(6):936–46.

26. Shaw DS, Sitnick SL, Reuben J, et al. Transactional effects among maternal depression, neighborhood deprivation, and child conduct problems from early childhood through adolescence: a tale of two low-income samples. Dev Psychopathol 2016;28(3):819–36.

27. Lovejoy MC, Graczyk PA, O'Hare E, et al. Maternal depression and parenting behavior: a meta-analytic review. Clin Psychol Rev 2000;20(5):561–92.

28. Conger RD, Wallace LE, Sun Y, et al. Economic pressure in African-American families: a replication and extension of the family stress model. Dev Psychol 2002;38(2):179–93.

29. Shaw DS, Shelleby EC. Early-starting conduct problems: intersection of conduct problems and poverty. Annu Rev Clin Psychol 2014;10:503–28.

30. Lavigne JV, Gouze KR, Hopkins J, et al. A multidomain cascade model of early childhood risk factors associated with oppositional defiant disorder symptoms in a community sample of 6-year-olds. Dev Psychopathol 2015;28(4pt2):1547–62.

31. Shea SE, Coyne LW. Maternal dysphoric mood, stress, and parenting practices in mothers of Head Start preschoolers: the role of experiential avoidance. Child Fam Behav Ther 2011;33(3):231–47.
32. Patterson GR. Coercive family process. Eugene (OR): Castalia Publishing; 1982.
33. Smith JD, Dishion TJ, Shaw DS, et al. Coercive family process and early-onset conduct problems from age 2 to school entry. Dev Psychopathol 2014; 26(4 Pt 1):917–32.
34. Rubin KH, Burgess KB, Dwyer KM, et al. Predicting preschoolers' externalizing behaviors from toddler temperament, conflict, and maternal negativity. Dev Psychol 2003;39(1):164–76.
35. Cunningham CE, Boyle MH. Preschoolers at risk for attention-deficit hyperactivity disorder and oppositional defiance disorder: family, parenting and behavioral correlates. J Abnorm Child Psychol 2002;30(6):555–69.
36. Gardner F, Burton J, Klimes I. Randomised controlled trial of a parenting intervention in the voluntary sector for reducing child conduct problems: outcomes and mechanisms of change. J Child Psychol Psychiatry 2006;47(11):1123–32.
37. Volk HE, Neuman RJ, Todd RD. A systematic evaluation of ADHD and comorbid psychopathology in a population-based twin sample. J Am Acad Child Adolesc Psychiatry 2005;44(8):768–75.
38. Burke JD, Loeber R, Lahey BB, et al. Developmental transitions among affective and behavioral disorders in adolescent boys. J Child Psychol Psychiatry 2005; 46(11):1200–10.
39. Loeber R, Green SM, Keenan K, et al. Which boys will fare worse? Early predictors of the onset of conduct disorder in a six-year longitudinal study. J Am Acad Child Adolesc Psychiatry 1995;34(4):499–509.
40. Lynskey MT, Fergusson DM. Childhood conduct problems, attention deficit behaviors, and adolescent alcohol, tobacco, and illicit drug use. J Abnorm Child Psychol 1995;23(3):281–302.
41. Weeland J, Overbeek G, de Castro BO, et al. Underlying mechanisms of gene-environment interactions in externalizing behavior: a systematic review and search for theoretical mechanisms. Clin Child Fam Psychol Rev 2015;18(4): 413–42.
42. Heils A, Teufel A, Petri S, et al. Allelic variation of human serotonin transporter gene expression. J Neurochem 1996;66(6):2621–4.
43. Caspi A, McClay J, Moffitt TE, et al. Role of genotype in the cycle of violence in maltreated children. Science 2002;297(5582):851–4.
44. Byrd AL, Manuck SB. MAOA, childhood maltreatment, and antisocial behavior: meta-analysis of a gene-environment interaction. Biol Psychiatry 2014;75(1): 9–17.
45. Agnafors S, Sydsjö G, Comasco E, et al. Early predictors of behavioural problems in pre-schoolers – a longitudinal study of constitutional and environmental main and interaction effects. BMC Pediatr 2016;16:76.
46. Fergusson DM, Horwood LJ, Miller AL, et al. Life Stress, 5-HTTLPR and mental disorder: findings from a 30 year longitudinal study. Br J Psychiatry 2011; 198(2):129–35.
47. Nordermeer SD, Luman M, Oosterlaan J. A systematic review and meta-analysis of neuroimaging in oppositional defiant disorder and conduct disorder taking attention-deficit hyperactivity disorder into account. Neuropsychol Rev 2016; 26(1):44–72.
48. Rogers JC, De Brito SA. Cortical and subcortical gray matter volume in youths with conduct problems: a meta-analysis. JAMA Psychiatry 2016;73(1):64–72.

49. Fairchild G, Passamonti L, Hurford G, et al. Brain structure abnormalities in early-onset and adolescent-onset conduct disorder. Am J Psychiatry 2011;168(6): 624–33.

50. Thijssen S, Ringoot AP, Wildeboer A, et al. Brain morphology of childhood aggressive behavior: a multi-informant study in school-age children. Cogn Affect Behav Neurosci 2015;15(3):564–77.

51. Fairchild G, Van Goozen SH, Stollery S, et al. Fear conditioning and affective modulation of the startle reflex in male adolescents with early-onset or adolescence-onset conduct disorder and healthy control subjects. Biol Psychiatry 2008;63(3):279–85.

52. Matthys W, Vanderschuren LJ, Schutter DJ. The neurobiology of oppositional defiant disorder and conduct disorder: altered functioning in three mental domains. Dev Psychopathol 2013;25(1):193–207.

53. Singer T, Seymour B, O'Doherty J, et al. Empathy for pain involves the affective but not sensory components of pain. Science 2004;303(5661):1157–62.

54. Phelps EA, LeDoux JE. Contributions of the amygdala to emotion processing: from animal models to human behavior. Neuron 2005;48(2):175–87.

55. Skogan AH, Zeiner P, Egeland J, et al. Inhibition and working memory in young preschool children with symptoms of ADHD and/or oppositional-defiant disorder. Child Neuropsychol 2014;20(5):607–24.

56. Schoemaker K, Bunte T, Wiebe S, et al. Executive function deficits in preschool children with ADHD and DBD. J Child Psychol Psychiatry 2012;53(2):111–9.

57. Fairchild G, van Goozen SH, Stollery SJ, et al. Decision making and executive function in male adolescents with early-onset or adolescence-onset conduct disorder and control subjects. Biol Psychiatry 2009;66(2):162–8.

58. Hobson CW, Scott S, Rubia K. Investigation of cool and hot executive function in ODD/CD independently of ADHD. J Child Psychol Psychiatry 2011;52(10): 1035–43.

59. Baker E, Shelton KH, Baibazarova E, et al. Low skin conductance activity in infancy predicts aggression in toddlers 2 years later. Psychol Sci 2013;24(6): 1051–6.

60. Posthumus JA, Bocker KB, Raaijmakers MA, et al. Heart rate and skin conductance in four-year-old children with aggressive behavior. Biol Psychol 2009; 82(2):164–8.

61. Van Goozen SH, Snoek H, Matthys W, et al. Evidence of fearlessness in behaviorally disordered children: a study on startle reflex modulation. J Child Psychol Psychiatry 2004;45(4):884–92.

62. Steiner H. Practice parameters for the assessment and treatments of children and adolescents with conduct disorder. J Am Acad Child Adolesc Psychiatry 1997; 36(10):122S–39S.

63. Ivanova MY, Achenbach TM, Rescorla LA, et al. Syndromes of preschool psychopathology reported by parents in 23 societies. J Am Acad Child Adolesc Psychiatry 2010;49(12):1215–24.

64. Egger HL, Erkanli A, Keeler G, et al. Test-retest reliability of the preschool age psychiatric assessment (PAPA). J Am Acad Child Adolesc Psychiatry 2006; 45(5):538–49.

65. Egger HL, Angold A. The Preschool Age Psychiatric Assessment (PAPA): a structured parent interview for diagnosing psychiatric disorders in preschool children. In: DelCarmen-Wiggins R, Carter AS, editors. Handbook of infant, toddler and preschool mental health assessment. New York: Oxford; 2004. p. 223–46.

66. Wakschlag LS, Hill C, Carter AS, et al. Observational assessment of preschool disruptive behavior, part I: reliability of the Disruptive Behavior Diagnostic Observation Schedule (DB-DOS). J Am Acad Child Adolesc Psychiatry 2008;47(6): 622–31.

67. Wakschlag LS, Briggs-Gowan MJ, Hill C, et al. Observational assessment of preschool disruptive behavior, part II: validity of the Disruptive Behavior Diagnostic Observation Schedule (DB-DOS). J Am Acad Child Adolesc Psychiatry 2008; 47(6):632–41.

68. Bunte TL, Shoemaker K, Hessen DH, et al. Clinical usefulness of the Kiddie-Disruptive Behavior Disorder Schedule in the diagnosis of DBD and ADHD in preschool children. J Abnorm Child Psychol 2013;41(5):681–90.

69. PetitClerc A, Briggs-Gowan MJ, Estabrook R, et al. Contextual variation in young children's observed disruptive behavior on the DB-DOS: implications for early identification. J Child Psychol Psychiatry 2015;56(9):1008–16.

70. Eyberg SM, Nelson MM, Boggs SR. Evidence-based psychosocial treatments for children and adolescents with disruptive behavior. J Clin Child Adolesc Psychol 2008;37(1):215–37.

71. Kazdin AE. Parent management training: evidence, outcomes and issues. J Am Acad Child Adolesc Psychiatry 1997;36(10):1349–56.

72. Furlong M, McGilloway S, Bywater T, et al. Cochrane Review: behavioural and cognitive-behavioural group-based parenting programmes for early-onset conduct problems in children aged 3 to 12 years. Evid Based Child Health 2013;8(2):318–692.

73. Forgatch MS, DeGarmo DS, Beldvas ZG. An efficacious theory-based intervention for stepfamilies. Behav Ther 2005;36(4):357–65.

74. Brinkmeyer MY, Eyberg SM. Parent-child interaction therapy for oppositional children. In: Kazdin AE, Weisz JR, editors. Evidence-based psychotherapies for children and adolescents. New York: Guilford Press; 2003. p. 204–23.

75. Abrahamse ME, Junger M, Chavannes EL, et al. Parent-child interaction therapy for preschool children with disruptive behavior problems in The Netherlands. Child Adolesc Psychiatry Ment Health 2012;6(1):24.

76. Solomon M, Ono M, Timmer S, et al. The effectiveness of parent-child interaction therapy for families of children on the autism spectrum. J Autism Dev Disord 2008;38(9):1767–76.

77. Timmer SG, Urquiza AJ, Zebell NM, et al. Parent-child interaction therapy: application to maltreating parent-child dyads. Child Abuse Negl 2005;29(7):825–41.

78. Comer JS, Furr JM, Cooper-Vince C, et al. Rationale and considerations for the internet-based delivery of parent-child interaction therapy. Cogn Behav Pract 2015;22(3):302–16.

79. Menting TA, de Castro O, Matthys W. Effectiveness of the incredible years parent training to modify disruptive and prosocial child behavior: a meta-analytic review. Clin Psychol Rev 2013;33(8):901–12.

80. Posthumus JA, Raaijmakers MAJ, Maassen GH, et al. Sustained effects of Incredible Years as a preventive intervention in preschool children with conduct problems. J Abnorm Child Psychol 2012;40(4):487–500.

81. Reid MJ, Webster-Stratton C, Hammond M. Follow-up of children who received the Incredible Years intervention for oppositional-defiant disorder: maintenance and prediction of 2-year outcome. Behav Ther 2003;34:471–91.

82. Webster-Stratton C, Hammond M. Treating children with early-onset conduct problems: a comparison of child and parent training interventions. J Consult Clin Psychol 1997;65(1):93–109.

83. Gross D, Fogg L, Webster-Stratton C, et al. Parent training of toddlers in day care in low-income urban communities. J Consult Clin Psychol 2003;71(2):261–78.

84. Lau AS, Fung JJ, Yung V. Group parent training with immigrant Chinese families: enhancing engagement and augmenting skills training. J Clin Psychol 2010; 66(8):880–94.

85. Reid MJ, Webster-Stratton C, Beauchaine TP. Parent training in head start: a comparison of program response among African-American, Asian-American, Caucasian, and Hispanic mothers. Prev Sci 2002;2(4):209–27.

86. Nixon RD, Sweeney L, Erickson DB, et al. Parent-child interaction therapy: a comparison of standard and abbreviated treatments for oppositional defiant preschoolers. J Consult Clin Psychol 2003;71(2):251–60.

87. Berkovits MD, O'Brien KA, Carter CG, et al. Early identification and intervention for behavior problems in primary care: a comparison of two abbreviated versions of parent-child interaction therapy. Behav Ther 2010;41(3):375–87.

88. Enebrink P, Högström J, Forster M, et al. Internet-based parent management training: a randomized controlled study. Behav Res Ther 2012;50(4):240–9.

Depression and Anxiety in Preschoolers
A Review of the Past 7 Years

Diana J. Whalen, PhD*, Chad M. Sylvester, MD, PhD,
Joan L. Luby, MD

KEYWORDS

- Preschool depression • Preschool anxiety • Early onset • Mental disorder • Review

KEY POINTS

- Empirical work increasingly validates and clarifies the clinical characteristics of internalizing disorders in preschool-aged children.
- Studies using structural and functional neuroimaging have highlighted neural differences among children with preschool-onset internalizing disorders, and these differences are strikingly similar to those found in adolescents and adults with internalizing disorders.
- Several evidence-based treatments have shown promise for preschool-onset internalizing disorder and additional research is currently underway to further validate these treatment options.

INTRODUCTION

A little more than a decade ago the concept of a preschooler with depression and/or anxiety disorders was not taken seriously. Many people think that early childhood is a time of happiness, joy, and freedom from this kind of adult-level burden. Others suggest that preschoolers do not have the emotional or intellectual capacity to even harbor such intense feelings. However, since that time, hundreds of articles have been published defining, describing, and validating preschool-onset internalizing disorders

Conflict of Interest: Dr J.L. Luby has received royalties from Guilford Press. Drs C.M. Sylvester and D.J. Whalen report no biomedical financial interests or potential conflicts of interest.
Disclosure: This work was supported by the National Institutes of Health (R01MH098454-01A1 to J.L. Luby). Dr D.J. Whalen's work was supported by NIH grant T32 MH100019 (principal investigators [PIs]: Barch and J.L. Luby) and L30 MH108015 (PI: D.J. Whalen). Dr C.M. Sylvester's work was supported by NIH grant K23MH109983, the Taylor Institute, and the McDonnell Foundation.
Department of Psychiatry, Washington University School of Medicine, 4444 Forest Park, Suite 2100, St Louis, MO 63108, USA
* Corresponding author.
E-mail address: diana.whalen@wustl.edu

and linking these early disorders to differences in behavior and brain functioning later in life. The scientific community has come to accept that many disorders of childhood and adolescence may have their onset as early as preschool. This article focuses on advances made toward elucidating the nature of preschool-onset depression and anxiety disorders, specifically focusing on diagnostic assessment/comorbidities, prevalence, risk factors, neurobiological correlates, and prognosis/treatment. Because other recent articles and reviews[1–5] have been published in this area, this article focuses on work conducted over the last 7 years.

With wider acceptance of preschool internalizing disorders came controversy over how to correctly differentiate depression and anxiety, as well as how to accurately diagnose these disorders in such young children. Research on this topic has traditionally been split between two approaches:

1. A broad, two-dimensional grouping of symptoms into categories such as internalizing and externalizing (eg, Child Behavior Checklist [CBCL] score)
2. A more categorically defined taxonomy of specific symptoms and disorders (eg, Diagnostic and Statistical Manual of Mental Disorders [DSM]–5).

There are strengths and weakness to both approaches. However, one primary challenge is the limited ability of preschoolers to verbalize their own emotional states related to these symptoms. In addition, there are also high levels of comorbidity between the internalizing disorders as well as between internalizing and externalizing disorders in childhood.[6–8] Another potential problem to the categorically based approaches is the duration of symptoms that are often required to meet formal criteria for DSM-5 diagnosis. Certain disorders require durations that are developmentally inappropriate given the child's age. For instance, a 6-month duration for a child 3 or 4 years old represents a significant proportion of the child's life, and therefore may not be a developmentally appropriate threshold. In addition, given greater affective variation and shifting of mental state early in development, there is some evidence that young children have periods of brightening (eg, in major depressive disorder [MDD]) that may mitigate the presentation of persistent symptoms for several weeks.[9]

The remainder of this article first describes the literature on preschool internalizing disorders, defined broadly and typically comprising symptoms of depression and anxiety together. Next, it focuses on reviewing the literature that has assessed preschool-onset depression and anxiety as specific and discrete disorders.

RESEARCH ON PRESCHOOL INTERNALIZING DISORDERS

Literature examining internalizing disorders in early childhood has lagged far behind the literature for externalizing disorders, in part because of the nature of symptom presentation. For instance, a shy, withdrawn child is less likely to attract attention and disrupt social activities. Internalizing disorders are theorized to exist on a continuum, with early differences detectable even in infancy.[10] However, work in this area continues to grow. One benefit of this more dimensional approach to assessment is that depression and anxiety are often intimately linked at this young age with high rates of comorbidity. Dimensional approaches account for this and provide children with a score indicating higher or lower internalizing symptoms. In much of the literature to date, symptoms are assessed using the CBCL[11] and/or the Strengths and Difficulties Questionnaire (SDQ[12]).

Sterba and colleagues[13] modeled the course of maternal-reported internalizing symptoms on the CBCL in 1364 children from ages 2 to 11 years. Two-thirds of these children were grouped in a low, stable class of internalizing symptoms, indicating that, over time, their symptoms remained below clinical thresholds. However, there were also groups of children who maintained increased symptoms across the years, and those who showed initial declines in symptoms during the preschool period, followed by increases at school age. These findings highlight both the high prevalence rates of significant internalizing symptoms in a community sample and the overall stability in young children's internalizing symptom trajectories over time. Using the DSM nosology and a structured interview (eg, Preschool Age Psychiatric Assessment [PAPA]), Sterba and colleagues[14] also studied differentiation among disorders in a community sample of preschoolers stratified by CBCL scores and found evidence for 3 distinguishable internalizing syndromes: social phobia, separation anxiety, and generalized anxiety/MDD. These findings mirror what is often seen in older children, in that Generalized Anxiety Disorder/MDD are highly correlated and unidimensional. Attempting to replicate the findings of Sterba and colleagues,[14] Strickland and colleagues[15] assessed a large, ethnically diverse community sample of preschoolers (n = 796) with the Children's Symptom Inventory. However, 4 distinct syndromes were identified: social phobia, separation anxiety, generalized anxiety, and MDD. The investigators suggest that the discrepant findings may be caused by the stratification used in the Sterba and colleagues[14] sample, as well as the slightly older range of ages in the replication sample.

Several psychosocial and child characteristics have been shown to be associated with risk for internalizing disorders in preschoolers, and many of these same risk factors correspond with risk for depression and anxiety as well. These risk factors include negative family environments, child temperament,[16] problematic peer relationships, and stressful life events. Depression and anxiety symptoms (measured together)[17] increased between 1.5 and 5 years of age, specifically for children in high-rising and moderate-rising trajectories. Difficult temperament at 5 months of age and maternal depression distinguished the high-rising trajectory from the lower-risk trajectories. In a large sample of German children (n = 1887), stressful life events predicted emotional and behavioral symptoms reported on the CBCL,[18] and the effect was particularly strong for children experiencing multiple stressful life events. Specifically, a parent restarting work, the move of a best friend, a family move, and death of a parent were associated with increased rates of internalizing disorders. Several studies have used data from the National Institute of Child Health and Human Development (NICHD) Study of Early Child Care and Youth Development, a longitudinal, multisite study of young children and their families to assess risk factors for internalizing mental disorder.[13,19,20] Each showed variability in the development and stability of internalizing disorders across time, as well as several risk factors that predicted trajectory membership. Davis and colleagues[19] found that a unique combination of high negative emotionality in children and high maternal warmth predicted trajectories of increasing internalizing symptoms across preschool through adolescence. Fanti and Henrich[20] found that, from ages 2 to 12 years, trajectories of pure internalizing symptoms were influenced by maternal history of depression, as well as greater risk for being asocial with peers at later ages.

Limited work has linked internalizing symptoms with differences in biological and neural indices. Cortisol reactivity to a laboratory challenge has been found to be dysregulated in preschoolers with internalizing symptoms, particularly among girls.[21] One study used both cross-sectional and longitudinal analyses to evaluate the role of social and neuroendocrinological risk factors (eg, cortisol) in the development of internalizing symptoms at preschool.[22] Both negative peer relations and family environments were concurrently associated with internalizing symptoms in preschoolers, with increases in cortisol level during a stressful task moderating the relationship between negative family environment and internalizing symptoms.

Few attempts have been made to evaluate treatment in broadly defined preschool internalizing disorders. One study found that a brief intervention delivered to parents of preschool children at risk for internalizing disorders showed benefits for girls into middle adolescence.[23] Given the high prevalence rates of internalizing disorders in young children and the strong likelihood of continuation throughout development, future work should focus on treatment evaluations and recommendations for these syndromes.

ASSESSMENT OF PRESCHOOL DEPRESSION

DSM-5 makes no distinction between childhood and adult forms of depression, with the disorder being characterized by the same core symptoms and across the lifespan. Symptoms include sadness/irritability, loss of pleasure/anhedonia, concentration difficulty, negative self-evaluations/guilt, recurrent thoughts about death/suicide, fatigue, and changes in appetite. Until recently, diagnoses of clinical depression in preschoolers have historically been met with skepticism and unease. Recent research has focused on describing, validating, and identifying specific, developmentally appropriate diagnostic criteria for application to preschool children.[6,24] Research conducted by Luby and colleagues[25,26] suggests that some adjustments to the current criteria for depression may be indicated, including the addition of a developmental adjustment to the death preoccupation symptom (eg, persistent engagement in activities or play themes with death or suicide) as well as lessening the duration criteria. In addition, this research found that the symptom of anhedonia in preschoolers marked a more severe subtype of depression that differentiated depressed preschoolers from both psychiatric and healthy control groups.[27] The symptom of anhedonia was the most specific for preschool MDD because reports of anhedonia were not seen in any healthy or attention-deficit/hyperactivity disorder (ADHD)/oppositional defiant disorder (ODD) preschoolers in the sample.[26] Luby and colleagues[25,27,28] have published extensively on the reliability and validity of these adjusted criteria for preschool children in 2 unique samples.[9] Furthermore, data from numerous national and international sites have validated the construct of preschool depression[29–31] using similar structured assessment measures.

There are several methods available to assess for preschool depression from a DSM framework. These methods include both screening checklists and structured interviews. One method that has been successfully used to screen for depression in preschool children is the Preschool Feelings Checklist,[32] which is a 16-item yes-or-no questionnaire that is suitable for use in a variety of settings, such as community-based centers and primary care offices, with established reliability.[32] A score of 3 or greater on this checklist typically indicates depressive symptoms at clinically significant levels, and signals that further clinical evaluation is warranted. This tool offers a major public health benefit, namely the ability to quickly screen for depression in young children in a variety of settings. Other more generic screening tools that also include depression subscales are the CBCL[11] and the SDQ.[12] The most widely used structured interview for assessing preschool depression to date is the PAPA.[33,34] The PAPA consists of a series of developmentally appropriate questions assessing the DSM criteria for childhood depression, with information being obtained from parents of children in this young age range. Other work has also used the Diagnostic Interview Schedule for Children, Parent Scale, Young Child.[35] A new version of the Kiddie Schedule for Affective Disorders Early Childhood has also recently been developed and is in use in several ongoing studies.[36]

PREVALENCE AND COURSE OF PRESCHOOL DEPRESSION

The population prevalence of preschool-onset depression remains understudied, given the recent acceptance by the scientific and clinical community of this phenomenon. Further, there have been few epidemiologic studies using developmentally appropriate diagnostic interviews.[7,34,37] Egger and Angold[6] found rates of preschool depression ranging from 0% to 2.1% depending on the sample and assessment measure used. These prevalence rates for preschool depression ($\sim$2%) were later replicated in 2 different community samples in 2009[7] and 2011.[38] Recently, Wichstrøm and colleagues[8] assessed a community sample of Norwegian children (n = 2475) using a structured diagnostic tool, the PAPA,[33,34] to determine the prevalence of psychiatric disorders in preschoolers. The prevalence rate in this sample was approximately 2%, similar to studies conducted in the United States.

Because the investigation of preschool-onset depression is still fairly new, there is little information regarding the stability and course of preschool depression into later childhood.[14,39,40] Consistent with homotypic continuity, preschool depression predicts MDD later in childhood and adolescence.[39,41,42] However, evidence also suggests that preschool depression predicts anxiety disorders and ADHD in later childhood as well.[39,43] Using structured clinical interviews across time, one study found gender differences in depressive symptom severity from preschool through early adolescence.[44] Specifically, boys in the high-severity class showed an increase in symptoms from preschool through early school age followed by a decline in later school age, whereas girls in the high-severity latent class remained stable and high in depressive symptoms across time. Early childhood social adversity, familial history of affective disorder, preschool-onset ODD/CD, and school-age functional impairment differentiated high-risk trajectory classes among both boys and girls.[44]

FACTORS ASSOCIATED WITH PRESCHOOL DEPRESSION

Factors and mechanisms contributing to preschool-onset depression remain understudied, particularly compared with known risk factors and mechanisms of childhood and adolescent depression. These factors encompass a variety of domains, including constructs both within child, family, and broader environmental systems.[45]

In addition to the anhedonia research described earlier, pathologic guilt[46–48] and irritability[49,50] have also emerged as key markers of preschool depression. Pathologic guilt is defined as a very low threshold for experiencing guilt following a transgression and may manifest as preoccupied, delayed recovery from guilty feelings, even for situations in which the child is not responsible.[46] This type of guilt occurring during the preschool years was found to be associated with smaller anterior insula volumes, a region known to be associated with guilt processing, measured at school age, which were predictive of a recurrence of depression.[51] Irritability has been defined as a low frustration tolerance characterized by anger and temper outbursts. Data from a large community sample of preschoolers also show that irritability measured at age 3 years predicted both depression and ODD at age 6 years,[50] even after accounting for overlapping items between irritability and psychiatric diagnoses. Furthermore, in the same sample, irritability continued to predict greater functional impairment and treatment use at age 9 years, although it did not continue to predict depression at age 9 years.[50] Changes in sleep and increased fatigue are also commonly reported symptoms of preschool depression.[46,50] However, sleep patterns have also been shown to be a risk factor for preschool depression and anxiety. Specifically, parent-reported sleep onset latency and the child's refusal to sleep alone independently predicted both preschool-onset depression and anxiety severity across time.[52] This work suggests that 2 common sleep problems may be important to target in early interventions for preschool depression.

Surprisingly little work has focused on thoughts of death and suicidal ideation (SI) in preschool-onset depression.[53–55] In part, the lack of research has been attributed to the belief that young children do not possess a mature, coherent conceptualization of death and dying. In addition, the meaning of death-related and suicidal statements and actions by young children is unclear; perhaps they represent a more general signal of distress, rather than an explicit wish to die. In one of the only studies of such behavior in preschool children younger than 7 years, Whalen and colleagues[53] evaluated the clinical significance of suicidality in a sample of 306 children between the ages of 3 and 7 years enrolled in a longitudinal investigation of preschool depression. Preschool SI was concurrently associated with several child mental disorders, including depression, anxiety disorders, ADHD, ODD, and CD, as well as demographic variables, including male gender and maternal psychiatric mental disorder. Preschool SI was the strongest predictor of later, school-age SI, even when controlling for psychiatric disorders at both time points.[53] Thus, the continuity of SI into later childhood suggests that, much like preschool-onset depression, preschool-onset SI may not be a developmentally transient phenomenon.

Other work has focused on the heritability/genetics[56–59] associated with early-onset depression and, more specifically, a large body of literature has linked parental history of depression and related mental disorder to preschool-onset depression in their children.[29,41,42,60,61] For example, a recent epidemiologic study found 2 distinct pathways linking prenatal and postnatal maternal depression to adolescent depressive symptoms: one pathway through preschool irritability symptoms and another through preschool anxiety/depressive symptoms.[42] The investigators suggest that prenatal maternal depressive symptoms may lead to an intrauterine environment that is not conducive to healthy fetal development, thereby increasing risk for atypical development in childhood. Further, it is well documented that postnatal maternal depressive symptoms negatively affect the mother's ability to provide sensitive and responsive caregiving, increasing the risk for problematic outcomes in her children.

Early childhood temperament has emerged as a risk factor for depression both in preschool and at older ages.[17,19,29,41,42,60,62,63] For example, in a multimethod, multi-informant, longitudinal study of preschoolers, early childhood temperament (age 3 years) was assessed using the Laboratory Temperament Assessment Battery, with each child participating in a standardized set of 12 tasks designed to elicit positive and negative affectivity, as well as inhibitory control.[29] Observed inhibitory control prospectively predicted the onset of depression by age 6 years. Interesting statistical interactions also emerged between early child temperament, early life stress, and parental mood disorders. Specifically, early life stress seemed to more greatly affect children with low temperamental fear/inhibition and without a history of parental mood/anxiety disorder to predict the onset of depression.

Research stemming from the Preschool Depression Study (PDS), a longitudinal study of preschool depression that has also included multiple waves of neuroimaging,[47] has uncovered several unique psychosocial and health factors associated with preschool-onset depression. For instance, children diagnosed with preschool-onset depression and/or anxiety disorders were no more likely than healthy preschoolers to be involved in relational aggression as an aggressor or victim at preschool or school age.[64] However, children with a preschool-onset depression and/or anxiety diagnosis were more than 6 times as likely to be classified as aggressive-victim at school age compared with healthy preschoolers. This finding held even after controlling for prior aggressor/victim status as well as current psychiatric symptoms and functional impairment. This finding suggests that preschool-onset psychiatric disorders may be a pathway toward poor peer relationships at school age. Growth mixture modeling was also used to create physical health trajectories in the PDS sample.[65] Two unique trajectories were found:

1. A stable low group with few physical health problems
2. A high, increasing group of children who experienced higher and increasing physical health problems over time

Preschool psychiatric diagnoses, including depression, were found to predict membership in the high, increasing latent trajectory class. Furthermore, preschool psychiatric disorders mediated relations between adversity and physical health, suggesting a strong influence of early symptoms on co-occurring and later physical health problems. In addition, preschoolers in this study were grouped according to the intensity of their tantrum behaviors: normative, excessive without aggression, and excessive with aggression.[66] Preschoolers with a diagnosis of MDD were much more likely to engage in self-injurious behavior during a tantrum episode than healthy preschoolers as well as preschoolers with other disruptive behavior diagnoses.

Moving to factors outside the child, family stress/conflict,[17,60,67] parenting practices,[60] and neglect[68] have all been shown to be associated with preschool-onset depression. In a diverse community sample of n = 796 4-year-olds, multiple risk factors encompassing several domains were assessed and then incorporated into models to determine unique correlates of depressive versus anxiety symptoms.[60] The best-fitting model specified that family stress/conflict had direct effects on child symptoms of depression and anxiety, as well as indirect effects on these symptoms through pathways incorporating parenting depressive symptoms and parenting practices. Of interest is that distal risk factors, such as socioeconomic status and family stress/conflict affected child symptoms through long mediational chains with variables that were more proximal to the child (eg, temperament).

NEUROBIOLOGICAL CORRELATES OF PRESCHOOL DEPRESSION

A particularly exciting and innovative area is investigation of neural indicators as predictors of preschool depression as well as the ways in which preschool depression alters neurocircuitry. There have been several studies that investigated neural correlates of currently depressed preschoolers[69,70] and in children/adolescents with a history of preschool depression.[51,71–79] For example, one study used functional MRI (fMRI) to examine functional brain activity and its relationship to emotion regulation in n = 23 currently depressed preschoolers aged 4 to 6 years and n = 31 matched, healthy preschoolers.[69] The investigators found evidence for increased amygdala activity during a face-viewing task in depressed compared with healthy preschoolers. This finding mirrors what has been shown in older children and adolescents with depression and suggests that disrupted amygdala functioning may be a neural biomarker for depression. Neurobiological alterations have also been shown in older children/adolescents with a history of preschool-onset depression. Findings from the PDS sample indicate greater activation to sad faces in the bilateral frontal cortex, amygdala, claustrum hippocampal, and parahippocampal gyrus,[71] as well as less activity in regions of the prefrontal cortex following a sad mood induction[75] among children with a history of preschool-onset depression. This same sample also showed smaller left hippocampal volumes and significant negative correlations between right hippocampal volume and left amygdala activation to negatively valenced faces,[76] a pattern often seen in childhood and adolescent MDD. Alterations have also been shown in subgenual cingulate connectivity,[73] default mode network connectivity,[72] and functional connectivity of the amygdala.[74] Children in the PDS study have completed up to 3 fMRI scans, allowing for trajectories of development in specific brain regions to be modeled. Recently, Luby and colleagues[77] examined the impact of early childhood depression on trajectories of cortical gray matter development across the 3 fMRI scans. Experiencing preschool-onset depression led to alterations in neural development, specifically cortical gray matter volume loss and thinning over time. Taken together, this body of work provides strong evidence for significant neurobiological alterations in currently depressed as well as previously depressed preschoolers that continues throughout childhood and into adolescence.

Other work has focused on neural reactivity assessed using event-related potentials (ERPs) in preschoolers with depression[80] and using ERP as an indicator of risk for depression.[63] For example, children (n = 84) participating in a large ongoing randomized controlled trial, the Parent-Child Interaction Therapy–Emotion Development (PCIT-ED), for preschool-onset MDD (PO-MDD) completed a guessing game while ERPs were recorded.[80] Of these, n = 53 depressed preschoolers (aged 4–7 years) and n = 25 matched, healthy control children had usable data. Depressed children had reduced reward positivity, an ERP component that indexes responses to positive outcomes compared with healthy children. This reduction is consistent with findings from samples of depressed adolescents and adults, and offers the first evidence for similar reward-related neural dysfunction at a much younger age, highlighting the importance of reward processing in understanding the pathophysiology of depression.

In addition to neurologic correlates, physiologic correlates have also been studied and linked to PO-MDD. In one study, N = 166 4-year-old children participating in an ongoing longitudinal study of temperament and risk for depression provided a morning or evening cortisol sample.[62] Observational assessments of temperament and parenting practices were conducted as well as clinical interviews assessing maternal history of depression and life stress. Findings indicate that increased waking cortisol level was associated with maternal history of depression and lower child positive emotionality before the onset of depression. This finding suggests that increased waking cortisol level may be a vulnerability marker for later depression, particularly because it is highly related to other prominent risk factors, such as parental history and temperament.

TREATMENT OF PRESCHOOL DEPRESSION

Evidence-based options for the treatment of preschool depression include both parenting interventions and psychotherapeutic interventions. Again, work from Luby and colleagues[26,81,82] has been at the forefront of this area.[83] There are several psychotherapies designed for other psychiatric disorders in preschool children; however, these do not have empirical validation for the treatment of depression. For example, play therapy is widely used with very young children; this approach is often used for a host of problems presenting in early childhood, but empirical evidence showing efficacy is lacking. Other techniques based on cognitive-behavioral principles have also been applied to treat internalizing symptoms in young children, with some forms designed and tested for posttraumatic stress disorder.[84,85] However, to date there have been no specific adaptations made to treat preschool depression. Given the limited empirical validity of treatments for preschool-onset depression, Luby and colleagues[82] developed the PCIT-ED to specifically address the emotion development impairments hypothesized to characterize early-onset depression. PCIT-ED includes

3 modules conducted over 14 sessions. PCIT targets the parent-child relationship using behavioral and play therapy techniques to enhance relationship quality and parents' ability to set nurturing and effective limits with the child. This therapy seems to be a promising treatment of PO-MDD.[81,83]

Although the literature contains some case reports of the use of antidepressants in preschool children, no large-scale empirical studies that investigate the safety and efficacy of these medications have been conducted in children less than 7 years of age. Further, there is some evidence that young children are more prone to some of the activating side effects of antidepressant medications.[86] Based on this, the use of medications is not recommended as a first or second line of treatment of preschool depression and should be considered only in severe and treatment-resistant cases. If medication is used, patients should be closely monitored by a child psychiatrist.

ASSESSMENT OF PRESCHOOL ANXIETY DISORDERS

DSM-5 defines anxiety disorders as "disorders that share features of excessive fear and anxiety and related behavioral disorders."[87] DSM-5 describes 11 different anxiety disorders, and the 4 most common anxiety disorders experienced in the preschool period are:

- Separation anxiety disorder (excessive fear surrounding separation from caregivers)
- Social phobia (excessive fear of negative social evaluation)
- Generalized anxiety disorder (excessive anxious anticipation of future events)
- Specific phobia (excessive fear of specific stimuli, such as dogs or heights)

Several studies have confirmed that anxiety symptoms in preschoolers tend to cluster into the specific categories listed earlier and support the use of these different diagnoses in preschoolers rather than 1 nonspecific anxiety disorder diagnosis.[15,88,89] Notably, posttraumatic stress disorder and obsessive-compulsive disorder are no longer classified as anxiety disorders and are not considered here.

When considering whether a child has a preschool anxiety disorder, it is critical to distinguish symptoms that cross the clinical threshold from normative situational fear. Fear is a normative, adaptive emotional response to perceived threats in the environment. The fear response includes physiologic responses such as increased heart rate and overt behavioral manifestations such as fearful expressions or crying; these responses serve important adaptive functions to promote fight or flight in response to threats as well as providing cues to caregivers to promote protective behaviors. Normative fear follows a well-defined developmental trajectory that is preserved across cultures: stranger anxiety emerges at around age 9 months, whereas separation anxiety occurs in the first year or two of life.[90,91]

Anxiety disorders are distinguished from normal fear and anxiety based on high levels of distress and functional impairment. Of note, fear and anxiety may be expressed differently in preschoolers compared with adults and may be expressed as crying, anger, avoidance, freezing, clinging, or tantrums. Impairment in preschool anxiety disorders can take several forms, including high levels of distress, avoidance of important activities such as school or peer interactions, and disruption of family functioning. Several studies using objective measures have discovered that, in many cases, preschool anxiety disorders can be highly impairing[38,92] and are even more impairing in the context of comorbid depression[93] or ODD.[94]

Because of the high degree of variability in expression of anxiety during the preschool period and because of the difficulty in distinguishing normative from clinically significant fear, it is important to use a multimodal approach to diagnosing preschool anxiety disorders. Ideally, the assessment of preschoolers includes parent-report and teacher-report symptom questionnaires,[11,89] diagnostic interviews with the child and parent,[6,95] and direct observation of the child in situations that are expected to provoke mild fear.[96] As with other preschool psychiatric assessments, it is also important to obtain a comprehensive assessment of medical, social, school, and familial factors.

PREVALENCE OF PRESCHOOL ANXIETY DISORDERS

Most studies estimate the prevalence of preschool anxiety disorders in the range of 10% to 20%,[6,7,37,38,92,94,97–99] although some studies cite prevalences as low as 1.5%[8] and others report prevalences of more than 20%.[100] The wide variation likely reflects variation in assessment tools (clinical interview, parental report, direct observation) and geographic location, and demographic differences between study samples. Despite this variation, anxiety disorders are widely acknowledged as the most prevalent class of psychiatric illness during the preschool period and across the lifespan, and retrospective studies report the median age of onset for anxiety disorders at around 6 years of age.[97,101,102] Altogether, these data suggest that anxiety disorders are the most common type of psychiatric illness for all age groups, and symptoms usually start during or near the preschool period. In contrast with older children and adults,[101,102] most studies during the preschool period do not find that prevalence rates for anxiety disorders differ based on sex[7,97,103–105] or ethnicity.[7,103,106] Preschoolers with anxiety disorders are more likely to have other anxiety disorders,[38,100] depression,[38] ADHD,[7] and ODD[7,38,94] relative to peers, with up to 30% to 50% of preschoolers with anxiety disorder having some other nonanxious psychiatric disorder.[92]

RISK FACTORS FOR PRESCHOOL ANXIETY DISORDERS

Heritability estimates for preschool anxiety disorders range widely, from 40% to 65%.[107] These estimates are lower than for other psychiatric disorders such as autism, schizophrenia, ADHD, and bipolar disorder,[108] suggesting a strong influence of both genetics and environment in determining risk for preschool anxiety disorders.

Temperament, defined as early-appearing, traitlike individual differences in emotional, attentional, and motor reactivity to novel stimuli,[109] is one of the most potent known risk factors for developing an anxiety disorder across the lifespan, including during the preschool period. Behavioral inhibition (BI) is a temperament that can be measured during the first year of life and is associated with high reactivity and negative emotional response to novel stimuli such as strangers or new toys. BI has consistently been identified as a strong risk factor for developing an anxiety disorder as a preschooler[100,103,105,110] and beyond.[111,112] In addition to BI, the temperaments of low positive affectivity,[103] low sociability, low exuberance,[113] high negative affect, and low effortful control[60] have also been associated with risk for preschool anxiety disorders.

Several family-based factors have also been associated with risk for preschool anxiety disorders; these factors may operate through a combination of genetic and environmental influences. Parental history of internalizing difficulties, including high anxiety,[105] an anxiety disorder,[103] or depression,[60,103] is a risk factor for preschool anxiety disorders. Parental anxiety and depression could be associated with preschool anxiety through genetic transmission, parenting techniques, observation of parental anxiety, or other mechanisms.[114,115] Beyond family history, parents who are younger,[38] poorer,[38,60] and less educated[103] are more likely to have children with preschool anxiety disorders. Family structure is also related to risk, because children who do not live with both biological parents and children with more siblings in the household[92] are more likely to develop preschool anxiety disorders relative to peers. Life stressors additionally confer risk for preschool anxiety disorders,[103,116] and preschoolers with high levels of conflict in the home are more likely to experience significant anxiety relative to preschoolers in low-conflict homes.[60]

Variation in parenting styles is also associated with variation in risk for preschool anxiety disorders. The parenting style with the least risk for preschool anxiety is authoritative: high in both warmth and control.[103] This type of parent is sensitive and empathic to the child's fears, but still gently and firmly encourages gradual exposure to feared stimuli (such as peer interactions). Parents who are less supportive of their children's emotions or more permissive in allowing their children to avoid feared stimuli are more likely to have a child with a preschool anxiety disorder.[103,117,118] Similarly, overprotective parenting is associated with increased risk for preschool anxiety disorders.[106,110,116] Overprotective parenting may be associated with anxiety disorders because children are not given the opportunity to master feared situations such as separating from caregivers or communicating with peers.

TREATMENT OF PRESCHOOL ANXIETY DISORDERS

Evidence-based options for treatment of preschool anxiety disorders include a variety of parenting[119] and psychotherapeutic interventions. Several studies support the use of cognitive behavior therapy (CBT)[120–124] with heavy parental involvement during treatment. Including the parent in sessions may increase preschoolers' comfort and aid in extending therapeutic techniques outside the therapy session. In addition to CBT, evidence also supports the use of modified versions of PCIT in the treatment of preschool anxiety disorders.[125,126] A combination of training in parenting skills, cognitive restructuring, and exposure has been shown to reduce progression to anxiety disorders in preschoolers at high risk based on having high BI.[127]

In contrast with a strong evidence base for psychotherapeutic interventions, there is limited support for the use of medication for preschool anxiety disorders. In general, medication should be reserved for highly impaired children who are not candidates for therapy or who fail other interventions. A recent review describes 11 preliminary studies of medication in preschool depressive and anxiety disorders and suggests that medications may be beneficial in some instances.[128]

CASE STUDY

W.H. is a 4.5-year-old white boy who for the last 6 months has displayed frequent sadness and irritability with minor frustrations or having preferences not met (eg, being given the wrong-color cup). He expresses a persistent negative self-view and thinks he is not as good as other children at sports and that no one likes him (when there is no evidence that this is true). He has on several occasions been so upset about this that he has stated that he wished he was dead. When he breaks a rule, he apologizes excessively to his mother after he is caught. He has a great deal of difficulty separating from his mother to go to preschool every morning and elaborate good-bye rituals have been necessary with many reassurances. He has a family history of affective disorders in relatives but has no other medical or developmental problems. He is from an intact family but there is a great deal of marital conflict, which he worries about.

This case provides a typical picture of depression with associated separation anxiety in a preschool child. Persistent negative self-appraisals as well as excessive guilt are the markers most suggestive of depression, because the irritability evident in this case is a more nonspecific marker. Parent-child psychotherapy that focuses on the relationships and enhancing more adaptive emotion processing would be a first line of treatment in this case.

SUMMARY

This article reviews recent literature on preschool-onset depression and anxiety, with a focus on assessment, prevalence, risk factors, and treatment options. A surprising amount of research has been conducted on preschool-onset internalizing disorders over the last 10 years; the field seems to be moving toward general acceptance and recognition for these constellations of symptoms in young children. Despite this growth in research, much work still needs to be done to further elucidate the causes, risks, and protective factors for preschool-onset internalizing disorders. More specifically, as outlined by Hankin,[5] there is still a great need for developmental, theoretic models to incorporate research findings from multiple levels of analysis, including neurobiological, genetic, environmental, to more effectively highlight key causal and risk factors contributing to preschool internalizing symptoms. In addition, these types of models will uncover the protective factors that shield young children from these early-onset disorders, leading to more effective and targeted treatments.

In addition, this article highlights the need for and importance of longitudinal studies focused on early-onset internalizing disorders. These types of studies likely need to begin during infancy to capture the prodromal period for early-onset internalizing disorders. Given the vast differences already seen in physiologic, neurobiological, emotional, and social functioning among preschoolers with and without internalizing disorders, research is now needed to investigate these areas at younger ages, before the onset of disorder. In addition, as stated earlier, they need to include assessments in various domains of functioning.

Along this line, the unique pathways differentiating trajectories of and risk factors for preschool-onset anxiety disorders and depression remain unclear. It seems that there is a general set of risk factors that are related to both anxiety disorders and depression in preschoolers, with some additional evidence supporting the distinctiveness of particular risk factors, such as guilt, for depression and unique symptom profiles differentiating depression and anxiety. This issue is further complicated by the high rates of comorbidity between anxiety and depression in this age range (as well as throughout childhood) and the well-documented multifinality in outcomes among children with early-onset depression and anxiety. Beginning to answer these exciting but fundamental questions on preschool internalizing disorders will significantly challenge researchers and clinicians for the remainder of the decade.

ACKNOWLEDGMENTS

The authors would like to extend their appreciation to Shana Sanchez, BA, for her assistance with the preparation of this article.

REFERENCES

1. Tandon M, Cardeli E, Luby J. Internalizing disorders in early childhood: a review of depressive and anxiety disorders. Child Adolesc Psychiatr Clin N Am 2009; 18(3):593–610.
2. Sylvester C, Pine DS. Anxiety disorders. In: Luby J, editor. Handbook of preschool mental health: development, disorders, and treatment. 2nd edition. New York: Guilford Publications; 2016. p. 137–64.

3. Luby JL, Belden AC. Depressive disorders. In: Luby JL, editor. Handbook of preschool mental health: development, disorders, and treatment. 2nd edition. New York: Guildford Press; 2016. p. 164–87.
4. Dougherty LR, Leppert KA, Merwin SM, et al. Advances and directions in preschool mental health research. Child Dev Perspect 2015;9(1):14–9.
5. Hankin BL. Depression from childhood through adolescence: risk mechanisms across multiple systems and levels of analysis. Curr Opin Psychol 2015;4:13–20.
6. Egger HL, Angold A. Common emotional and behavioral disorders in preschool children: presentation, nosology, and epidemiology. J Child Psychol Psychiatry 2006;47(3–4):313–37.
7. Lavigne JV, LeBailly SA, Hopkins J, et al. The prevalence of ADHD, ODD, depression, and anxiety in a community sample of 4-year-olds. J Clin Child Adolesc Psychol 2009;38(3):315–28.
8. Wichstrøm L, Berg-Nielsen TS, Angold A, et al. Prevalence of psychiatric disorders in preschoolers. J Child Psychol Psychiatry 2012;53(6):695–705.
9. Gaffrey MS, Belden AC, Luby JL. The 2-week duration criterion and severity and course of early childhood depression: implications for nosology. J Affect Disord 2011;133(3):537–45.
10. Colder CR, Mott JA, Berman AS. The interactive effects of infant activity level and fear on growth trajectories of early childhood behavior problems. Dev Psychopathol 2002;(1):1–23.
11. Achenbach TM, Rescorla LA. Manual for the ASEBA preschool forms & profiles: an integrated system of multi-informant assessment; child behavior checklist for ages 1 1/2-5; language development survey; Caregiver-Teacher report form. Burlington (VT): University of Vermont; 2000.
12. Goodman R. The strengths and difficulties questionnaire: a research note. J Child Psychol Psychiatry 1997;38(5):581–6.
13. Sterba SK, Prinstein MJ, Cox MJ. Trajectories of internalizing problems across childhood: heterogeneity, external validity, and gender differences. Dev Psychopathol 2007;19(2):345–66.
14. Sterba S, Egger HL, Angold A. Diagnostic specificity and nonspecificity in the dimensions of preschool psychopathology. J Child Psychol Psychiatry 2007; 48(10):1005–13.
15. Strickland J, Keller J, Lavigne JV, et al. The structure of psychopathology in a community sample of preschoolers. J Abnorm Child Psychol 2011;39(4): 601–10.
16. De Pauw SS, Mervielde I, Van Leeuwen KG. How are traits related to problem behavior in preschoolers? Similarities and contrasts between temperament and personality. J Abnorm Child Psychol 2009;37(3):309–25.
17. Côté SM, Boivin M, Liu X, et al. Depression and anxiety symptoms: onset, developmental course and risk factors during early childhood. J Child Psychol Psychiatry 2009;50(10):1201–8.
18. Furniss T, Beyer T, Müller JM. Impact of life events on child mental health before school entry at age six. Eur Child Adolesc Psychiatry 2009;18(12):717–24.
19. Davis S, Votruba-Drzal E, Silk JS. Trajectories of internalizing symptoms from early childhood to adolescence: associations with temperament and parenting. Soc Dev 2015;24:3.
20. Fanti KA, Henrich CC. Trajectories of pure and co-occurring internalizing and externalizing problems from age 2 to age 12: findings from the National Institute of Child Health and human development study of early child care. Dev Psychol 2010;46(5):1159–75.

21. Kryski KR, Smith HJ, Sheikh HI, et al. HPA axis reactivity in early childhood: associations with symptoms and moderation by sex. Psychoneuroendocrinology 2013;38(10):2327–36.

22. von Klitzing K, Perren S, Klein AM, et al. The interaction of social risk factors and HPA axis dysregulation in predicting emotional symptoms of five- and six-year-old children. J Psychiatr Res 2012;46(3):290–7.

23. Rapee RM. The preventative effects of a brief, early intervention for preschool-aged children at risk for internalising: follow-up into middle adolescence. J Child Psychol Psychiatry 2013;54(7):780–8.

24. Egger HL, Emde RN. Developmentally sensitive diagnostic criteria for mental health disorders in early childhood: the Diagnostic and Statistical Manual Of Mental Disorders—IV, the Research Diagnostic Criteria—Preschool Age, and the Diagnostic Classification of Mental Health and Developmental Disorders of Infancy and Early Childhood—Revised. Am Psychol 2011;66(2):95–106.

25. Luby JL, Heffelfinger A, Mrakotsky C, et al. Preschool major depressive disorder: preliminary validation for developmentally modified DSM-IV criteria. J Am Acad Child Adolesc Psychiatry 2002;41(8):928–37.

26. Luby JL, Heffelfinger A, Mrakotsky CC, et al. The clinical picture of depression in preschool children. J Am Acad Child Adolesc Psychiatry 2003;42(3):340–8.

27. Luby JL, Mrakotsky C, Heffelfinger A, et al. Characteristics of depressed preschoolers with and without anhedonia: evidence for a melancholic depressive subtype in young children. Am J Psychiatry 2004;161(11):1998–2004.

28. Luby JL, Belden A. Depressive-symptom onset during toddlerhood in a sample of depressed preschoolers: implications for future investigations of major depressive disorder in toddlers. Infant Ment Health J 2012;33(2):139–47.

29. Bufferd SJ, Dougherty LR, Olino TM, et al. Predictors of the onset of depression in young children: a multi-method, multi-informant longitudinal study from ages 3 to 6. J Child Psychol Psychiatry 2014;55(11):1279–87.

30. Fuhrmann P, Equit M, Schmidt K, et al. Prevalence of depressive symptoms and associated developmental disorders in preschool children: a population-based study. Eur Child Adolesc Psychiatry 2013;23(4):219–24.

31. Wichstrøm L, Berg-Nielsen TS. Psychiatric disorders in preschoolers: the structure of DSM-IV symptoms and profiles of comorbidity. Eur Child Adolesc Psychiatry 2014;23(7):551–62.

32. Luby JL, Heffelfinger A, Koenig-McNaught AL, et al. The preschool feelings checklist: a brief and sensitive screening measure for depression in young children. J Am Acad Child Adolesc Psychiatry 2004;43(6):708–17.

33. Egger HL, Ascher B, Angold A. The preschool age psychiatric assessment: version 1.4. Center for Developmental Epidemiology, Department of Psychiatry and Behavioral Sciences. Durham (NC): Duke Univ Med Cent; 2003.

34. Egger HL, Erkanli A, Keeler G, et al. Test-retest reliability of the Preschool Age Psychiatric Assessment (PAPA). J Am Acad Child Adolesc Psychiatry 2006; 45(5):538–49.

35. Fisher P, Lucas C. Diagnostic interview schedule for children (DISC-IV)-young child. New York: Columbia Univ; 2006.

36. Gaffrey MS, Luby JL. Kiddie schedule for affective disorders and schizophrenia - early childhood version (K-SADS-EC). St Louis (MO): Washington University; 2012.

37. Keenan K, Shaw DS, Walsh B, et al. DSM-III-R disorders in preschool children from low-income families. J Am Acad Child Adolesc Psychiatry 1997;36(5): 620–7.

38. Bufferd SJ, Dougherty LR, Carlson GA, et al. Parent-reported mental health in preschoolers: findings using a diagnostic interview. Compr Psychiatry 2011; 52(4):359–69.
39. Luby JL, Gaffrey MS, Tillman R, et al. Trajectories of preschool disorders to full DSM depression at school age and early adolescence: continuity of preschool depression. Am J Psychiatry 2014;171(7):768–76.
40. Luby JL, Si X, Belden AC, et al. Preschool depression: homotypic continuity and course over 24 months. Arch Gen Psychiatry 2009;66(8):897–905.
41. Reinfjell T, Kårstad SB, Berg-Nielsen TS, et al. Predictors of change in depressive symptoms from preschool to first grade. Dev Psychopathol 2016;28(4 Pt 2): 1517–30.
42. Whelan YM, Leibenluft E, Stringaris A, et al. Pathways from maternal depressive symptoms to adolescent depressive symptoms: the unique contribution of irritability symptoms. J Child Psychol Psychiatry 2015;56(10):1092–100.
43. Bufferd SJ, Dougherty LR, Carlson GA, et al. Psychiatric disorders in preschoolers: continuity from ages 3 to 6. Am J Psychiatry 2012;169(11):1157–64.
44. Whalen DJ, Luby JL, Tilman R, et al. Latent class profiles of depressive symptoms from early to middle childhood: predictors, outcomes, and gender effects. J Child Psychol Psychiatry 2016;57(7):794–804.
45. Navsaria N, Gilbert KE, Lenze SN, et al. Effects of early environment and caregiving: risk and protective factors in developmental psychopathology. In: Luby JL, editor. Handbook of preschool mental health: development, disorders, and treatment. 2nd edition. New York: Guilford Press; 2016. p. 27–136.
46. Luby JL, Belden A, Sullivan J, et al. Shame and guilt in preschool depression: evidence for elevations in self-conscious emotions in depression as early as age 3. J Child Psychol Psychiatry 2009;50(9):1156–66.
47. Luby JL, Belden AC, Pautsch J, et al. The clinical significance of preschool depression: impairment in functioning and clinical markers of the disorder. J Affect Disord 2009;112(1–3):111–9.
48. Luby JL. Preschool depression the importance of identification of depression early in development. Curr Dir Psychol Sci 2010;19(2):91–5.
49. Dougherty LR, Smith VC, Bufferd SJ, et al. Preschool irritability predicts child psychopathology, functional impairment, and service use at age nine. J Child Psychol Psychiatry 2015;56(9):999–1007.
50. Dougherty LR, Smith VC, Bufferd SJ, et al. Preschool irritability: longitudinal associations with psychiatric disorders at age 6 and parental psychopathology. J Am Acad Child Adolesc Psychiatry 2013;52(12):1304–13.
51. Belden AC, Barch DM, Oakberg TJ, et al. Anterior insula volume and guilt: neurobehavioral markers of recurrence after early childhood major depressive disorder. JAMA Psychiatry 2015;72(1):40–8.
52. Whalen DJ, Gilbert KE, Barch DM, et al. Variation in common preschool sleep problems as an early predictor for depression and anxiety symptom severity across time. J Child Psychol Psychiatry 2017;58(2):151–9.
53. Whalen DJ, Dixon-Gordon K, Belden AC, et al. Correlates and consequences of suicidal cognitions and behaviors in children ages 3 to 7 years. J Am Acad Child Adolesc Psychiatry 2015;54(11):926–37.e2.
54. Whalen DJ, Belden AC, Luby JL, et al. Dr. Whalen et al. reply. J Am Acad Child Adolesc Psychiatry 2016;55(3):243–5.
55. Zeanah CH, Gleason MM. Suicidality in very young children. J Am Acad Child Adolesc Psychiatry 2015;54(11):884–5.

56. Kovacs M, Lopez-Duran N. Prodromal symptoms and atypical affectivity as predictors of major depression in juveniles: implications for prevention. J Child Psychol Psychiatry 2010;51(4):472–96.

57. Dempster EL. Evidence of an association between the vasopressin V1b receptor gene (AVPR1B) and childhood-onset mood disorders. Arch Gen Psychiatry 2007;64(10):1189.

58. Strauss J, Barr CL, George CJ, et al. Brain-derived neurotrophic factor variants are associated with childhood-onset mood disorder: confirmation in a Hungarian sample. Mol Psychiatry 2005;10(9):861–7.

59. Bogdan R, Agrawal A, Gaffrey MS, et al. Serotonin transporter-linked polymorphic region (5-HTTLPR) genotype and stressful life events interact to predict preschool-onset depression: a replication and developmental extension. J Child Psychol Psychiatry 2014;55(5):448–57.

60. Hopkins J, Lavigne JV, Gouze KR, et al. Multi-domain models of risk factors for depression and anxiety symptoms in preschoolers: evidence for common and specific factors. J Abnorm Child Psychol 2013;41(5):705–22.

61. Rogers CE, Lenze SN, Luby JL. Late preterm birth, maternal depression, and risk of preschool psychiatric disorders. J Am Acad Child Adolesc Psychiatry 2013;52(3):309–18.

62. Dougherty LR, Klein DN, Olino TM, et al. Increased waking salivary cortisol and depression risk in preschoolers: the role of maternal history of melancholic depression and early child temperament. J Child Psychol Psychiatry 2009; 50(12):1495–503.

63. Shankman SA, Klein DN, Torpey DC, et al. Do positive and negative temperament traits interact in predicting risk for depression? A resting EEG study of 329 preschoolers. Dev Psychopathol 2011;23(2):551–62.

64. Belden AC, Gaffrey MS, Luby JL. Relational aggression in children with preschool-onset psychiatric disorders. J Am Acad Child Adolesc Psychiatry 2012;51(9):889–901.

65. Whalen DJ, Belden AC, Tillman R, et al. Early adversity, psychopathology, and latent class profiles of global physical health from preschool through early adolescence. Psychosom Med 2016;78(9):1008–18.

66. Belden AC, Thomson NR, Luby JL. Temper tantrums in healthy versus depressed and disruptive preschoolers: defining tantrum behaviors associated with clinical problems. J Pediatr 2008;152(1):117–22.

67. Luby JL, Belden AC, Spitznagel E. Risk factors for preschool depression: the mediating role of early stressful life events. J Child Psychol Psychiatry 2006; 47(12):1292–8.

68. Bennett DS, Sullivan MW, Lewis M. Neglected children, shame-proneness, and depressive symptoms. Child Maltreat 2010;15(4):305–14.

69. Gaffrey MS, Barch DM, Singer J, et al. Disrupted amygdala reactivity in depressed 4- to 6-year-old children. J Am Acad Child Adolesc Psychiatry 2013;52(7):737–46.

70. Gaffrey MS, Luby JL, Belden AC, et al. Association between depression severity and amygdala reactivity during sad face viewing in depressed preschoolers: an fMRI study. J Affect Disord 2011;129(1–3):364–70.

71. Barch DM, Gaffrey MS, Botteron KN, et al. Functional brain activation to emotionally valenced faces in school-aged children with a history of preschool-onset major depression. Biol Psychiatry 2012;72(12):1035–42.

72. Gaffrey MS, Luby JL, Botteron K, et al. Default mode network connectivity in children with a history of preschool onset depression. J Child Psychol Psychiatry 2012;53(9):964–72.

73. Gaffrey MS, Luby JL, Repovš G, et al. Subgenual cingulate connectivity in children with a history of preschool-depression. Neuroreport 2010;21(18):1182–8.

74. Luking KR, Repovs G, Belden AC, et al. Functional connectivity of the amygdala in early-childhood-onset depression. J Am Acad Child Adolesc Psychiatry 2011; 50(10):1027–41.e3.

75. Pagliaccio D, Luby J, Gaffrey M, et al. Anomalous functional brain activation following negative mood induction in children with pre-school onset major depression. Dev Cogn Neurosci 2012;2(2):256–67.

76. Suzuki H, Botteron KN, Luby JL, et al. Structural-functional correlations between hippocampal volume and cortico-limbic emotional responses in depressed children. Cogn Affect Behav Neurosci 2012;13(1):135–51.

77. Luby JL, Belden AC, Jackson JJ, et al. Early childhood depression and alterations in the trajectory of gray matter maturation in middle childhood and early adolescence. JAMA Psychiatry 2016;73(1):31–8.

78. Belden AC, Pagliaccio D, Murphy ER, et al. Neural activation during cognitive emotion regulation in previously depressed compared to healthy children: evidence of specific alterations. J Am Acad Child Adolesc Psychiatry 2015; 54(9):771–81.

79. Marrus N, Belden A, Nishino T, et al. Ventromedial prefrontal cortex thinning in preschool-onset depression. J Affect Disord 2015;180:79–86.

80. Belden AC, Irvin K, Hajcak G, et al. Neural correlates of reward processing in depressed and healthy preschool-age children. J Am Acad Child Adolesc Psychiatry 2016;55(12):1081–9.

81. Luby J, Lenze S, Tillman R. A novel early intervention for preschool depression: findings from a pilot randomized controlled trial. J Child Psychol Psychiatry 2012;53(3):313–22.

82. Luby JL. Treatment of anxiety and depression in the preschool period. J Am Acad Child Adolesc Psychiatry 2013;52(4):346–58.

83. Lenze SN, Pautsch J, Luby J. Parent–child interaction therapy emotion development: a novel treatment for depression in preschool children. Depress Anxiety 2011;28(2):153–9.

84. Scheeringa MS, Weems CF, Cohen JA, et al. Trauma-focused cognitive-behavioral therapy for posttraumatic stress disorder in three-through six year-old children: a randomized clinical trial. J Child Psychol Psychiatry 2011; 52(8):853–60.

85. Salloum A, Wang W, Robst J, et al. Stepped care versus standard trauma-focused cognitive behavioral therapy for young children. J Child Psychol Psychiatry 2016;57(5):614–22.

86. Gleason MM, Egger HL, Emslie GJ, et al. Psychopharmacological treatment for very young children: contexts and guidelines. J Am Acad Child Adolesc Psychiatry 2007;46(12):1532–72.

87. American Psychiatric Association. Diagnostic and statistical manual of mental disorders (DSM-5®). Washington, DC: American Psychiatric Association; 2013.

88. Spence SH, Rapee R, McDonald C, et al. The structure of anxiety symptoms among preschoolers. Behav Res Ther 2001;39(11):1293–316.

89. Edwards SL, Rapee RM, Kennedy SJ, et al. The assessment of anxiety symptoms in preschool-aged children: the revised Preschool Anxiety Scale. J Clin Child Adolesc Psychol 2010;39(3):400–9.

90. Gullone E. The development of normal fear: a century of research. Clin Psychol Rev 2000;20(4):429–51.
91. Beesdo K, Knappe S, Pine DS. Anxiety and anxiety disorders in children and adolescents: developmental issues and implications for DSM-V. Psychiatr Clin North Am 2009;32(3):483–524.
92. Franz L, Angold A, Copeland W, et al. Preschool anxiety disorders in pediatric primary care: prevalence and comorbidity. J Am Acad Child Adolesc Psychiatry 2013;52(12):1294–303.e1.
93. von Klitzing K, White LO, Otto Y, et al. Depressive comorbidity in preschool anxiety disorder. J Child Psychol Psychiatry 2014;55(10):1107–16.
94. Martín V, Granero R, Ezpeleta L. Comorbidity of oppositional defiant disorder and anxiety disorders in preschoolers. Psicothema 2014;26(1):27–32.
95. Birmaher B, Ehmann M, Axelson DA, et al. Schedule for affective disorders and schizophrenia for school-age children (K-SADS-PL) for the assessment of preschool children – a preliminary psychometric study. J Psychiatr Res 2009; 43(7):680–6.
96. Mian ND, Carter AS, Pine DS, et al. Development of a novel observational measure for anxiety in young children: the Anxiety Dimensional Observation Scale. J Child Psychol Psychiatry 2015;56(9):1017–25.
97. Petresco S, Anselmi L, Santos IS, et al. Prevalence and comorbidity of psychiatric disorders among 6-year-old children: 2004 Pelotas Birth Cohort. Soc Psychiatry Psychiatr Epidemiol 2014;49(6):975–83.
98. Lavigne JV, Gibbons RD, Christoffel KK, et al. Prevalence rates and correlates of psychiatric disorders among preschool children. J Am Acad Child Adolesc Psychiatry 1996;35(2):204–14.
99. Earls F. Application of DSM-III in an epidemiological study of preschool children. Am J Psychiatry 1982;139(2):242–3.
100. Paulus FW, Backes A, Sander CS, et al. Anxiety disorders and behavioral inhibition in preschool children: a population-based study. Child Psychiatry Hum Dev 2015;46(1):150–7.
101. Kessler RC, Berglund P, Demler O, et al. Lifetime prevalence and age-of-onset distributions of DSM-IV disorders in the national comorbidity survey replication. Arch Gen Psychiatry 2005;62(6):593–602.
102. Merikangas KR, He J, Burstein M, et al. Lifetime prevalence of mental disorders in U.S. adolescents: results from the National Comorbidity Survey Replication–Adolescent Supplement (NCS-A). J Am Acad Child Adolesc Psychiatry 2010; 49(10):980–9.
103. Dougherty LR, Tolep MR, Bufferd SJ, et al. Preschool anxiety disorders: comprehensive assessment of clinical, demographic, temperamental, familial, and life stress correlates. J Clin Child Adolesc Psychol 2013;42(5):577–89.
104. Gleason MM, Zamfirescu A, Egger HL, et al. Epidemiology of psychiatric disorders in very young children in a Romanian pediatric setting. Eur Child Adolesc Psychiatry 2011;20(10):527–35.
105. Shamir-Essakow G, Ungerer JA, Rapee RM. Attachment, behavioral inhibition, and anxiety in preschool children. J Abnorm Child Psychol 2005;33(2):131–43.
106. Hudson JL, Dodd HF, Lyneham HJ, et al. Temperament and family environment in the development of anxiety disorder: two-year follow-up. J Am Acad Child Adolesc Psychiatry 2011;50(12):1255–64.e1.
107. Eley TC, Bolton D, O'Connor TG, et al. A twin study of anxiety-related behaviours in pre-school children. J Child Psychol Psychiatry 2003;44(7):945–60.

108. McGrath LM, Weill S, Robinson EB, et al. Bringing a developmental perspective to anxiety genetics. Dev Psychopathol 2012;24(4):1179–93.

109. Rothbart MK. Temperament, development, and personality. Curr Dir Psychol Sci 2007;16(4):207–12.

110. Vreeke LJ, Muris P, Mayer B, et al. Skittish, shielded, and scared: relations among behavioral inhibition, overprotective parenting, and anxiety in native and non-native Dutch preschool children. J Anxiety Disord 2013;27(7):703–10.

111. Clauss JA, Blackford JU. Behavioral inhibition and risk for developing social anxiety disorder: a meta-analytic study. J Am Acad Child Adolesc Psychiatry 2012;51(10):1066–75.e1.

112. Rapee RM. Preschool environment and temperament as predictors of social and nonsocial anxiety disorders in middle adolescence. J Am Acad Child Adolesc Psychiatry 2014;53(3):320–8.

113. Dougherty LR, Bufferd SJ, Carlson GA, et al. Preschoolers' observed temperament and psychiatric disorders assessed with a parent diagnostic interview. J Clin Child Adolesc Psychol 2011;40(2):295–306.

114. Rachman S. Neo-conditioning and the classical theory of fear acquisition. Clin Psychol Rev 1991;11(2):155–73.

115. Field AP, Lawson J. Fear information and the development of fears during childhood: effects on implicit fear responses and behavioural avoidance. Behav Res Ther 2003;41(11):1277–93.

116. Edwards SL, Rapee RM, Kennedy S. Prediction of anxiety symptoms in preschool-aged children: examination of maternal and paternal perspectives. J Child Psychol Psychiatry 2010;51(3):313–21.

117. Braungart-Rieker JM, Hill-Soderlund AL, Karrass J. Fear and anger reactivity trajectories from 4 to 16 months: the roles of temperament, regulation, and maternal sensitivity. Dev Psychol 2010;46(4):791–804.

118. Lewis-Morrarty E, Degnan KA, Chronis-Tuscano A, et al. Maternal over-control moderates the association between early childhood behavioral inhibition and adolescent social anxiety symptoms. J Abnorm Child Psychol 2012;40(8): 1363–73.

119. Kennedy SJ, Rapee RM, Edwards SL. A selective intervention program for inhibited preschool-aged children of parents with an anxiety disorder: effects on current anxiety disorders and temperament. J Am Acad Child Adolesc Psychiatry 2009;48(6):602–9.

120. Hirshfeld-Becker DR, Masek B, Henin A, et al. Cognitive behavioral therapy for 4- to 7-year-old children with anxiety disorders: a randomized clinical trial. J Consult Clin Psychol 2010;78(4):498–510.

121. Donovan CL, March S. Online CBT for preschool anxiety disorders: a randomised control trial. Behav Res Ther 2014;58:24–35.

122. Schneider S, Blatter-Meunier J, Herren C, et al. Disorder-specific cognitive-behavioral therapy for separation anxiety disorder in young children: a randomized waiting-list-controlled trial. Psychother Psychosom 2011;80(4):206–15.

123. Monga S, Young A, Owens M. Evaluating a cognitive behavioral therapy group program for anxious five to seven year old children: a pilot study. Depress Anxiety 2009;26(3):243–50.

124. Freeman J, Sapyta J, Garcia A, et al. Family-based treatment of early childhood obsessive-compulsive disorder: the Pediatric Obsessive-Compulsive Disorder Treatment Study for Young Children (POTS Jr)–a randomized clinical trial. JAMA Psychiatry 2014;71(6):689–98.

125. Carpenter AL, Puliafico AC, Kurtz SM, et al. Extending parent-child interaction therapy for early childhood internalizing problems: new advances for an overlooked population. Clin Child Fam Psychol Rev 2014;17(4):340–56.

126. Comer JS, Puliafico AC, Aschenbrand SG, et al. A pilot feasibility evaluation of the CALM Program for anxiety disorders in early childhood. J Anxiety Disord 2012;26(1):40–9.

127. Rapee RM, Kennedy SJ, Ingram M, et al. Altering the trajectory of anxiety in at-risk young children. Am J Psychiatry 2010;167(12):1518–25.

128. Barterian JA, Rappuhn E, Seif EL, et al. Current state of evidence for medication treatment of preschool internalizing disorders. ScientificWorldJournal 2014; 2014:286085.

Attention Deficit Hyperactivity Disorder in Preschool-Age Children

Mini Tandon, DO, Alba Pergjika, MD, MPH*

KEYWORDS

- Preschool children • Attention deficit hyperactivity disorder • Assessment
- Treatment

KEY POINTS

- Preschool children with attention deficit hyperactivity disorder are at greater risk of placement in special education classes and use more special needs services.
- The etiology of attention deficit hyperactivity disorder is multifactorial and highly genetic.
- Assessment tools for diagnosis of attention deficit hyperactivity disorder vary. The foundational assessments include a psychiatric and medical assessment.
- Behavioral intervention lasting at least 8 weeks is recommended before initiating a pharmacologic agent, although the lack of availability of nonpharmacologic intervention is noteworthy.
- In preschool children, data suggest that stimulants such as methylphenidates are less efficacious and cause side effects more commonly than in school age and older children.

INTRODUCTION

Attention deficit hyperactivity disorder (ADHD) is a neurodevelopmental disorder and one of the most common psychiatric disorders in childhood. Preschool children with ADHD are at greater risk of placement in special education classes and use more special needs services. Prevalence of ADHD in preschool-age children is similar to that in school-age children. Estimates vary at 2% to 5.7%, with a male/female ratio of 5:1.[1,2] A diagnosis of ADHD in later preschool years shows more stability than in earlier years. Comorbid disruptive disorders are predictors of continuity of ADHD within the preschool years.[3] Preschoolers with ADHD are more likely to meet criteria for comorbid oppositional defiant disorder (ODD) (8 times), conduct disorder (CD) (26 times), and depressive symptoms (9 times).[1] Older preschoolers with ADHD have shown deficits

Disclosures: Royalties, Dr M. Tandon has a copyright on a children's book.
Division of Child and Adolescent Psychiatry, Washington University School of Medicine, 660 South Euclid Avenue, Campus Box 8134, St Louis, MO 63110, USA
* Corresponding author.
E-mail address: pergjikaa@psychiatry.wustl.edu

in age-appropriate performance-based measures, and most continue to have symptoms into adulthood.[4] Given findings for validity, stability, and correlated deficits, the field has moved progressively forward from whether ADHD exists among preschool-aged children.

The etiology of ADHD is multifactorial and highly genetic. Perinatal stress, low birth weight, traumatic brain injury, maternal smoking and alcohol use during pregnancy, lead exposure, severe early deprivation, and familial loading may all contribute to risk (child has >50% chance of having ADHD if a parent has been diagnosed with the disease). First-degree relatives of those with ADHD are 2 to 8 times more likely than relatives of unaffected individuals to have ADHD. Heritability of 71% to 90% has been found in twin studies internationally for ADHD combined and inattentive types. However, gene-environment interaction cannot be ruled out, and adoption studies of individuals with ADHD are scarce.[5]

The core symptoms of ADHD are associated with dysregulation of neural symptoms affecting the neurotransmitters dopamine and norepinephrine in the frontal lobes. Regulation of these neurotransmitters is the target of pharmacotherapy.[6] However, the neuronal circuitry involved in the ADHD brain is much more complex. Neuroimaging findings are nonspecific. They include smaller total cerebral, cerebellar, corpus callosum, frontal lobe, and caudate volumes and lower levels of dopamine transporter in the nucleus accumbens (reward center).[7] Preschool boys with higher hyperactivity and inattentiveness have lower sympathetic and higher parasympathetic activity.[6] Girls are underrepresented in structural imaging studies.[7]

The most basic elements for assessment of ADHD include a comprehensive psychiatric and medical assessment. The psychiatric assessment will determine whether age-inappropriate symptoms of inattention, hyperactivity, and impulsivity are present for at least 6 months in multiple settings and affect functioning or development. Preschool-age–specific assessments that have proven validity include the ADHD Rating Scale IV,[8] The Vanderbilt ADHD Teacher and Parent Rating Scales,[9] Conners Comprehensive Behavior Rating Scales,[10] and Conner's Teacher Rating Scale-Revised[11]—a brief, age-specific version of the Conners Teacher Rating Scale. Child Behavior Checklist (CBCL/1.5-5) for preschoolers has empirically proven validity and reliability in rating and internalizing and externalizing symptoms and includes an attention domain.[12] The CBCL/1.5-5 and Strengths and Difficulties Questionnaire have an internal consistency of 0.58%. The Connors Continuous Performance Test was found to have poor to slight utility in the assessment of ADHD symptoms in children.[13]

Parent-teacher agreement across ages and types of behavior has not been consistent.[14] Dysfunction has to be present across domains for a diagnosis of ADHD. In certain studies, there is poor parent-teacher agreement: global ADHD symptoms are reported at a higher rate by parents compared with teachers. This could be because of the characteristics of the sample, parents' understanding of developmentally appropriate behavior, difference in structure and expectations across settings, or normal preschool-age development. The hyperactive-impulsive symptoms reported by parents in clinical settings can resemble those reported by parents most often in nonclinical study samples.[14] A similar disagreement exists between parents themselves. Parenting stress is a predictive factor, accounting for 25% of the variance.[12] Mothers with elevated stress rate more externalizing behavior problems than fathers with similar levels of stress. The parental discrepancies did not apply to internalizing symptoms.

Developmentally, preschool-age children are undergoing significant changes, including learning to sustain attention and inhibit impulses, testing limits, and looking for more opportunities for independence. Developmental modifications to the diagnostic criteria may help the validity of the assessment tools.[15] Clinically, differences in symptom reporting can also provide an opportunity for further inquiry into potential situational factors.[14] Mothers may spend more time with preschool-age children. Maternal stress could be caused by difficulties coping with the child's ADHD. Maternal ADHD has been associated with maladaptive parenting and poor child behavioral treatment response, although mild symptoms have not limited such benefits in some studies.[16,17] Evidence is mixed regarding the degree to which treatment of maternal ADHD influences children's behavior or parenting. Some studies found that treatment of mothers improves their perceptions of parenting practices, reduces parental negative talk during non-homework tasks, and decreases reported child inappropriate behavior.[18,19] Others suggested no significant effects.[18] A 2016 sequential multiple assessment randomized trial (SMART) pilot study is underway to provide answers to how best to sequence maternal treatment of ADHD.[16] The children included will be between ages 3 and 8 years. Although the results of this study will not exclusively apply to preschool-age children, they will provide invaluable information. In the meantime, obtaining information from both parents or caregivers, not solely mothers, and administering parenting stress questionnaires will further inform the assessment, especially for externalizing symptoms when assessing preschool children.[12] Teachers' reporting of the presence of symptoms may increase confidence in the developmental inappropriateness of the behaviors.

TREATMENT OF ATTENTION DEFICIT HYPERACTIVITY DISORDER

The American Academy of Child and Adolescent Psychiatry (AACAP) published a treatment algorithm for preschoolers with ADHD in 2007. Behavioral interventions for at least 8 weeks are recommended before initiating a pharmacologic agent when behavior therapy fails.[20]

EVIDENCE-BASED NONPHARMACOLOGIC APPROACHES IN TREATMENT OF ATTENTION DEFICIT HYPERACTIVITY DISORDER
Evidence-based Behavioral Intervention for Attention Deficit Hyperactivity Disorder

Parent behavior training (PBT) is recommended as the first-line treatment of ADHD in preschool children. Data suggest that stimulants such as methylphenidate (MPH) are less efficacious and cause side effects more commonly in this population.[2,21] The most cited PBTs in the last 25 years are:

- Positive Parenting Program (Triple P)
- Incredible Years Parenting Program (Incredible Years)
- Parent-Child Interaction Therapy (PCIT)
- The New Forest Parenting Programme (NFPP)

Standardization is achieved with use of a manual. No discernible advantage to any specific PBT program has been found. There is a dose effect with greater benefit associated with increased number of sessions attended by parents. Benefits are sustained 6 months after the completion of the program.[21] A summary of each program is provided below.

PBT is designed to help parents manage a child's problem behaviors with effective discipline strategies by using rewards and nonpunitive consequences. The goal is to promote a positive relationship between child and parent.[21] Structured parent training, a type of PBT, over an 8-week period, is effective in improving both clinical and direct observational measures of ADHD behaviors in preschoolers when compared with parent counseling and support (PC&S) only.[22] Preschoolers receive 8 one-hour weekly visits by 2 specially trained therapists at their home. Based on a treatment manual (Information Manual for Professionals Working with Families with Hyperactive Children Ages 2–9), mothers, not fathers, have received the training in all cases. The initial sessions include maternal education of ADHD, emphasis on the importance of praise, and introduction to a behavioral diary. The diary is used in subsequent sessions to discuss parent's feelings about the behavior that week and emphasize behavioral strategies: clear messages, routines, countdowns, reminders, limit setting, and avoiding confrontations. These messages are reinforced weekly, in addition to learning to avoid threats and discussing temper tantrums. Quiet time and time out concepts are introduced in week 4. Week 5 is used to review the progress and inquire about parent's ability to implement the strategies and their own coping mechanisms. Weeks 6 and 7 include 15-minute observations of parent-child interaction. Feedback is provided regarding quality of interaction and importance of implementing previously discussed behavioral techniques. The last session focuses on 1 or 2 areas of concern. Parents in the PC&S receive support and can use a diary for guidance, but no training is provided. The improvements in ADHD symptoms in the PC&S group approached significance, but the effect size of the parent training intervention was twice as much as that in the PC&S group. The effects of parent training were maintained for 15 weeks after treatment.[22]

Triple P was developed by Sanders in 1999. The goal was to develop effective evidence-based parenting interventions that may prevent conduct problems at a population level.[23] It is not specific to preschoolers with ADHD. The program targets disruptive behaviors that are also found in ADHD. Triple P has 5 different levels of support for parents: communication strategies, a one-time assistance to parents with minimal concerns for their child's behavior, targeted counseling for mild to moderate child behavioral difficulties, positive parenting skills for children with severe behavioral difficulties, and intensive support when concerns are complex. Parents can access this support via self-directed programs, telephone-assisted, group, and individual ways. The program seeks to find the minimally sufficient condition that, when changed, significantly alters the child's risk for conduct problem development. Different variants of Triple P have been compared among each other and with waiting list preschoolers with ADHD. The enhanced version of behavioral family interventions, for example, includes 2 extra sessions, for a total of 12 sessions compared with 10 in the standard behavioral family interventions, comprising partner support training and coping skills training. Partner support training and coping skills training are 2 evidence-based adjunctive interventions that address family risk factors of marital conflict and parental adjustment, respectively. The program is 15 to 17 weeks long. Both enhanced behavioral family interventions and standard behavioral family interventions are associated with significantly fewer observed child negative behaviors, significantly lower level of mother-reported disruptive child behavior, and improvement in parenting skills, efficacy, and satisfaction when compared with the waiting list group. Postintervention, in this study of 87 preschoolers (age 3) with comorbid ADHD and disruptive behavior, no significant difference was found between the 2 groups on the Inattentive Behavior or Conduct Problem Behavioral factors. However, these findings have public health implications because any of the parent programs are cost effective and the outcomes are maintained at 1- and 3-year follow-up.[23,24]

The NFPP was specifically developed to address the self-regulation deficiency abilities of preschoolers with ADHD.[2] Similar to the structured parent training program, NFPP is 8 weeks long, with weekly 90-minute session delivered by a single practitioner. The program is delivered at home and not in a clinical setting, which is different from some of other PBT interventions. Supporting the child's development through parental scaffolding is a key component of the NFPP. In addition to behavioral strategies, the program includes games and activities that target the self-regulatory and attention deficits that cause impairment in children with ADHD. NFPP claims to target ADHD processes. It is expected to be more effective than current treatments for preschool ADHD.

Forehand and colleagues[25] compared 2 PBT programs in a sample of preschoolers with ADHD and comorbid ODD to see whether the presence of ODD influenced the outcome of the PBT. NFPP was used to treat ADHD, and Helping the Noncompliant Child (HNC) targeted ODD symptoms. Helping the Noncompliant Child was more effective than NFPP with disruptive behavior in the presence of comorbid ODD. However, it was equally effective across ADHD only and comorbid ADHD diagnosis. A secondary analysis of this study found that 44.6% of the 130 three- to 4-year-old children with ADHD had comorbid ODD. NFPP was more effective with disruptive behaviors when children had a diagnosis of ADHD only, based on parent report. Although teachers reported fewer disruptive behaviors, they did not reach significance. An interesting point about bias was raised by the authors. It is possible that the halo effect contributes to improvements in behavior rated by parents versus teachers.

Emotion regulation is often deficient in children with ADHD. This limits their executive functioning skills like behavioral inhibition and attentional flexibility, thus hindering their ability to adapt to their environment. In adolescents, emotion dysregulation mediates the relationship between ADHD and depressive symptoms.[1] Parent-child interaction therapy (PCIT) is an evidence-based intervention for young children with ODD/CD, which, when paired with an emotional development (ED) strategy, was found to be significantly more effective than psychoeducation alone on executive functioning and emotion regulation.[26] PCIT, by itself, effectively treats risk factors associated with preschool ADHD, such as ineffective parenting, maternal depression, and child comorbid internalizing and externalizing symptoms. The results can last 3 to 6 years posttreatment.[1] An updated form of PCIT, PCIT–Emotional Development (PCIT-ED) treats preschoolers with depressive symptoms by teaching parents to be emotional coaches for their children and increase their emotional regulation. The ED module is 8 sessions long and focusses on parents' own abilities to regulate their emotions during parent-child encounters, teaching children emotion identification and age appropriate relaxation skills, teaching parents labeling of emotions as they are expressed by children in real time, and live coaching of use of ED skills. It may be a promising intervention for treatment of preschool depression. When PCIT-ED was applied to 6 children with ADHD, whose ages ranged from 3 to 7 years, emotion coaching of children's excessive guilt and anhedonia were not found to be as relevant. Based on the observation and parents' feedback of PCIT-ED, PCIT–emotional coaching was developed. It is meant to address parents' major concerns of expressions of anger and frustration, lack of responsibility for children's actions, and what is viewed as too little guilt, rather than fear, sadness, or excessive guilt. Therefore, PCIT–emotional coaching emphasizes parent responses to child emotions, parent discussion of child emotions, and parents' own emotion expression via modeling. This is a novel strategy in treating emotional dysregulation in preschoolers with ADHD, and further studies need to be developed. The overarching target of PCIT-ED is not treatment of ADHD but improvement of parent-child interactions, treatment of comorbidities, and reduction of ADHD-related impairment.[1]

Community Parent Education Program

The Community Parent Education Program (COPE) is a Canadian manual-based parent education program that was created by Cunningham and colleagues[27] to target severe externalizing behavioral problems in children with ADHD, ODD, and CD. Similar to other parenting programs, it is based on social learning models. What distinguishes it from other parenting programs is that it is large group and community based, which increases the likelihood of parental adherence. Groups can have up to 25 to 30 parents. Weekly 2-hour sessions over 10 weeks are held by trained group leaders. The groups are participant driven. Each meeting is structured in 10 phases:

- Informal social activities
- Review of homework in subgroups
- Large-group discussions of homework projects
- Solutions to videotaped vignettes of a problematic situation
- Discussions of proposed solutions
- The modeling of a group's solution by trained leaders
- Subgroup brainstorm applications
- Dyad strategy rehearsals
- Homework planning
- A summary of a session

New strategies are taught in each session. COPE has been found effective in reducing child behavioral problems as rated by parents when parents experience decrease in parental stress. These findings have also been replicated overseas but not in preschool children. In Finland, COPE was found to be as effective as parenting programs in reducing behavior problems in school-age children. COPE is more consistently effective in reducing comorbid behavior and social functioning compared with ADHD symptoms.[27]

The Incredible Years (IY) Preschool Basic parenting program is a manual-based program that aims to teach parents how to recognize and treat their children's emotional and behavioral problems for those who are at risk of conduct problems.[28] The program consists of 8 to 12 weeks of 2- to 2.5-hour parenting sessions. Besides teaching positive parenting, the program uses techniques to help parents via modeling, discussing previous experiences with and feelings about raising their children, and analyzing video material of family behavior. The IY organization has developed programs for babies (0–12 months), toddlers (1–3 years), and school-age children. Advanced programs can be recommended for an additional 9 to 12 weeks in which the focus is problem solving by both parents and children. ADHD symptoms and oppositional problems significantly decreased from pre-intervention to 12-month follow-up with large effect sizes (between 0.17 and 0.44) in a Portuguese study. Even though most of the preschoolers in the study continued to have ADHD symptoms in the clinical range, the symptom reduction post-IY was significant. As in other parenting programs, mothers' self-reported sense of parenting competence and efficacy significantly increase after participation in IY.[28]

Combination PBT and school- or day care–based interventions have also been studied. Parental attendance at 5 or more sessions has been associated with greater improvement in child behavior. However, the trials offer inconsistent results. Some studies show that children improved more when they received a combination of interventions and others found no added benefit compared with psychoeducation.[21]

As shown above, parent behavioral interventions effectively address disruptive behaviors in preschool children with ADHD. However, convenience, transportation, socioeconomic status, and child care can interfere with consistent and sufficient participation. Telephone and internet-assisted parent training programs have been implemented, and their efficacy is now being studied in Canada and Finland.[29,30] The Finnish study was conducted over a 12-month period. It included weekly 45-minute telephone coaching sessions and 11 weekly online sessions that targeted interventions for disruptive behavior in 4-year-old children. The children did not have ADHD diagnosed, but the screening criteria at a primary health care clinic indicated a high level of disruptive behavior (score >5 points on the conduct problem scale of the Strengths and Difficulties Questionnaire lasting 6 months). The parent had reported that their 4-year-old child had difficulties in one single question. At baseline, externalizing symptoms were rated at 19.8, total at 44.6, and internalizing at 10.6 in the CBCL/1.5-5. Parents developed skills to strengthen the parent-child relationship, reinforce positive behavior, reduce conflict, manage daily transitions, and include prosocial behavior. About 7 to 10 months after randomization, the intervention group received 2 booster coaching sessions. Total, externalizing, and internalizing symptoms of CBCL/1.5-5 improved significantly and achieved statistical significance. However, some of the symptom domains such as attention and ADHD did not reach significance, and there were several study limitations.[30] The Canadian trials included preschool and school-age children with ADHD, anxiety disorders, and ODD with almost half of them having comorbid diagnosis. Handbooks and videos of Strongest Families Smart Website were distributed to participant families. Families also received weekly telephone coaching. Assessments were blindly conducted and evaluated at 120, 240, and 365 days after randomization. In the overall analysis, significantly more children were diagnosis free at 240 and 365 days after randomization ($P<.001$).[29] These findings suggest an interesting public health intervention that can reach a large portion of the population.[30]

Two independent meta-analyses that were conducted in 2014 and 2016 found that parent-administered behavior interventions led to a moderate reduction in both ADHD symptoms and conduct problems, which are maintained for preschool children.[31,32] Although the studies were not specific to preschool age children (ages ranged from 33–144 months), the 2014 review included several studies on preschoolers. In conjunction with other research, medication did not enhance improvements in ADHD symptoms, and the strength of the association was further increased when medication was removed.[32,33] Parent training was a core therapeutic intervention, which improved appropriate use of positive strategies such as praise and encouragement. Parents also had improved self-concept—possibly because their interventions were validated by experienced therapists or because of positive effects of applied behavioral strategies. The severity of child ADHD or parental mental illness was not accounted for in the analysis, different parent interventions were implemented in each study, and the studies included comorbid conduct or oppositional defiant disorders and not ADHD alone. A more standardized parent intervention program may be warranted, although all have proven similar efficacy.[32] Because treatment delivery effectiveness was measured via parental ratings, the role of bias cannot be underestimated. Although the behavioral interventions also improved parental self-esteem, there was no improvement in parental well-being. There was a moderate but not statistically significant improvement in parental stress. Teacher ratings and academic and social outcomes would provide important objective data and should be included in future research.

Neurofeedback

Neurofeedback is based on the principle that the brain emits different types of waves depending on concentration state. The goal is to teach self-regulation using operant reinforcement procedures by using electroencephalogram indices of interest that are converted into visual or acoustic signals and feedback automatically in real time to the patient.[34] For example, cortical activity may be represented by the speed of a ball presented on a computer screen. Learning occurs when the ball rises, falls, or advances more quickly in response to patient's regulated changes in brain activity. The 2 neurofeedback approaches that have been used to treat ADHD are frequency band training (targeting the frontal lobes) and slow cortical potential training. A meta-analysis of randomized controlled trials examined the effects of neurofeedback (specifically frequency band training) on ADHD symptoms and neuropsychological deficits in children and adolescents with ADHD ages 3 to 18 years.[32] Only 2 of the 13 studies included children who were 6 years old, and both studies placed the 6-year-old children in the control group.[35,36] Therefore, a conclusion about efficacy of neurofeedback in preschool children cannot be made. Overall, this meta-analysis does not support neurofeedback as an effective treatment for ADHD in children.

EVIDENCE-BASED PHARMACOLOGIC TREATMENT FOR ATTENTION DEFICIT HYPERACTIVITY DISORDER

The main neurotransmitters implicated in the pathophysiology of ADHD are dopamine and norepinephrine. Cognitive deficits may be emerging from dysfunctions in the fronto- striatal brain and associated with dopaminergic mesocortical areas. Dysfunctions in reward and motivational processes could be caused by impaired signaling in the mesolimbic dopaminergic system. The default mode network (DMN) has been increasingly studied. The DMN includes brain regions that are active when a person is awake and alert but not actively engaged but deactivated during tasks. In the ADHD brain, there are thought to be DMN deficits at rest and during a task, leading to decreased inhibition and executive functioning impairment. How medications affect the DMN is an important investigative next step.[37]

Stimulants (MPHs, amphetamines) and nonstimulants (guanfacine, atomoxetine) are used to reduce ADHD symptoms by enhancing the synaptic levels of dopamine and norepinephrine in the brain. The US Food and Drug Administration (FDA) has only approved the short-acting stimulant formulations amphetamine salt combo, dextroamphetamine (two different brand names, Zenzedi and ProCentra), and amphetamine sulfate for treatment of ADHD in children.[20]

Psychostimulants have been the first-line medication for treatment of ADHD and the most commonly prescribed ones for decades in school-age children even though practice parameters recommend behavioral interventions first. Their efficacy has been well documented in several trials as has their relative safety. The Preschool ADHD Treatment study (PATS) funded by the National Institutes of Mental Health was a multicenter, randomized, efficacy trial designed to evaluate the short-term efficacy and long-term safety of immediate-release MPH specifically in preschoolers ages 3 to 5 years with severe ADHD that was unresponsive to a 10-week psychosocial intervention.[38] The PATS trial evaluated the effects of MPH on preschoolers' social skills, classroom behavior, emotional status, and parenting stress. In the parallel group trial (best dose vs placebo), which ran for 5 weeks, doses of methylphenidate were 2.5, 5, and 7.5 mg 3 times a day with an average of 14.22 ± 8.1 mg/d.[39] Only 21% of the preschoolers on best-dose MPH and 13% on placebo achieved remission. In the maintenance phase of PATS (40 weeks), mean dose of MPH increased to 19.98 ± 9.56 mg/d, which was associated with improvements in children's parent-rated social skills and teacher-rated social competence and a significant decrease in emotional outbursts and crying. At 3- and 6-year naturalistic follow-up, about 1 child in 4 was off medications, and 1 in 10 was on an antipsychotic. At each follow-up point, 60% and 70%, respectively, were on an indicated ADHD medication: monotherapy or combined atomoxetine, stimulant, and antipsychotic.[40] In school-age children, a 2015 systemic review concluded that MPH use is associated with improvement in ADHD teacher-rated symptoms corresponding to -9.6 points on the ADHD rating scale.[41] The mean age was 9.7 years (ages 3–18) with 2 trials including participants who were 19 to 21 years old. There were several subgroup analyses, including trials of preschool-age children (2–6 years) that showed that age did not significantly influence the intervention effect. This particular study found that it was underpowered to identify a difference in serious adverse events.[41]

The safety of MPHs has been investigated extensively. In the PATS study, tolerability of MPH was assessed by examining the percentage of children who did not drop out of the study based on medication-induced side effects.[42] The FDA definition of a serious side effect is a seizure or an adverse effect that significantly affects functioning and presents a serious medical threat. A loss of greater than 10% of baseline weight is considered severe by the FDA, and loss of less than 2 pounds is considered nonreportable. Annual growth rates were 20.3% less than expected for height and 55.2% for weight in preschoolers who were prescribed MPH in the PATS study.[43] About 11% of preschoolers (N = 183) who were on MPH for a year discontinued treatment, and about 30% experienced moderate-to-severe side effects. Parents rated the adverse effects (AE), demonstrated in **Table 1**, statistically more often in the MPH group then placebo. There were no significant differences in AE frequencies between dose conditions.[42]

Three of 8 severe AEs met the FDA criteria for serious. They were experienced by different preschoolers and included a possible seizure, hospitalizations for abdominal migraine disorder in a child with prestudy hospitalization for the same, and *Mycoplasma* pneumonia during titration. The side effects reported during the titration phase included tics, formication, rash, seizure, and insomnia. In the maintenance phase, the AEs were appetite loss, irritability and 1 instance of insomnia, tics, weight loss, depression, anxiety, social isolation, and scalding self. The risk of slowed growth rate needs to be balanced against possible and expected benefits when prescribing to preschoolers.[42]

Other medications besides stimulants have been studied in preschoolers with ADHD. Atomoxetine is a noradrenergic reuptake inhibitor that is FDA approved for treatment of ADHD in children and adolescents but not preschoolers. An 8-week, double-blind, placebo-controlled, randomized clinical trial in preschoolers ages 5 to 6 years (N = 101) comparing atomoxetine (dose 1.8 mg/kg/d) with placebo was found to be well tolerated.[44] It reduced core ADHD symptoms based on parent and teacher reports; however, there was no overall clinical and functional improvement based on Clinical Global Impression severity and Clinical Global Impression improvement scales. The preschoolers in the atomoxetine group continued to be significantly impaired by the end of the study.[44] For preschoolers with significant externalizing symptoms, second-generation antipsychotics have also been used for symptom management. Risperidone has been studied more widely. A 6-week, double-blind clinical study comparing risperidone (0.5–1.5 mg/d) with MPH (5–20 mg/d) in preschoolers with

Table 1 Total daily dose				
	Decreased Appetite	Sleep Disturbance	Weight Loss	% of Subjects With Moderate-to-Severe AE
Placebo	—	—	—	15–20
TDD MPH 3.75 mg	—	—	—	16–21
TDD MPH 7.5 mg	—	—	—	19–24
MPH 15 mg	$\chi^2 = 5.4$, P<.03	$\chi^2 = 5.4$, P<.03	—	25–30
MPH 22.5 mg	—	—	$\chi^2 = 4.0$, P<.05	25–30

Abbreviation: TDD, total daily dose.

Data from Wigal T, Greenhill L, Chuang S, et al. Safety and tolerability of methylphenidate in preschool children with ADHD. J Am Acad Child Adolesc Psychiatry 2006;45(11):1294–303.

ADHD found that they both significantly improved ADHD symptoms based on Conners and parent ADHD rating scales. There was no significant difference in symptom improvement between the 2 groups. Metabolic side effects were not measured, and this was a relatively short study with a small number of patients (N = 38).[45] When risperidone (mean, 1.05 ± 0.51 mg/d) and aripiprazole (mean, 4.69 ± 1.25 mg/d) were compared in preschoolers with comorbid ADHD and disruptive behavior disorder, about a third of preschoolers in each group experienced significant improvement in ADHD and ODD symptoms.[46] The most common side effects for risperidone included daytime drowsiness and anorexia,[45] elevated prolactin level (22.38 ± 3.61), and increased weight (1.25 ± 0.68 kg).[46] Abilify (aripiprazole) also caused weight gain (1.2 ± 1.13 kg), but this was not significantly more than the risperidone group. Prolactin level increased significantly less (1.37 ± 0.87) in the Abilify (aripiprazole) group than in the risperidone group as expected.[46]

EVIDENCE-BASED COMBINATION BEHAVIORAL AND MEDICATION TREATMENT FOR ATTENTION DEFICIT HYPERACTIVITY DISORDER

The National Institute of Mental Health Multimodal Treatment Attention Deficit Hyperactivity Disorder study and the Multimodal Psychosocial Treatment study have significantly advanced the treatment of ADHD in 7- to 9-year-olds by examining single and combined effects of pharmacologic and behavioral treatments.[47] Pelham and colleagues'[33] contribution to existing treatment literature was to study the sequence in which the 2 evidence-based modalities for ADHD are implemented via a SMART in children ages 5 to 12, over a school year. The initial dose of the medication that was used in the study was an 8-hour stimulant equivalent to 0.15 mg/kg MPH on a twice a day basis. The initial behavioral plan included 8 sessions of group parent training plus a daily report card at school with home rewards concurrent with group social skills training for children. The adaptive medication treatment included increasing school dose and adding evening/weekend doses. The adaptive behavioral intervention included classroom assistance, tutoring, and overall more assistance for the children in the classroom and at home. Three aims were identified. **Table 2** summarizes the study aims and the concurrent findings.

An explanation for the significant differences in effect in behavioral strategy first (BehFirst) versus medication strategy first (MedFirst) can be attributed to the fact that BehFirst parents attended most of the parent sessions, whereas only some of the parents in the medicine then behavior (MB) group attended the sessions. Suboptimal engagement and attendance in behavioral treatments for ADHD have been reported in other research as well. Even though this study includes children older than the preschool age of interest group, it still offers significant implications that the sequencing of the intervention is paramount to desired effect.[33] This is especially true in preschoolers, as practice parameters recommend behavioral interventions first.

Nutrition, Exercise, and Sleep

The FDA maintains that artificial food dyes are safe for children, and more than 3000 food additives are allowed for use in the United States. This use differs from that of other countries such as Canada and the European Union where about 500 are allowed. However, since the 1970s, studies have published reports of associations between artificial colors and preservatives and hyperactive behavior in children.[48] Studies focusing on preschoolers specifically are scarce. A 2007 European study found that a diet that included artificial colors or a sodium benzoate preservative or both resulted in increased hyperactivity in 3-year-olds from a general population

Table 2
Summary of study aims and findings of treatment sequencing for childhood ADHD–Pelham et al study

Study Aims	Study Findings
Does it produce better outcomes to initiate treatment with a low-dose stimulant or behavioral intervention?	BehFirst and intensifying behavioral intervention (BB) children displayed significantly fewer rule violations per hour than MedFirst children in comparison to both increase medication dose (MM) protocol and add behavior modification to medication (MB) protocol. BehFirst group showed a trend of fewer out-of-class disciplinary events than the MedFirst group but failed to reach statistical significance.
What is the most effective treatment pattern and conditional secondary/adaptive treatment?	The best of the 4 treatment protocols (BM, BB, MB, MM) was the one that started with behavioral treatment and then added medication (B-then-M) in case of insufficient response. The worst protocol was M-then-B. For insufficient responders to first-stage medication treatment, increasing medication dose was superior to adding behavioral treatment.
What improves endpoint results more if there is insufficient response to initial treatment, enhancing the primary treatment modality or adding the second one?	B-then-B was significantly superior on the primary outcome (classroom rule violations), disciplinary actions, and teacher and parent ratings. For insufficient responders to first-stage behavioral treatment adding second-stage behavioral treatment resulted in significantly fewer violations than did adding medication.

Data from Pelham WE, Fabiano GA, Waxmonsky JG, et al. Treatment sequencing for childhood ADHD: a multiple-randomization study of adaptive medication and behavioral interventions. J Clin Child Adolesc Psychol 2016;45(4):396–415.

sample.[49] It is postulated that an individually constructed elimination diet might be effective for treatment of ADHD in children whose ADHD is triggered by foods. IgE is implicated in typical food allergies, but IgG may be implicated in reactions to foods that are not mediated by IgE. Some research has focused on studying a correlation between foods high in IgG and exacerbation of ADHD symptoms.[50] Elimination diets, removing specific foods from the diet in an attempt to reduce exposure to potential allergens that could influence ADHD, have been studied for years.[48] A 2011 study of children ages 4 to 8, not specific to preschoolers, found that a restriction/elimination diet was effective for ADHD in 60% of the sample but that IgG levels did not provide additional insight into which children should be treated.[50] Food intolerance rather than food allergy could be the case instead.[48] Specific compounds have not been identified as the culprit either.[49] A broad range of substances, including monosodium glutamate, preservatives, caffeine, food colors, and chocolate, were eliminated in a study of preschool boys with ADHD. As a result, about half of the preschoolers exhibited 50% improvement in the Abbreviated Symptom Questionnaire score, a 10-item version of the Conners Rating Scale. There was also an improvement in nighttime awakenings in this population.[51] In the school-age population, when combining both general elimination diets and studies specific to eliminating food color, the effect sizes have been small ($d = 0.2$ to $d = 0.4$). Research findings agree that an elimination diet (food restriction or food elimination diet) tested over a 2- or 4-week period may produce small aggregate effects in the likelihood of a positive response in a vulnerable subpopulation of some school-age children; their characteristics are yet to be determined. How to implement the elimination diet in everyday practice poses another challenge for both clinicians and families, but nutritional counseling should be included.[48]

Omega-3 fatty acid supplementation has also been studied as an alternative treatment for ADHD. Increased omega-3 fatty acid concentrations in cell membranes can affect serotonin and dopamine neurotransmission specifically in the frontal cortex. Omega-3 fatty acids can also potentially reduce oxidative stress, which is shown to be higher in ADHD. Therefore, supplementation with omega-3 fatty acids has been studied in several double-blind, placebo-controlled trials, which have shown mixed results. A 2011 meta-analysis of school-age children found that omega-3 fatty acids with high dose of eicosapentaenoic acid were modestly effective in treatment of ADHD in this population when compared with pharmacologic interventions (effect size = 0.31) and no significant difference was found when given as monotherapy versus augmentation to other ADHD treatments.[52] A 2014 review found that there is Center for Evidence-Based Medicine level-1 evidence that shows efficacy of omega-3 fatty acids at doses 1 to 2 mg daily for treatment of ADHD in school-age children.[53] No preschoolers were included in these reviews, and use of these supplements cannot be generalized to them. Some findings suggest reduced magnesium levels in patients with ADHD, but this is not well investigated in preschoolers. There is Center for Evidence-Based Medicine level-4 evidence that magnesium supplementation may be beneficial in treating ADHD, with no randomized, placebo-controlled trials demonstrating such efficacy. Children whose families are considering nutritional interventions must be screened for nutritional deficiencies.[53]

Sleep problems are hypothesized to be related with pathogenesis of ADHD. Disturbances in sleep may lead to excessive daytime sleepiness, which can be associated with disinhibition, hyperarousal, maladaptive emotional regulation processes, and issues with executive functioning, which mimic ADHD.[53,54] Greater internalizing symptoms, aggression, and somatic complaints can be present years later in preschoolers with chronic sleep issues. Sleep onset latency, refusal to sleep alone, and nighttime awakenings in children ages 3 to 6 were found to be a predictor of depression and anxiety across time but not ADHD.[54]

The impact of exercise on overall health has been well studied, with meta-analyses looking at the effects of exercise in ADHD symptoms. The literature indicates that repeated physical activity may improve measures of executive functioning, especially spatial span and working memory. One study in preschoolers found significant negative relation between physical activity in kindergarten and ADHD severity in first grade, as rated by both parents and teachers.[55]

SUMMARY

AACAP practice guidelines recommend behavioral interventions for a short period before initiating pharmacologic treatment in preschoolers with ADHD when behavior therapy fails. Research indicates that all the behavioral treatment strategies that exist show similar efficacy. However, in a recent study published in the *Journal of Child and Adolescent Psychopharmacology*, most child and adolescent psychiatrists (CAP) of the 339 board-certified CAPs asked, did not follow the guidelines.[20] Physical safety was the major contributing factor to this decision, suggesting that a sense of urgency may lead physicians to use stimulants as first-line treatment versus behavior therapy. Another possibility is that preschoolers may have not responded to behavior therapy by the time they see a child and adolescent psychiatrist. Many regions report a notable lack of behavioral interventionists available for this young age.

AACAP guidelines also recommend MPH as first-line stimulant medication largely based on the results of PATS. However, only slightly more than half of CAPs used MPH. The rest of the CAPs may be using the FDA-approved short-acting formulations instead, as they have been approved for use in children as young as 3 years, albeit with limited evidence. None of the long-acting stimulants have been approved in children younger than age 6 years.[20] Previous failed medication trials or lack of tolerability could also be a factor. Given the increased sensitivity to side effects with MPH use in the preschool population and the efficacy of behavioral interventions, attempts should be made, whenever possible, at behavioral interventions first.

REFERENCES

1. Chronis-Tuscano A, Lewis-Morrarty E, Woods KE, et al. Parent–Child interaction therapy with emotion coaching for preschoolers with attention-deficit/hyperactivity disorder. Cogn Behav Pract 2016;23(1):62–78.

2. Lange AM, Daley D, Frydenberg M, et al. The effectiveness of parent training as a treatment for preschool attention-deficit/hyperactivity disorder: study protocol for a randomized controlled, multicenter trial of the new forest parenting program in everyday clinical practice. JMIR Res Protoc 2016;5(2):e51.

3. Tandon M, Si X, Luby J. Preschool onset attention-deficit/hyperactivity disorder: course and predictors of stability over 24 months. J Child Adolesc Psychopharmacol 2011;21(4):321–30.

4. Tandon M, Si X, Belden A, et al. Attention-deficit/hyperactivity disorder in preschool children: an investigation of validation based on visual attention performance. J Child Adolesc Psychopharmacol 2009;19(2):137–46.

5. Thapar A, Cooper M, Eyre O, et al. Practitioner review: what have we learnt about the causes of ADHD? J Child Psychol Psychiatry 2012;54(1):3–16.

6. Wang TS, Huang WL, Kuo TB, et al. Inattentive and hyperactive preschool-age boys have lower sympathetic and higher parasympathetic activity. J Physiol Sci 2012;63(2):87–94.

7. Valera EM, Faraone SV, Murray KE, et al. Meta-analysis of structural imaging findings in attention-deficit/hyperactivity disorder. Biol Psychiatry 2007;61(12):1361–9.

8. Zhang S, Faries DE, Vowles M, et al. ADHD rating scale IV: psychometric properties from a multinational study as clinician-administered instrument. Int J Methods Psychiatr Res 2005;14(4):186–201.

9. Wolraich ML. Psychometric properties of the vanderbilt ADHD diagnostic parent rating scale in a referred population. J Pediatr Psychol 2003;28(8):559–68.

10. Subcommittee on Attention-Deficit/Hyperactivity Disorder; Steering Committee on Quality Improvement and Management, Wolraich M, Brown L, et al. ADHD: clinical practice guideline for the diagnosis, evaluation, and treatment of attention-deficit/hyperactivity disorder in children and adolescents. Pediatrics 2011;128(5):1007–22.

11. Purpura DJ, Lonigan CJ. Conners' teacher rating scale for preschool children: a revised, brief, age-specific measure. J Clin Child Adolesc Psychol 2009;38(2):263–72.

12. van der Veen-Mulders L, Nauta MH, Timmerman ME, et al. Predictors of discrepancies between fathers and mothers in rating behaviors of preschool children with and without ADHD. Europ Child Adolesc Psychiatry 2016;26(3):265–376.

13. Edwards MC, Gardner ES, Chelonis JJ, et al. Estimates of the validity and utility of the Conners' continuous performance test in the assessment of inattentive and/or hyperactive-impulsive behaviors in children. J Abnorm Child Psychol 2007;35(3): 393–404.

14. Murray DW, Kollins SH, Hardy KK, et al. Parent versus teacher ratings of attention-deficit/hyperactivity disorder symptoms in the preschoolers with attention-deficit/hyperactivity disorder treatment study (PATS). J Child Adolesc Psychopharmacol 2007;17(5):605–19.

15. Posner K, Melvin GA, Murray DW, et al. Clinical presentation of attention-deficit/ Hyperactivity disorder in preschool children: the preschoolers with attention-deficit/Hyperactivity treatment study (PATS). J Child Adolesc Psychopharmacol 2007;17(5):547–62.

16. Chronis-Tuscano A, Wang CH, Strickland J, et al. Personalized treatment of mothers with ADHD and their young at-risk children: a SMART pilot. J Clin Child Adolesc Psychol 2016;45(4):510–21.

17. Sonuga-Barke EJ, Daley D, Thompson M. Does maternal ADHD reduce the effectiveness of parent training for preschool children's ADHD? J Am Acad Child Adolesc Psychiatry 2002;41(6):696–702.

18. Chronis-Tuscano A, Rooney M, Seymour KE, et al. Effects of maternal stimulant medication on observed parenting in mother–child dyads with attention-deficit/ hyperactivity disorder. J Clin Child Adolesc Psychol 2010;39(4):581–7.

19. Waxmonsky JG, Waschbusch DA, Babinski DE, et al. Does pharmacological treatment of ADHD in adults enhance parenting performance? Results of a double-blind randomized trial. CNS Drugs 2014;28(7):665–77.

20. Chung J, Tchaconas A, Meryash D, et al. Treatment of attention-deficit/hyperactivity disorder in preschool-age children: child and adolescent psychiatrists' adherence to clinical practice guidelines. J Child Adolesc Psychopharmacol 2016;26(4): 335–43.

21. Charach A, Carson P, Fox S, et al. Interventions for preschool children at high risk for ADHD: a comparative effectiveness review. Pediatrics 2013;131(5): e1584–604.

22. Sonuga-Barke EJ, Daley D, Thompson M, et al. Parent-based therapies for preschool attention-deficit/hyperactivity disorder: a randomized, controlled trial with a community sample. J Am Acad Child Adolesc Psychiatry 2001;40(4): 402–8.

23. Sanders MR, Bor W, Morawska A. Maintenance of treatment gains: a comparison of enhanced, standard, and self-directed triple p-positive parenting program. J Abnormal Child Psychol 2007;35(6):983–98.

24. Bor W, Sanders MR, Markie-Dadds C. The effects of triple p-positive parenting program on preschool children with co-occurring disruptive behavior and attentional/hyperactive difficulties. J Abnormal Child Psychol 2002;30(6):571–87.

25. Forehand R, Parent J, Sonuga-Barke E, et al. Which type of parent training works best for preschoolers with Comorbid ADHD and ODD? A secondary analysis of a randomized controlled trial comparing generic and specialized programs. J Abnormal Child Psychol 2016;44(8):1503–13.

26. Luby J, Lenze S, Tillman R. A novel early intervention for preschool depression: findings from a pilot randomized controlled trial. J Child Psychol Psychiatry 2011;53(3):313–22.

27. Thorell LB. The community parent education program (COPE): treatment effects in a clinical and a community-based sample. Clin Child Psychol Psychiatry 2009;14(3):373–87.

28. Azevedo AF, Seabra-Santos MJ, Gaspar MF, et al. A parent-based intervention programme involving preschoolers with AD/HD behaviours: are children's and mothers' effects sustained over time? Eur Child Adolesc Psychiatry 2013;23(6): 437–50.
29. McGrath PJ, Lingley-Pottie P, Thurston C, et al. Telephone-based mental health interventions for child disruptive behavior or anxiety disorders: randomized trials and overall analysis. J Am Acad Child Adolesc Psychiatry 2011;50(11):1162–72.
30. Sourander A, McGrath PJ, Ristkari T, et al. Internet-assisted parent training intervention for disruptive behavior in 4-year-old children. JAMA Psychiatry 2016; 73(4):378.
31. Daley D, van der Oord S, Ferrin M, et al. Behavioral interventions in attention-deficit/hyperactivity disorder: a meta-analysis of randomized controlled trials across multiple outcome domains. J Am Acad Child Adolesc Psychiatry 2014; 53(8):835–47, 847.e1–5.
32. Coates J, Taylor JA, Sayal K. Parenting interventions for ADHD: a systematic literature review and meta-analysis. J Attention Disord 2014;19(10):831–43.
33. Pelham WE, Fabiano GA, Waxmonsky JG, et al. Treatment sequencing for CHILDHOOD ADHD: a multiple-randomization study of adaptive medication and behavioral interventions. J Clin Child Adolesc Psychol 2016;45(4):396–415.
34. Cortese S, Ferrin M, Brandeis D, et al. Neurofeedback for attention-deficit/hyperactivity disorder: meta-analysis of clinical and neuropsychological outcomes from randomized controlled trials. J Am Acad Child Adolesc Psychiatry 2016;55(6):444–55.
35. Arnold LE, Lofthouse N, Hersch S, et al. EEG Neurofeedback for ADHD: double-blind sham-controlled Randomized pilot feasibility trial. J Attention Disord 2012; 17(5):410–9.
36. Bakhshayesh AR, Hänsch S, Wyschkon A, et al. Neurofeedback in ADHD: a single-blind randomized controlled trial. Eur Child Adolesc Psychiatry 2011; 20(9):481–91.
37. Albrecht B, Uebel-von Sandersleben H, Gevensleben H, et al. Pathophysiology of ADHD and associated problems—starting points for NF interventions? Front Hum Neurosci 2015;9:359.
38. March JS. The preschool ADHD treatment study (PATS) as the culmination of twenty years of clinical trials in pediatric psychopharmacology. J Am Acad Child Adolesc Psychiatry 2011;50(5):427–30.
39. Abikoff HB, Vitiello B, Riddle MA, et al. Methylphenidate effects on functional outcomes in the preschoolers with attention-deficit/hyperactivity disorder treatment study (PATS). J Child Adolesc Psychopharmacol 2007;17(5):581–92.
40. Vitiello B, Lazzaretto D, Yershova K, et al. Pharmacotherapy of the preschool ADHD treatment study (PATS) children growing up. J Am Acad Child Adolesc Psychiatry 2015;54(7):550–6.
41. Storebø OJ, Krogh HB, Ramstad E, et al. Methylphenidate for attention-deficit/hyperactivity disorder in children and adolescents: cochrane systematic review with meta-analyses and trial sequential analyses of randomized clinical trials. BMJ 2015;351:h5203.
42. Wigal T, Greenhill L, Chuang S, et al. Safety and tolerability of methylphenidate in preschool children with ADHD. J Am Acad Child Adolesc Psychiatry 2006;45(11): 1294–303.
43. Swanson J, Greenhill L, Wigal T, et al. Stimulant-related reductions of growth rates in the PATS. J Am Acad Child Adolesc Psychiatry 2006;45(11):1304–13.

44. Kratochvil CJ, Vaughan BS, Stoner JA, et al. A double-blind, placebo-controlled study of atomoxetine in young children with ADHD. Pediatrics 2011;127(4): e862–8.

45. Arabgol F, Panaghi L, Nikzad V. Risperidone versus methylphenidate in treatment of preschool children with attention-deficit hyperactivity disorder. Iran J Pediatr 2015;25(1):e265.

46. Hasanpour-Dehkordi A, Safavi P, AmirAhmadi M. Comparison of risperidone and aripiprazole in the treatment of preschool children with disruptive behavior disorder and attention deficit-hyperactivity disorder: a randomized clinical trial. J Adv Pharm Technol Res 2016;7(2):43.

47. Pliszka S, AACAP Work Group on Quality Issues. Practice parameter for the assessment and treatment of children and adolescents with attention-deficit/hyperactivity dsorder. J Am Acad Child Adolesc Psychiatry 2007;46(7):894–921.

48. Nigg JT, Holton K. Restriction and elimination diets in ADHD treatment. Child Adolesc Psychiatr Clin N Am 2014;23(4):937–53.

49. McCann D, Barrett A, Cooper A, et al. Food additives and hyperactive behaviour in 3-year-old and 8/9-year-old children in the community: a randomized, double-blinded, placebo-controlled trial. The Lancet 2007;370(9598):1560–7.

50. Pelsser LM, Frankena K, Toorman J, et al. Effects of a restricted elimination diet on the behaviour of children with attention-deficit hyperactivity disorder (INCA study): a randomized controlled trial. The Lancet 2011;377(9764):494–503.

51. Kaplan BJ, McNicol J, Conte RA, et al. Dietary replacement in preschool-aged hyperactive boys. Pediatrics 1989;83(1):7–17.

52. Bloch MH, Qawasmi A. Omega-3 fatty acid Supplementation for the treatment of children with attention-deficit/Hyperactivity disorder symptomatology: systematic review and meta-analysis. J Am Acad Child Adolesc Psychiatry 2011;50(10): 991–1000.

53. Bloch MH, Mulqueen J. Nutritional supplements for the treatment of ADHD. Child Adolesc Psychiatr Clin N Am 2014;23(4):883–97.

54. Whalen DJ, Gilbert KE, Barch DM, et al. Variation in common preschool sleep problems as an early predictor for depression and anxiety symptom severity across time. J Child Psychol Psychiatry 2017;58(2):151–9.

55. Barnard-Brak L, Davis T, Sulak T, et al. The association between physical education and symptoms of attention deficit Hyperactivity disorder. J Phys Act Health 2011;8(7):964–70.

Intellectual Disability and Language Disorder

Natasha Marrus, MD, PhD[a],*, Lacey Hall, MS[b]

KEYWORDS

- Intellectual disability • Global developmental delay • Language disorder
- Early intervention • Multidisciplinary care

KEY POINTS

- Intellectual disability (ID) and language disorders are neurodevelopmental conditions arising in early childhood.
- Child psychiatrists are likely to encounter children with ID and language disorders because both are strongly associated with challenging behaviors and mental disorders.
- Because early intervention is associated with optimal outcomes in ID and language disorders, child psychiatrists must be aware of their signs and symptoms, particularly as related to delays in cognitive and adaptive function.
- Optimal management of both ID and language disorders requires a multidisciplinary, team-based, and family centered approach. Child psychiatrists play an important role on this team, given their expertise with contextualizing and treating challenging behaviors.

INTRODUCTION

Among parents' foremost developmental concerns are cognitive delays, in particular delays in language and adaptive function. Both are features of intellectual disability (ID), or, when language is specifically affected, language disorders. Child psychiatrists frequently encounter these conditions, particularly because they are associated with an increased risk of challenging behaviors and mental disorder. In working with affected children and their families, child psychiatrists should be prepared to identify relevant signs and symptoms, manage psychiatric comorbidities, refer to specialists for comprehensive assessment and multidisciplinary treatments, and foster family-centered care. Child psychiatrists thus play an important role in addressing the multifaceted nature of these conditions and in optimizing independence and functional outcomes.

[a] Department of Psychiatry, Division of Child and Adolescent Psychiatry, Washington University in St Louis, 660 South Euclid Avenue, Box 8504, St Louis, MO 63110, USA; [b] Department of Psychology, St. Jude Children's Research Hospital, 262 Danny Thomas Place, Memphis, TN 38105, USA
* Corresponding author.
E-mail address: Natasha@wustl.edu

Child Adolesc Psychiatric Clin N Am 26 (2017) 539–554
http://dx.doi.org/10.1016/j.chc.2017.03.001
1056-4993/17/© 2017 Elsevier Inc. All rights reserved.

childpsych.theclinics.com

INTELLECTUAL DISABILITY

ID is a neurodevelopmental disorder characterized by 3 features[1]:

- Deficits in cognition
- Deficits in adaptive function
- Onset during the developmental period

Collective attitudes toward ID have shifted from a model of static deficiencies to a more dynamic, strength-based perspective, and so-called mental retardation, the prior diagnostic term, has fallen out of favor. The introduction of the term "Intellectual Disability" in Diagnostic and Statistical Manual of Mental Disorders, Fifth edition (DSM-5) was presaged by Rosa's Law, a 2010 federal statute requiring that ID replace mental retardation in health, legal, and educational policy (P.L. 111–256). Also, in contrast with DSM-4–Text Revision, absolute intelligence quotient (IQ) cutoffs no longer define severity; mild, moderate, severe, or profound ID is now classified by level of adaptive functioning within a range of IQ scores. Adaptive functioning encompasses 3 domains:

- The conceptual domain, which includes language, knowledge, and memory
- The social domain, which includes empathy, social judgment, and rule-following ability
- The practical domain, which includes self-care, organization, and daily living skills

Estimates of ID range between 1% and 3%, with a male/female ratio of 1.6:1.[2] Causes of ID include genetic abnormalities, as well as prenatal, perinatal, and postnatal environmental factors[3,4] (**Fig. 1**). Suspicion of ID can arise during infancy, although children less than 5 years of age are typically diagnosed with global

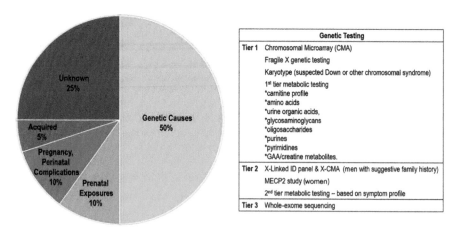

Fig. 1. Causes of ID and their respective percentages[4] are shown, together with a list of currently recommended genetic testing. Several non-genetic factors also lead to ID, including congenital infections, exposures to teratogens or toxins, prematurity, hypoxia, trauma, intracranial hemorrhage, central nervous system infection or malignancy, psychosocial deprivation, malnutrition, or acquired hypothyroidism. CpG, cytosine-phosphate-guanine; GAA, guanidinoacetate; MECP2, methyl-CpG binding protein 2. (*Information from* Moeschler JB, Shevell M. Comprehensive evaluation of the child with intellectual disability or global developmental delays. Pediatrics 2014;134(3):e903–18; and Pivalizza P, Lalani SR. Intellectual disability in children: evaluation for a cause. UpToDate: Waltham (MA); 2016.)

developmental delay, which requires delays in 2 or more functional domains associated with intellectual and adaptive impairment and which shows some correlation with ID. ID can be determined with greater certainty by age 5 years, when cognitive abilities become more stable. Children with less severe ID may not be diagnosed until school age, when academic demands highlight weaknesses in cognition.[5] Outcomes vary depending on severity: individuals with mild ID may achieve some signs of independence, such as having a job or starting a family,[6] although more severe ID requires long-term community supports for housing, occupational activities, and recreational activities.

Evaluation

A comprehensive history entails a birth/prenatal history; family history; 3-generation pedigree; and information on the course and timing of delays in language, motor, social-emotional, and adaptive functioning.[7] Children with ID may have a history of delays in talking, sitting up, crawling, or walking; immature play and social interaction; and poor comprehension, learning, and problem solving. Screening tools, such as the Ages and Stages Questionnaire,[8] can usefully clarify the extent of these concerns (see Ref.[9] for other examples). Frequent neurologic comorbidities, such as seizures and motor signs (eg, spasticity, ataxia, hypotonia), as well as developmental regression, should be assessed. Physical examination includes a complete neurologic examination, measurement of head circumference, and attention to features associated with genetic syndromes, such as facial dysmorphisms and skin findings.[3] A comprehensive evaluation of intellectual and adaptive functioning through neuropsychological testing is ultimately necessary for diagnosis.

Medical work-up includes testing for genetic syndromes, metabolic disorders, acquired hypothyroidism, and lead exposure.[3] When a genetic syndrome or metabolic disorder is suspected, referral to a geneticist is recommended to ensure the most comprehensive testing. A neurology referral is recommended for any neurologic concerns. Brain MRI is advised if microcephaly, macrocephaly, seizures, or neurologic signs are present.[7,10] Children with ID are more likely to have other medical conditions, including cataracts, vision and hearing impairments, congenital heart disease, constipation, obesity, and sleep disorders, which may prompt additional referrals. Such comorbidities not only affect overall function and quality of life but can also increase challenging behaviors.

Differential Diagnosis

The differential diagnosis for ID includes other neurodevelopmental disorders, which can also be comorbid with ID:

- Autism spectrum disorder (ASD), which has a similar prevalence to ID, and is characterized by impaired social communication, restricted interests, and repetitive behaviors. At least 25% of children with ASD have ID.[11]
- Language disorders, like ID, feature language delays. The occurrence of language delay should prompt investigation of other delays, so that ID is not overlooked.
- Epilepsy may manifest with delays and regression in core developmental domains, such as language. Behaviors suggestive of epilepsy include staring spells, shaking spells, and intermittent changes in levels of consciousness with associated automatisms (eg, blinking, lip smacking).

These potential diagnostic confounds highlight the importance of comprehensive evaluations and neuropsychological testing.

Challenging Behaviors, Comorbidity, and Management

Challenging behaviors are common in ID and can be more strongly associated with parental stress than the level of cognitive impairment.[12] These challenging behaviors may include noncompliance, property destruction, tantrums, "meltdowns", and physical aggression toward self or others. Although challenging behaviors occur in 4% to 9% of typically developing children, they occur in 25% of children with ID.[13] A major factor in ID stems from communication impairment, which limits the ability to express frustration and/or explain external factors or underlying physical or emotional distress. Children and adolescents with ID are also known to have a higher prevalence of psychiatric disorders, including attention-deficit/hyperactivity disorder (ADHD), mood disorders, anxiety disorders, and psychotic disorders.[14]

The psychopharmacologic evidence base is limited in ID, although there is support for judicious use of medication for disruptive behaviors and psychiatric comorbidities.[15,16] **Table 1** lists common medication classes, typical uses, side effects, and suggested monitoring. In preschoolers, behavioral treatment options are first line,

Table 1
Medications for intellectual disability

Medications by Class	Target Behaviors	Adverse Effects	Monitoring
Typical antipsychotics (eg, haloperidol, chlorpromazine)	Agitation, aggression, hyperactivity, self-injury	Extrapyramidal symptoms, tardive dyskinesia	AIMS
Atypical antipsychotics (eg, risperidone, aripiprazole, olanzapine)	Irritability, aggressiveness, hyperactivity, self-injurious behavior, repetitive behaviors	Weight gain, somnolence, increased risk of diabetes, extrapyramidal symptoms, akathisia, tardive dyskinesia	Blood glucose, HbA1c, lipids AIMS
Mood stabilizers (eg, lithium, valproic acid, carbamazepine)	Mood lability, aggression, impulsivity, self-injurious behavior	Lithium: tremor, renal and thyroid toxicity Valproate: tremor, sedation, weight gain Carbamazepine: nausea, vomiting	Renal and thyroid monitoring for lithium, liver function tests, CBC, and ammonia with valproic acid, regular drug levels for all 3
SSRIs (eg, fluoxetine, sertraline, fluvoxamine)	Depressed mood, anxiety, self-injurious behavior, repetitive behaviors	Activation, agitation, aggression, nausea	None specific
Stimulants (eg, methylphenidate)	Hyperactivity, inattention, impulsivity	Loss of appetite, insomnia, depressed mood	Height, weight, vital signs
Alpha-agonists (eg, clonidine, guanfacine)	Hyperactivity, inattention, impulsivity, tics	Hypotension, sedation, increased depression	Vital signs

Abbreviations: AIMS, Abnormal Involuntary Movement Scale; CBC, complete blood count; HbA1c, hemoglobin A1c; SSRI, selective serotonin reuptake inhibitor.

Data from Handen BL, Gilchrist R. Practitioner review: psychopharmacology in children and adolescents with mental retardation. J Child Psychol Psychiatry 2006;47(9):871–82.

given their effectiveness and more frequent medication side effects in younger children. Nevertheless, when safety or ability to engage in therapy are concerns, medication may be instrumental for successful implementation of a treatment plan and reducing caregiver stress. Medication is also an element of combined therapy (medication plus behavioral management), and psychiatrists can guide the appropriate balance of behavior and medication. Low starting doses are recommended, with slow titration, along with systematic evaluation of both positive and negative effects in the context of the entire treatment plan.

Among behavioral treatments, applied behavioral analysis (ABA) has a well-established evidence base.[17] ABA attempts to modify antecedents and/or consequences of specific behaviors, either to discourage a problematic behavior or encourage an alternative behavior. Functional behavioral analyses provide detailed measurement of potential instigators of challenging behavior, such as need for attention or help, escape from demands, attempt to get what is wanted, protest, or self-stimulation.[13] Behavioral planning is then tailored to the child's behavioral profile and developmental level. In addition to ABA, parent-training approaches (eg, Stepping Stones Triple P[18] and Parent-Child Interaction Therapy[19]) show evidence for improving disruptive behaviors in ID.

Promotion of Developmental Progress

Children with ID/global developmental delay benefit from intensive early intervention and multidisciplinary services.[20] Federal law under the Individuals with Disability Education Act mandates that state-run programs identify children with disabilities and provide developmental services. Before age 3 years, families receive an Individualized Family Service Plan (IFSP), which implements an individualized program of services and developmental therapies. These services and therapies may include speech and language therapy, occupational and physical therapy, psychological and behavioral services, medical services, nutrition counseling, assistive technology, family counseling and training, home visitation, and social services. The IFSP applies for ages 0 to 3 years, after which children who qualify for ongoing services are transitioned to an Individual Education Plan (IEP) with multidisciplinary preschool programming.

LANGUAGE DISORDERS

In DSM-5, language disorders are classified as communication disorders. Communication comprises all verbal and nonverbal input used to transmit information between individuals, including language and speech. Language involves conveying information through the form, content, and function of symbolic systems according to specified rules (see **Fig. 1**). Speech is the oral production of language. Delayed talking may thus reflect disturbances in speech, language, and/or communication. Historically, language disorders have been referred to by a variety of terms, including developmental language disorders and specific language impairment. The focus here is on early childhood features of language disorders per DSM-5, which implicate language form and function (**Fig. 2**).

Prevalence estimates for language disorder generally range between 3% and 8%,[21,22] with a male/female ratio of 1.33:1 in an epidemiologic sample.[21] Language disorders are heritable and generally seem to be polygenic, although some specific genetic factors, including the FOXP2 gene and linkage markers on chromosomes 3, 6, and 19, have been identified.[23] Language disorders can also be acquired secondary to infection, brain injury, neglect, and abuse.

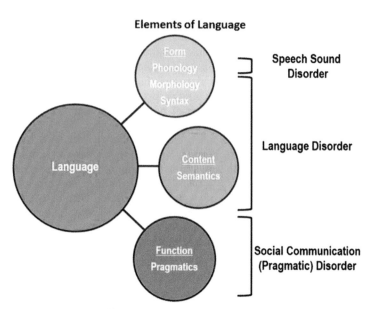

Fig. 2. Language disorders affect 1 or more fundamental aspects of language: form, content, and function. Deficits may involve morphology (understanding and use of the building blocks of words), syntax (grammar), and semantics (vocabulary). Phonology, the ability to distinguish and use speech sounds appropriately, is affected in speech sound disorder. Disorders of pragmatics, the use of language, are encompassed within social communication (pragmatic) disorder.

Early language difficulties are a risk factor for impaired literacy skills, memory skills, and nonverbal abilities,[24,25] although individual patterns of strengths and weaknesses in distinct aspects of language may vary over time. In some cases, so-called illusory recovery occurs,[26] whereby a child's language seems to normalize, but deficits return with subsequent increases in demands. In addition, rates of language growth may plateau by early adolescence, increasing the gap between children with and without language disorders.[27] Receptive language impairments have worse prognoses than expressive language impairments. Deficits of comprehension are less responsive to therapy and do not resolve spontaneously; they are linked to increased likelihood of social difficulties,[28] struggles with nonverbal reasoning,[29] and psychiatric conditions.[30]

Language Delay and Late Talkers Versus Language Disorder

Natural variability in language acquisition can make it challenging to assess early delays and to distinguish them from language disorders, which involve more persistent symptoms. Prevalence of late language emergence in 2-year-old children ranges between 10% and 20%,[31] and boys are 3 times more likely to be affected.[32,33] Most of these children do not ultimately have language disorders.[34] This late-talkers group may have only a few words at age 2 years, but matches peers in expressive language skills by age 3 years.[34,35]

Because only some children with late language emergence have language disorders, assessment and management of this group has been debated. Compared with children who develop language disorders, late talkers use more communicative gestures,[36] are less likely to have receptive language delay,[37] and show better recall of sentences on standardized testing.[38] Nonetheless, toddlers and preschoolers with late language emergence should be referred to a speech/language therapist, because they may be at risk for later language and literacy difficulties.[39] In the presence of associated risk factors for language disorders, such as ASD, global developmental delay, or hearing impairment, direct speech and language services are generally indicated. For children at lower risk, periodic monitoring is recommended, together with guidance for parents to provide indirect language stimulation (**Box 1**). If persistent delays or additional developmental concerns arise, a complete assessment and direct intervention may be warranted.

Evaluation

The history should review not only language development and milestones but also any other delays, challenging behaviors, mood and anxiety, and trauma that could result in developmental setbacks. In language disorders, progress is generally slow from the outset, and regression is uncommon, unlike in ASD.[40] Although speech delays frequently co-occur, they are not a hallmark. **Table 2** provides a description of typical language milestones and clinically significant red flags. Impaired receptive and expressive language commonly co-occur, and difficulties with comprehension, in particular, are a red flag for chronic language difficulties.[41] The mental status examination should note form, function, and use of language, including articulation, fluency, and tone; comprehension; the frequency and complexity of verbal communication; vocabulary; social reciprocity; and use and responsiveness to nonverbal communication, such as gestures, body language, and facial expression.

The utility of language screeners has been deemed inconclusive,[42] although, in cases of clinical suspicion, screeners can help index the level of concern. Two accessible parent-report measures are the MacArthur Communicative Development Inventory (M-CDI)[43] and the Language Development Survey (LDS).[31] The M-CDI features

---

Box 1
Indirect stimulation of language competence in young children

Responsiveness

- Provide responses directly related to a child's communication act or focus of attention.
- Follow the child's lead in play.
- Discuss what the child is doing versus asking lots questions.

Language modeling

- Imitate or expand the child's actions or words.
- Rephrase what the child says in grammatically correct form.
- Provide examples of using gestures and other nonverbal cues.

Reinforcement of communication

- Provide opportunities to communicate wants and choices rather than anticipate all the child's needs.
- Allow adequate time to initiate communication and respond.
- Praise communication attempts.

Data from American Speech-Language-Hearing Association (n.d.). Spoken language disorders (practice portal). Available at: www.asha.org/Practice-Portal/Clinical-Topics/Spoken-Language-Disorders/. Accessed October 1, 2016.

Table 2
Language milestones and red flags

	Milestones		Red Flags	
	Receptive	Expressive	Receptive	Expressive
12 mo	Recognizes words as symbols for objects, 3–50 words, recognizes name	First words, communicative games	Does not respond to name or gestures	No babbling, pointing, gesturing
18 mo	Words are understood outside context of routine games	50–100 words, intents include requesting, answering questions, acknowledging	Does not follow 1-step directions	No "Ma-ma," "Da-da," or other names
2 y	Single words for objects out of sight	200–300 words, 2-word utterances, telegraphic speech with few grammar markers, symbolic play, speech is 50% intelligible	Does not point to pictures or other body parts when named	Does not use at least 25 words
2.5 y	What/who/where questions	Use of questions, early emerging grammar, narratives are primarily labels and descriptions	Does not verbally respond or nod/ shake head to questions	Does not combine 2 words into unique phrases
3 y	"Why?" questions and basic spatial terms (in/on/under); simple time concepts (eg, tomorrow)	Simple sentences, narratives are sequences with them but no plot, speech is 75% intelligible	Does not understand prepositions or action words, does not follow 2-step instructions	Does not use at least 200 words, does not ask for things by name, repeats phrases in response to questions, unintelligible most of the time
4 y	"When/how?" questions, basic colors, shapes, sizes	Can tell a story, uses conjunctions to conjoin sentences; speech is 100% intelligible	Poor understanding of instructions or question words	Disordered speech, no phrases of 5–6 words, echolalia, unintelligible most of the time
5 y	Letter names and sounds; numbers and counting	Correct use of past tense; uses conjunction words (when, so, because, if); narratives are chains with some plot	Poor understanding of instructions or question words	Unintelligible most of the time, deletes parts of words, echolalia, cannot describe short sequences of events
Any age				Regression or loss of milestones

Data from Chapman R. Children's language learning: an interactionist perspective. J Child Psychol Psychiatry 2000;41:33–54; and Miller J. Assessing language production in children. Boston (MA): Allyn & Bacon; 1981.

long and short versions (requiring 20 and 5 minutes, respectively) for ages between 8 and 36 months. The LDS, which applies up to 42 months, is embedded in the Child Behavior Checklist, which conveniently queries general behavioral concerns. It is also worthwhile to screen for anomalous social development, given the association of language delay and ASD. Two of the most common brief ASD screeners are the Modified Checklist for Autism (M-CHAT), for ages 16 to 30 months,[44] and the Social Communication Questionnaire, for ages 4 years and older.[45]

Medical work-up first involves ruling out hearing conditions, and referral for an audiological evaluation is an important initial step. An oral-motor evaluation should be considered if there are phonological concerns, or the child has feeding difficulties or drooling. For laboratory testing, a complete blood count may be considered to evaluate for anemia, which has been associated with developmental delay, as well as lead testing.[46] Genetic testing is not routine, because there are no common, strongly associated genetic markers of language disorders,[47] but a genetics referral is advised for features suggesting a genetic syndrome (discussed earlier). In cases of regression or concern for seizures, rapid referral to a neurologist is warranted.

Differential Diagnosis

Several conditions may present with communication difficulties in early childhood; in some cases, these are comorbid with language disorders, so a speech/language referral remains indicated:

- Hearing impairment: as mentioned earlier, this possibility should be considered early in the evaluation. For children with ID and impaired language, there is a risk of reduced hearing over time, and hearing should therefore be monitored.
- ID: language delays frequently occur in ID, although only a subset of individuals ultimately show deficiencies consistent with a language disorder. Marked language problems in individuals with ID should receive comprehensive evaluation and treatment.
- ASD: language delay and disorders are common in ASD, even when accounting for pragmatic language issues, which are universal. Consideration of ASD is important given the strong benefit of early intervention for ASD.
- ADHD: inattention and impulsivity may detract from opportunities to learn and practice language skills, particularly as related to pragmatics. Children with ADHD also have higher rates of language disorders.
- Selective mutism: in this condition, poor language output manifests in specific environments; for example, at school but not at home. Selective mutism is conceptualized as an anxiety disorder, although speech/language issues often co-occur.

Challenging Behavior and Comorbidities

Similar to children with ID, children with language disorders are at increased risk of challenging behaviors and psychiatric comorbidities. Among children with a language disorder, 40% to 75% show challenging behaviors[48] and 30% to 50% have psychiatric disorders,[49,50] most commonly ADHD, anxiety disorders, conduct disorders, and mood disorders. Conversely, research suggests that 40% of children with psychiatric diagnoses also have a language impairment.[51] Work by Beitchman and colleagues[52] showed that increased rates of psychiatric diagnoses continue up to early adulthood, and decreased psychiatric comorbidity was associated with special education.[53]

Common challenging behaviors include both internalizing and externalizing symptoms. Hyperactivity and attentional difficulties are frequently observed,[54,55] as well as shyness, social withdrawal, and poor self-esteem.[56] Socioemotional deficits may also be present, including difficulty inferring emotional reactions[57] and regulating emotions.[58] As children get older, they may struggle with forming and maintaining close relationships,[59] and are more likely to be bullied[60] and experience abuse.[61]

Management

Psychiatrists play an important role in managing psychiatric comorbidities, as well as monitoring progress and coordinating care. In addition to making speech/language referrals, they can assist families in obtaining an evaluation for an IFSP or IEP and advocate for further services or educational accommodations. Because psychiatrists are in a position to correlate language function with psychiatric symptoms, they can provide important contextual information about the relationship between a child's language function and associated behavioral concerns. This information may result in more appropriately structured and targeted behavioral interventions and reduce misattributions of challenging behavior.[62]

Language Interventions: Principles, Approaches, and Modalities

Language intervention is intended to enhance language output and comprehension, ensure access to academic content, and advance communication to the next developmental level. Principles of effective intervention include language facilitation in the context of communication; dynamic, generalizable interventions; regular assessment of response; and adaptation of treatment goals and strategies according to individual learning style, progress, and needs.[63] Early intervention is recommended, because accelerated language growth tends to occur earlier versus later in childhood,[41,64] and interventions implemented at younger ages[65] as well as interventions of longer duration have been shown to be more effective.[66] A meta-analysis of speech/language therapies supported efficacy in expressive, but not receptive, language impairment, and treatments of more than 8 weeks showed better results.[67]

Language interventions encompass a variety of approaches, treatment types, and modalities (Table 3). Therapy should be based on the child's specific needs and learning style, as identified by standardized testing, parental concerns, and teacher input. Targets are identified and learned through drill, repetition, and carryover tracking. For preschoolers, goals include augmenting vocabulary, conceptual understanding, and sentence variety and complexity. Associated communication targets may involve improving intelligibility and phonological awareness, as well as conversational and narrative skills. Social skills should also be emphasized, given the known interrelationship of social and language function.

In preschoolers with emerging language skills, parent-mediated interventions are often implemented. These interventions confer similar benefit to direct approaches by speech/language pathologists,[67] are well suited to language facilitation in a variety of naturalistic environments, and offer many opportunities for language input. Among therapeutic modalities, augmentative and alternative communication has accumulated a large body of evidence, especially in children with developmental delays.[68] Some concern has been expressed that augmentative forms of communication may replace speech entirely and therefore restrict children's communicative development; however, prevailing evidence suggests that augmentative communication promotes language development.

Table 3
Overview of evidence-based aspects of language interventions

	Key Features	Comments
Approach		
Clinician directed	• Clinician specifies treatment type, goals, and reinforcement	• Less naturalistic • Maximize practice of specific targets
Child directed	• Clinician provides naturalistic opportunities for a child response • Clinician follows the child's lead	• Useful when poor compliance with clinician-directed approaches • Useful for unassertive communicators
Parent mediated	• Parents use direct, individualized intervention practices with the child • Increased opportunity for language input	• Cost-effective • Growing evidence for early intervention
Treatment Type		
Behavioral therapies	• Use behavioral learning principles • Increase desired behaviors • Decrease inappropriate behaviors	• Instructional: discrete trial training • Play-based: pivotal response training • Often used in ASD and DD
Milieu therapy	• Therapist elicits and reinforces targeted responses • Naturalistic settings • Child may select topic to initiate interaction	• Evidence in several groups: late talkers, ASD, ID, children from high-risk and low-income families
Relationship-based approaches	• Promotes parent-child interactions • Common in early intervention programs	• Greenspan/DIR/Floortime encourages interaction through play • Used in ASD
Modalities		
Augmentative alternative communication	• Supplemental methods to replace speech • Can address impaired production or comprehension	• Aided symbols: PECS and speech generating devices • Unaided symbols: manual signs • Strong evidence in ASD and ID
Computer-based instruction	• Computer programs teach language skills	• Advantage of higher number of trials than with therapist • Example: Fast ForWord
Video modeling	• Videos show desired behaviors • Learners are videotaped • Practice videos are reviewed	• Parent-mediated example: Hanen Program

Abbreviations: DD, developmental delay; DIR, Developmental Individual-difference Relationship; PECS, Picture Exchange Communication System.
Data from American Speech-Language-Hearing Association (n.d.). Spoken language disorders (practice portal). Available at: www.asha.org/Practice-Portal/Clinical-Topics/Spoken-Language-Disorders/. Accessed October 1, 2016.

SUMMARY

Common Aspects of Managing Intellectual Disability and Language Disorders

Management of ID and language disorders shares several overarching features and principles. Because comprehensive assessments from other specialties are needed for diagnosis, sound clinical judgment must be exercised regarding referrals and following up on recommendations. The long-term impact and early emergence of these conditions is especially challenging for families; sensitivity and clarity are thus vital when delivering these diagnoses. Surveillance often occurs via a multidisciplinary team of speech and language pathologists, behavioral therapists, occupational and physical therapists, educators, social workers, and others. Maintaining clear communication and a strength-based perspective is important for implementation of therapies that promote ongoing learning and gains in adaptive function. In addition, the importance of culturally sensitive, family-centered care is increasingly emphasized. By respectfully listening to families, psychiatrists can ensure that their preferences and priorities contribute to treatment planning.

Future Directions

Although early childhood mental health and neurodevelopmental disorders are increasingly recognized, concerns remain for delays in diagnosis.[69,70] Development of improved screeners and expanded training for child psychiatrists in neurodevelopmental disorders[71] are worthwhile public health considerations to promote earlier identification and management. Further research on evidence-based treatment is also a priority, because extant literature frequently involves small samples or less rigorous study designs. Translational research in genetics, as well as neuroscience, will be important to elucidate mechanisms by which cognitive impairments interact with risk for mental disorder, thereby improving diagnostic sensitivity, treatments, and prevention.

REFERENCES

1. American Psychiatric Association. Diagnostic and statistical manual of mental disorders. 5th edition. Arlington (VA): American Psychiatric Association; 2013.
2. Leonard H, Wen X. The epidemiology of mental retardation: challenges and opportunities in the new millennium. Ment Retard Dev Disabil Res Rev 2002;8(3): 117–34.
3. Pivalizza P, Seema L. Intellectual disability in children: evaluation for a cause. In: Post TW, editor. UpToDate. Waltham (MA); 2016.
4. Toth K, de Lacy N, King BH. Intellectual disability. In: Dulcan MK, editor. Dulcan's textbook of child and adolescent psychiatry. 2nd edition; 2016.
5. Reschly DJ. Documenting the developmental origins of mild mental retardation. Appl Neuropsychol 2009;16(2):124–34.
6. Hall I, Strydom A, Richards M, et al. Social outcomes in adulthood of children with intellectual impairment: evidence from a birth cohort. J Intellect Disabil Res 2005; 49(Pt 3):171–82.
7. Curry CJ, Stevenson RE, Aughton D, et al. Evaluation of mental retardation: recommendations of a consensus conference: American College of Medical Genetics. Am J Med Genet 1997;72(4):468–77.
8. Squires J, Bricker D, Twombly E. The ASQ User's Guide for the Ages and Stages Questionnaire: a parent - completed, child monitoring system. 2nd edition. Baltimore (MD): Paul Brookes Publishing; 1990.

9. Mackrides PS, Ryherd SJ. Screening for developmental delay. Am Fam Physician 2011;84(5):544–9.
10. Moeschler JB, Shevell M. Comprehensive evaluation of the child with intellectual disability or global developmental delays. Pediatrics 2014;134(3):e903.
11. Chakrabarti S, Fombonne E. Pervasive developmental disorders in preschool children. JAMA 2001;285(24):3093–9.
12. Baker BL, McIntyre LL, Blacher J, et al. Pre-school children with and without developmental delay: behaviour problems and parenting stress over time. J Intellect Disabil Res 2003;47(Pt 4–5):217–30.
13. Harris JC. Intellectual disability: a guide for families and professionals. New York: Oxford University Press; 2010.
14. Einfeld SL, Ellis LA, Emerson E. Comorbidity of intellectual disability and mental disorder in children and adolescents: a systematic review. J Intellect Dev Disabil 2011;36(2):137–43.
15. McQuire C, Hassiotis A, Harrison B, et al. Pharmacological interventions for challenging behaviour in children with intellectual disabilities: a systematic review and meta-analysis. BMC Psychiatry 2015;15:303.
16. Handen BL, Gilchrist R. Practitioner review: psychopharmacology in children and adolescents with mental retardation. J Child Psychol Psychiatry 2006;47(9): 871–82.
17. Beavers GA, Iwata BA, Lerman DC. Thirty years of research on the functional analysis of problem behavior. J Appl Behav Anal 2013;46(1):1–21.
18. Tellegen CL, Sanders MR. Stepping Stones Triple P-Positive Parenting Program for children with disability: a systematic review and meta-analysis. Res Dev Disabil 2013;34(5):1556–71.
19. Bagner DM, Eyberg SM. Parent-child interaction therapy for disruptive behavior in children with mental retardation: a randomized controlled trial. J Clin Child Adolesc Psychol 2007;36(3):418–29.
20. Sturmey P, Didden R. Evidence-based practice and intellectual disabilities. West Sussex (United Kingdom): Wiley-Blackwell; 2014.
21. Tomblin JB, Records NL, Buckwalter P, et al. Prevalence of specific language impairment in kindergarten children. J Speech Lang Hear Res 1997;40(6): 1245–60.
22. Law J, Boyle J, Harris F, et al. Prevalence and natural history of primary speech and language delay: findings from a systematic review of the literature. Int J Lang Commun Disord 2000;35(2):165–88.
23. Newbury DF, Monaco AP. Genetic advances in the study of speech and language disorders. Neuron 2010;68(2):309–20.
24. St Clair MC, Pickles A, Durkin K, et al. A longitudinal study of behavioral, emotional and social difficulties in individuals with a history of specific language impairment (SLI). J Commun Disord 2011;44(2):186–99.
25. Conti-Ramsden G, Durkin K, Simkin Z, et al. Specific language impairment and school outcomes. I: identifying and explaining variability at the end of compulsory education. Int J Lang Commun Disord 2009;44(1):15–35.
26. Scarborough HS, Dobrich W. Development of children with early language delay. J Speech Hear Res 1990;33(1):70–83.
27. Rice ML. Language growth and genetics of specific language impairment. Int J Speech Lang Pathol 2013;15(3):223–33.
28. Clegg J, Hollis C, Mawhood L, et al. Developmental language disorders–a follow-up in later adult life. Cognitive, language and psychosocial outcomes. J Child Psychol Psychiatry 2005;46(2):128–49.

29. Stothard SE, Snowling MJ, Bishop DV, et al. Language-impaired preschoolers: a follow-up into adolescence. J Speech Lang Hear Res 1998;41(2):407–18.
30. Snowling MJ, Bishop DV, Stothard SE, et al. Psychosocial outcomes at 15 years of children with a preschool history of speech-language impairment. J Child Psychol Psychiatry 2006;47(8):759–65.
31. Rescorla L. The Language Development Survey: a screening tool for delayed language in toddlers. J Speech Hear Disord 1989;54(4):587–99.
32. Zubrick SR, Taylor CL, Rice ML, et al. Late language emergence at 24 months: an epidemiological study of prevalence, predictors, and covariates. J Speech Lang Hear Res 2007;50(6):1562–92.
33. Roulstone S, Loader S, Northstone K, et al. The speech and language of children aged 25 months: descriptive data from the Avon Longitudinal Study of Parents and Children. Early Child Dev Care 2002;172(3):259–68.
34. Rescorla L. Late talkers: do good predictors of outcome exist? Dev Disabil Res Rev 2011;17(2):141–50.
35. Fischel JE, Whitehurst GJ, Caulfield MB, et al. Language growth in children with expressive language delay. Pediatrics 1989;83(2):218–27.
36. Thal DJ, Tobias S. Communicative gestures in children with delayed onset of oral expressive vocabulary. J Speech Lang Hear Res 1992;35(6):1281–9.
37. Thal D, Tobias S, Morrison D. Language and gesture in late talkers: a 1-year follow-up. J Speech Lang Hear Res 1991;34(3):604–12.
38. Everitt A, Hannaford P, Conti-Ramsden G. Markers for persistent specific expressive language delay in 3-4-year-olds. Int J Lang Commun Disord 2013;48(5):534–53.
39. Rescorla L. Language and reading outcomes to age 9 in late-talking toddlers. J Speech Lang Hear Res 2002;45(2):360–71.
40. Pickles A, Simonoff E, Conti-Ramsden G, et al. Loss of language in early development of autism and specific language impairment. J Child Psychol Psychiatry 2009;50(7):843–52.
41. Conti-Ramsden G, Durkin K. Language development and assessment in the preschool period. Neuropsychol Rev 2012;22(4):384–401.
42. Nelson HD, Nygren P, Walker M, et al. U.S. Preventive Services Task Force evidence syntheses, formerly systematic evidence reviews. Screening for speech and language delay in preschool children. Rockville (MD): Agency for Healthcare Research and Quality (US); 2006.
43. Fenson L, Dale PS, Reznick JS, et al. Variability in early communicative development. Monogr Soc Res Child Dev 1994;59:1–173.
44. Robins DL, Fein D, Barton ML, et al. The Modified Checklist for Autism in Toddlers: an initial study investigating the early detection of autism and pervasive developmental disorders. J Autism Dev Disord 2001;31(2):131–44.
45. Berument SK, Rutter M, Lord C, et al. Autism Screening Questionnaire: diagnostic validity. Br J Psychiatry 1999;175(5):444.
46. Sices L. Overview of expressive language delay ("late talking") in young children. In: Post TW, editor. UpToDate. Waltham (MA); 2016.
47. Bishop DV. What causes specific language impairment in children? Curr Dir Psychol Sci 2006;15(5):217–21.
48. Stevenson J, Richman N. Behavior, language, and development in three-year-old children. J Autism Child schizophr 1978;8(3):299–313.
49. Beitchman JH, Nair R, Clegg M, et al. Prevalence of psychiatric disorders in children with speech and language disorders. J Am Acad Child Psychiatry 1986;25(4):528–35.

50. Baker L, Cantwell DP. A prospective psychiatric follow-up of children with speech/language disorders. J Am Acad Child Adolesc Psychiatry 1987;26(4): 546–53.
51. Cohen NJ, Barwick MA, Horodezky NB, et al. Language, achievement, and cognitive processing in psychiatrically disturbed children with previously identified and unsuspected language impairments. J Child Psychol Psychiatry 1998; 39(6):865–77.
52. Beitchman JH, Wilson B, Johnson CJ, et al. Fourteen-year follow-up of speech/language-impaired and control children: psychiatric outcome. J Am Acad Child Adolesc Psychiatry 2001;40(1):75–82.
53. Bao L, Brownlie EB, Beitchman JH. Mental health trajectories from adolescence to adulthood: language disorder and other childhood and adolescent risk factors. Dev Psychopathol 2016;28(2):489–504.
54. Baker L, Cantwell DP. Attention deficit disorder and speech/language disorders. Compr Ment Health Care 1992;2(1):3–16.
55. Tirosh E, Cohen A. Language deficit with attention-deficit disorder: a prevalent comorbidity. J Child Neurol 1998;13(10):493–7.
56. Durkin K, Conti-Ramsden G. Young people with specific language impairment: a review of social and emotional functioning in adolescence. Child Lang Teach Ther 2010;26(2):105–21.
57. Ford JA, Milosky LM. Inferring emotional reactions in social situations differences in children with language impairment. J Speech Lang Hear Res 2003;46(1): 21–30.
58. Fujiki M, Brinton B, Clarke D. Emotion regulation in children with specific language impairment. Lang Speech Hear Serv Sch 2002;33(2):102–11.
59. Wadman R, Durkin K, Conti-Ramsden G. Close relationships in adolescents with and without a history of specific language impairment. Lang Speech Hear Serv Sch 2011;42(1):41–51.
60. Hughes S. Bullying: what speech-language pathologists should know. Lang Speech Hear Serv Sch 2014;45(1):3–13.
61. Brownlie EB, Jabbar A, Beitchman J, et al. Language impairment and sexual assault of girls and women: findings from a community sample. J Abnorm Child Psychol 2007;35(4):618–26.
62. Cohen NJ, Davine M, Horodezky N, et al. Unsuspected language impairment in psychiatrically disturbed children: prevalence and language and behavioral characteristics. J Am Acad Child Adolesc Psychiatry 1993;32(3):595–603.
63. Roth F, Worthington CK. Treatment resource manual for speech-language pathology. Clifton Park (NY): Cengage Learning; 2015.
64. Bishop DV, Edmundson A. Language-impaired 4-year-olds: distinguishing transient from persistent impairment. J Speech Hear Disord 1987;52(2):156–73.
65. Carter J, Musher K. Evaluation and treatment of speech and language disorders in children. In: Post TW, editor. UpToDate. Waltham (MA); 2016.
66. Law J, Garrett Z, Nye C. Speech and language therapy interventions for children with primary speech and language delay or disorder. Cochrane Database Syst Rev 2003;(3):CD004110.
67. Law J, Garrett Z, Nye C. The efficacy of treatment for children with developmental speech and language delay/disorder: a meta-analysis. J Speech Lang Hear Res 2004;47(4):924–43.
68. Schlosser RW, Raghavendra P. Evidence-based practice in augmentative and alternative communication. Augment Altern Commun 2004;20(1):1–21.

69. Prelock PA, Hutchins T, Glascoe FP. Speech-language impairment: how to identify the most common and least diagnosed disability of childhood. Medscape J Med 2008;10(6):136.
70. Glascoe FP. Screening for developmental and behavioral problems. Ment Retard Dev Disabil Res Rev 2005;11(3):173–9.
71. Marrus N, Veenstra-VanderWeele J, Hellings JA, et al. Training of child and adolescent psychiatry fellows in autism and intellectual disability. Autism 2014; 18(4):471–5.

The Early Origins of Autism

John N. Constantino, MD*, Natasha Marrus, MD, PhD

KEYWORDS

- Autism spectrum disorder • Diagnosis • Genetics • Early childhood development

KEY POINTS

- The autism spectrum disorders (ASDs) are strongly genetically determined, and the clinical identification of deleterious genetic variants that influence the development of ASD in individual patients is becoming increasingly achievable for personalized approaches to care, including specification of recurrence risk in families.
- The ability to reliably identify most cases of ASD far earlier than the average age of community diagnosis presents a novel opportunity for implementation of early intervention.
- New waves of necessary research on the efficacy of early intensive behavioral intervention, and on the development of personalized approaches whose specificity is predicated on knowledge of the particular mechanisms of causation of the condition in individual patients, will ultimately transform the clinical approach to these conditions in early childhood.

INTRODUCTION

The diagnostic conceptualization of autism has shifted with the publication of Diagnostic and Statistical Manual of Mental Disorders (DSM)–5; language deficits, previously a core feature of autism, are no longer an independent criterion domain; instead they are inextricably linked to the characteristic social impairments of autism in a construct referred to as social communication.[1] Asperger syndrome and pervasive developmental disorder (PDD) not otherwise specified, once subtypes of PDDs, have been eliminated as separate diagnoses; most individuals who previously held these diagnoses are now in the broader diagnostic category of autism spectrum disorders (ASDs), except for (usually) milder cases that better fit the new DSM-5 diagnosis of social communication disorder. These changes reflect major advances in knowledge about symptom structure, patterns of familial transmission in the ASDs, the importance of specifying degree of impairment in adaptive functioning (which is imperfectly correlated with symptom burden), and comorbidity of ASD with neuropsychiatric impairments that range from epilepsy to intellectual disability to

Disclosure: Dr Constantino receives royalties from Western Psychological Services for the commercial distribution of the Social Responsiveness Scale, a quantitative measure of autistic traits.
Washington University School of Medicine, 660 South Euclid Avenue, Campus Box 8504, St Louis, MO 63110, USA
* Corresponding author.
E-mail address: constantino@wustl.edu

Child Adolesc Psychiatric Clin N Am 26 (2017) 555–570
http://dx.doi.org/10.1016/j.chc.2017.02.008
1056-4993/17/© 2017 Elsevier Inc. All rights reserved.

childpsych.theclinics.com

attention-deficit/hyperactivity disorder (ADHD) or almost any psychiatric disorder. These comorbidities and the wide range of severity of symptom burden and impairment in adaptive functioning reflect the marked diversity of genetic pathways to ASD and other neurodevelopmental susceptibilities represented by individual children and families. This diversity presents unique challenges and opportunities for comprehensive intervention planning at each successive stage of development. Overwhelmingly, the ASDs are influenced by genetic factors,[2] as reflected in a sibling recurrence rate that is 20 times higher than the population prevalence, and in twin and family studies of ASD conducted around the world, now cumulatively totaling more than 4 million subjects.[3]

EPIDEMIOLOGY

ASD is a recent addition to the DSM, having been introduced in DSM-3 in 1980, and until a little more than decade ago was considered rare. Between 1992 and 2001, the prevalence was estimated at 12.7 in 10,000.[4] In the United States, the most recent prevalence estimate of 1 in 68 is an order of magnitude greater.[5] Several reasons for this steep upswing in prevalence are at play. First, diagnostic criteria have become progressively more inclusive. DSM-5 now defines ASD as a spectrum that explicitly encompasses a range of core symptom severity, in contrast with prior definitions, which often invoked significant cognitive and language delays.[1] A greater variety of standardized assessment tools, including rapid developmental screeners that facilitate earlier detection of risk, are now available. Increasing rates of research citations and media coverage have promoted awareness of ASD, among both parents and clinicians. Furthermore, diagnostic substitution, whereby the same developmental disability receives a different diagnosis, previously contributed to reduced ASD diagnoses, particularly with respect to historical diagnoses of intellectual disability.[6,7]

Throughout the diagnostic evolution of ASD, one consistent epidemiologic feature has been the male/female sex ratio of 4:1. Observations of quantitative trait distributions and recurrence studies in later-born infant siblings confirm that this pronounced disparity is evident by the second year of life.[8] Failure to incorporate sex-specific norms in the diagnostic process has contributed to significant differences in the rates of community diagnosis for girls versus boys who manifest precisely the same level of quantitative symptom burden.[9–11] Furthermore, there is evidence that female sex can often moderate the phenotypic expression of inherited susceptibility to ASD and that a female protective effect is responsible for protecting young girls against the expression of inherited ASD susceptibility.[12–14]

Over the past decade it has become clear that social and cultural factors may influence the likelihood of individuals receiving a clinical diagnosis of ASD in the community.[15] For example, underdiagnosis has been linked to social disadvantage as related to parental education, income, socioeconomic status, and ethnic/minority status.[16–18]

Early Childhood Diagnosis

The largest body of evidence for diagnostic stability applies to children between 2 and 3 years of age. Diagnostic stability of more than 80% has repeatedly been shown among 2-year-olds 1 to 7 years from the initial diagnosis.[19–24] Factors associated with less stability of an ASD diagnosis include age less than 30 months at time of diagnosis,[23,25] lower severity of core symptoms,[26] and reliance on psychometric tools rather than clinical judgment to formulate a diagnosis.[20,22,27]

A related consideration is whether early evaluations for ASD in toddlers frequently miss diagnoses that can be identified later in the toddler period. In a recent longitudinal study of infant siblings at risk of ASD, Ozonoff and colleagues[21] found that almost half the children in the sample diagnosed with ASD at 36 months (when evaluated using a clinical best-estimate procedure) were not diagnosed when similarly assessed at 24 months. The investigators concluded that longitudinal follow-up and repeated screening in the first years of life is critical for children with early social-communicative deficits, because in some cases a diagnosis of ASD may not be detected at younger ages.

THE CURRENT DIAGNOSTIC PROCESS
Diagnostic Criteria

The full DSM-5 diagnostic criteria for ASD include:

A. Persistent deficits in social communication and social interaction across multiple contexts
B. Restricted, repetitive patterns of behavior, interests, or activities
C. Presence of symptoms that are present in the early developmental period
D. Clinically significant impairment in social, occupational, or other important areas of current functioning caused by the symptoms
E. The disturbances are not better explained by intellectual disability (intellectual developmental disorder) or global developmental delay (social communication should be less than that expected for general developmental level)

Furthermore, DSM-5 now calls for an improved understanding of both the individual's adaptive function and causal factors, which has been integrated through implementation of severity and clinical specifiers. The severity specifiers provide some characterization of adaptive function, which, like core symptom burden, is quantifiable. Clinical specifiers allow the listing of genetic or medical conditions that may be contributory, as well as clinical features that may help with future research into subcategories of ASD. An often-overlooked aspect of the characterization of severity in ASD is that the core symptom burden (criteria A and B) and impairment in social, occupational, or other important areas of adaptive functioning (criterion D) are only partially correlated; there are many clinical situations in which core ASD symptom burden is pronounced but impairment in adaptive functioning is mild, and vice versa. It can be well argued that most of the proven benefits of currently available interventions for autism are in the realm of adaptive functioning, not core symptom counts.[28] Improvements in adaptive functioning are achievable and critical for patients with ASD[29] but grossly underappreciated when measuring outcomes exclusively as a function of core symptom burden, as still often occurs in clinical trials. The hybrid severity index published in DSM-5 translates the effect of symptoms in each criterion domain (A and B) onto 3 broad categories of adaptive functioning, each of which is defined by descriptive scoring anchors that indicate the level of support that an affected individual requires.

Another noteworthy change in DSM-5 is that it is now deemed appropriate to diagnose ASD simultaneously with other psychiatric or developmental disorders (eg, ADHD) when there is ample evidence for comorbidity, in view of overwhelming evidence that many known, inherited causes of ASD are genetically independent (or partially independent) from the causes of other common neuropsychiatric disorders,[30] and it is therefore possible for an individual to be affected by more than 1 neuropsychiatric condition. This possibility also underscores the need to identify and treat comorbid disorders, many of which are more responsive to intervention than ASD, and have pronounced multiplier effects on the degree of impairment in adaptive functioning and/or capacity for a child with ASD to learn or respond to developmental therapy.

Clinical Assessment

Implied, but not explicit in the diagnostic criteria, are the elements of information gathering that are required to establish an ASD diagnosis:

1. Ascertainment of current symptoms sufficient to meet criteria A, B, and D
2. Acquisition of a developmental history consistent with an ASD (criterion C, provided by a primary caregiver of the child whenever possible)
3. Clinician confirmation

One aspect of assessing symptoms involves querying pathognomonic warning signs of ASD in the infant and toddler period. These warning signs include lack of protodeclarative pointing; lack of turn-taking, reciprocal games (eg, peekaboo); lack of symbolic interactive play (eg, feeding a baby doll); avoidance of eye contact; failing to respond to being called by name; stereotyped motor behaviors; and obsessive lining up of toys (Learn the Signs. Act Early, 2016. Available at: https://www.cdc.gov/ncbddd/actearly/milestones/index.html. Accessed March 13, 2017). Because the severity of current symptoms can vary as a function of environmental context and demands, appraisal of symptoms also requires caregivers to provide accounts of an affected child's behavior across multiple environments: to report on social interests and evolving capacity for peer relationships; to provide information on day-to-day social communication (including use of verbal and nonverbal language and communication, imagination, and play); to describe sensory responses and the frequency of repetitive or stereotypical behaviors of ASD, including behavioral rigidity; and to detail self-help skills and propensity for moodiness, tantrums, and outbursts.

Similarly, clinician confirmation relies on a diversity of prompts to elicit a child's highest capacity for social communication, and to introduce enough sensory arousal to elicit stereotyped responses if they are not immediately evident. Depending on the age of the child, this interaction can be a play-based assessment with toys commonly used by children within the local community or can be a more conversational interaction in which the child is asked about life at home and at school, friendships, and daily interactions with peers. Having made direct observations of the child and gathered adequate information to satisfy criteria A, B, and D, the clinician must determine that the clinical-level impairment in adaptive functioning is largely attributable to ASD and not to an alternative psychiatric, developmental, or neurologic disorder. For example, it is important for clinicians to rule out specific, potentially treatable causes of autistic syndromes, particularly in patients who are manifesting signs that may be caused or exacerbated by such conditions, including primarily epilepsies and metabolic disorders. Any suspicion of these warrants consultation and referral to a neurologist. For more detailed information on assessment algorithms, the authors refer readers to previously published sources[31,32]; a resource for assisting clinicians in the identification of rare, reversible causes of cognitive delay in early childhood can be found at http://treatable-id.net.

What becomes immediately evident in the diagnostic process, especially for milder ASD syndromes, is that fulfillment of diagnostic criteria is exquisitely sensitive to the notion of clinical threshold. There is an apparent tension between expert clinician judgment about where these thresholds should lie and the fundamental nature of the features described by criteria A, B, and D (their respective distributions, interrelations, and biological causes) that raises continuously evolving questions about how the clinical thresholds for these criteria should be established for diagnosis. Should they represent percentile cutoffs of the normal distribution (as dominates the diagnosis of intellectual disability)? Should absolute symptom burden or level of impairment of adaptive functioning dominate parameterization of the clinical threshold? In traditional ASD research, emphasis has unequivocally been on case designation and specification of symptom burden, although the introduction of severity specifiers in DSM-5 now provides readily implemented parameters of adaptive functioning for clinicians to use in the diagnostic process for ASD.

Differential Diagnosis

Although ASD is distinguished by a core disturbance in social communication, other psychiatric conditions may be associated with impairments in social skills, communication, or prominent restricted, repetitive behaviors. However, in these conditions, such symptoms occur secondarily. A careful developmental history is key to establishing whether these symptoms are attributable to ASD or another disorder and to appropriately guide strategies for intervention. In addition, the possibility of a psychiatric comorbidity should be considered, because this occurs in up to 72% of children with ASD.[33]

Intellectual disability

Intellectual disability is defined by standardized measurement of intelligence quotient (IQ; an index of an array of cognitive skills) and appraisal of impairment in adaptive functioning.[1] What commonly distinguishes children with intellectual disability alone from those with ASD alone is that they show interest in social engagement,[34] so that social overtures are responded to at a level consistent with their cognitive development. When social disturbances exceed what would be expected for cognitive delays, a comorbid diagnosis of ASD is invoked.

Specific language impairment

In language disorders, impaired communication stems primarily from issues with structural language (eg, vocabulary and grammar) rather than decreased social interest, as in ASD. Further, although language deficits may contribute to social awkwardness, social interest is generally intact. The related diagnosis of social communication disorder, introduced in DSM-5, describes deficits in the appropriate use of language, a subdomain of language known as pragmatics, which involves the ability to understand and implement social rules for verbal and nonverbal communication. Pragmatic language deficits are universal in ASD; however, children with social communication disorder are distinguished by the absence of restricted interests or repetitive behaviors.

Attention-deficit/hyperactivity disorder

Children with ADHD can show increased levels of autistic traits and often have difficulty with social skills. Conversely, many children with ASD appear physically restless, distracted, impulsive, and reactive, and some children with ASD will have comorbid ADHD. When hyperactivity, inattention, and impulsivity are predominantly linked to social situations, sensory overstimulation, rigidity, or intolerance of change, a diagnosis of ASD should be considered.

Anxiety disorders

Anxiety disorders are extremely common, and children with anxiety disorders may have impaired social skills and communication. On deeper examination, these are primarily related to inhibition and fearfulness (eg, as in the case of selective mutism) rather than a core deficit in social interest, awareness, or understanding. Furthermore, for children with obsessions and compulsions, their fixations and ritualized, compulsive behaviors are often ego-dystonic rather than self-stimulating, as is often the case with ASD.

Disruptive behavior disorders

Children with disruptive behavior disorders often appear uncooperative, defiant, and inclined to annoy others. In children with ASD, perceived noncompliance likely stems from core symptoms related to lack of social awareness, difficulty tolerating change or specific demands, or sensory defensiveness rather than purposeful defiance. Comorbid diagnoses in this category should therefore be rendered conservatively.

Standardized Measures of Symptom Burden

A range of screening and diagnostic instruments for ASD has been developed over the past 2 decades. The authors refer readers to 2 recent open-access reports that have synthesized the sizable literature on early diagnosis of ASD[32] and characterization of progress and outcomes in preschool children with ASD.[31]

The authors note that some of the more time-intensive instruments that have been relied on in traditional approaches to diagnostic assessment, and that have been increasingly adopted in the United States as prerequisites for both service eligibility and research participation, are expensive and difficult to acquire consistently in public health settings. When combined with rapidly obtainable information on developmental history and current symptoms in daily social contexts, standardized observational ratings by clinicians, without the need for extensive rater training, show tremendous promise for the diagnostic confirmation of ASD.[35]

Although there is, as expected, overlap in the concepts and the content of ASD ratings scales and diagnostic instruments, they differ in the aspect of the diagnostic process to which they apply (ie, developmental history vs current symptom ascertainment vs clinician confirmation), the populations for whom they are standardized, and the degree to which they are sensitive measures of subclinical variation in ASD traits. They also vary in terms of the need for trained raters, the time needed to train raters or to complete assessments, and the cost and feasibility of application in clinical settings. Among the most notable limitations is the degree to which the accuracy of many screening and diagnostic instruments has been validated in individuals with ASD with intellectual disability.

Quantitative approaches to the measurement of autistic traits

When standardized methods for quantitative assessment of ASD symptoms and traits have been applied to the general population, the unequivocal result from a host of studies, implementing numerous measurement instruments, is that the characteristic traits and features that characterize autism are continuously, not bimodally, distributed.[9,36–38] The authors recently showed this to be the case as early as the toddler period, using a novel video-referenced rating scale.[8] This instrument prompts caregivers to rate their child's social behavior against that of a typically developing child observed in a brief video, with the goal of improving on the ability of current ASD screeners to:

1. Measure early features of autistic syndromes typically first appreciable in clinical settings
2. Track developmental trajectories and monitor responses to interventions

In an epidemiologic sample of toddler twins aged 18 to 24 months, the authors found that levels of autistic traits in toddlers seem to be heritable, to correlate with level of ASD risk, and to have a continuous unimodal distribution (**Fig. 1**), recapitulating findings at older ages.

The continuous, heritable nature of autistic traits shown in general population studies is also confirmed by family studies of ASD. Standardized, quantitative measures show that subclinical autistic symptoms and traits occur among first-degree relatives of ASD-affected individuals with a frequency an order of magnitude higher than that observed in the general population.[39,40] Recently, very large genetic-epidemiologic studies have confirmed that the genetic susceptibilities to these

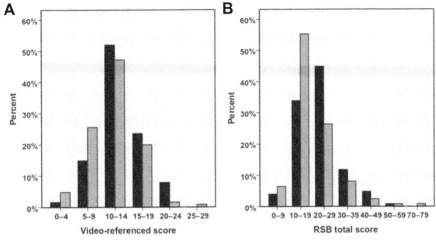

Fig. 1. Toddler scores (ages 18–21 months) on a video-referenced rating of reciprocal social behavior (RSB) are continuously distributed. Black bars represent male scores; gray bars represent female scores. (A) Scores for the 13 video-referenced items; (B) scores for all 44 questions, including 31 non–video-referenced items that query the caregiver's cumulative recall of the child's social behavior. The continuous distributions reflect the range of RSB present in toddlers. High scores indicate deficiencies in RSB and, in this general population sample, there is a preponderance of lower scores. Boys have, on average, significantly higher scores than girls (video-referenced, 13.5 [4.0] versus 11.4 [4.2]; RSB total, 24.1 [9.5] vs 18.9 [8.1]), consistent with measurements of RSB in later childhood and adulthood. One high-scoring outlier, representing the same individual, is present in both panels, and this child was ultimately diagnosed with ASD. (*Adapted from* Marrus N, Glowinski AL, Jacob T, et al. Rapid video-referenced ratings of reciprocal social behavior in toddlers: a twin study. J Child Psychol Psychiatry 2015;56(12):1342; with permission.)

subclinical syndromes show near-complete overlap with genetic underpinnings of the clinical-level syndromes,[41] strongly suggesting that the continuous distributions observed in nature relate to quantitative accumulation of causal susceptibility. Thus, although the diagnostic criteria for ASD do not yet consider percentile rank in the population distribution (as do diagnostic criteria for anorexia nervosa, hypertension, intellectual disability, and short stature), an increasingly compelling case can be made for parameterizing diagnostic thresholds in this manner.

Moreover, in the same way that height influences weight, the neurodevelopmental characteristics of intelligence, attention, structural language capacity, emotion regulation, and executive function can influence social communication, such that specification of the role of autistic symptoms in individual patients will requires the development of maps of the predictable relations between the variables (analogous to the height vs weight norms used in pediatric practice) to accurately ascertain the relative contribution of ASD symptoms to a given patient's neurodevelopmental syndrome.[42] This process is becoming especially relevant as clinicians understand more fully the biological influence (effect of inheritance) on each (separable) axis of human development, and recognize that even rare monogenic syndromes commonly have adverse influences on multiple domains of development (eg, effects of 16p11.2 rearrangements on intelligence, social responsiveness, and weight[43]); each is influenced by the mutation in a manner that represents a predictable shift against a (biparental) genetic and environmental background for that trait. In this way, rare syndromes can be more deeply understood, not simply by the variable and idiosyncratic array of deficits with which they are associated, but by how they influence such traits in the setting of the specific genetic and environmental background of an individual.

CAUSATION AND AN IMPENDING REVOLUTION IN AUTISM SPECTRUM DISORDER DIAGNOSIS

The past decade has witnessed an expansion in scientific discovery of the causes and biology of autism. Twin and family studies involving tens of thousands of individuals in ASD-affected families have overwhelmingly established the important role of genetic factors in the causation of most autistic syndromes,[3] and growing genetic evidence has implicated genes involved in synaptic development and plasticity.[44] In aggregate, this work suggests that developmental disruptions at multiple levels of neural architecture, from cellular connections to interregional neurocircuitry, lead to the emergence of ASD. Although neither a laboratory test nor a neural signature to date can reliably establish the presence of a nonsyndromic ASD, a rapidly increasing proportion of all cases (approaching a majority) can be attributed to the influence of deleterious molecular genetic variants or combinations of variants. It is expected that understanding these aspects of the genetics of autism will play a major part in revolutionizing diagnosis. The authors refer readers to Constantino and Charman[45] for an extensive recent review of the implications of advances in genetics on the diagnosis of ASD.

Resolution of many autistic syndromes with respect to the relative contribution of specific genetic variants also continues to illuminate understanding of the biology of autism comorbidities, such as ADHD, motor coordination impairment, epilepsy, intellectual disability, anxiety, and other mental disorders. Although none of these symptom clusters is specific to ASD, some mutations (eg, those associated with fragile X syndrome [FMR1], neurofibromatosis type 1 [NF1], tuberous sclerosis, and a host of newly discovered variants) have been associated with predictable profiles of comorbidity (whenever ASD arises) and therefore blur the distinction between core symptoms and associated symptoms, at least in the setting of these monogenic syndromes.[46,47]

In summary, advances in understanding the causes of autism (its genetic and population structure) suggest that diagnosis will ultimately benefit from further movement toward standardized quantitative characterization of the defining features of ASD, conducted simultaneously with (and controlling for) multiaxial characterization of those aspects of human development that influence the manifestation of autistic symptoms and impairments, and from the inclusion of genotype in taxonomic classification. For some putative causes of ASD, the conversion from statistical association in large genetic studies to knowledge of the specific impact of a deleterious variant in individual patients is still at an early stage.

Efforts to advance earlier diagnosis have also revealed neurocognitive signatures of early ASD risk that may yield a first generation of diagnostic biomarkers. Studies of infants at familial risk of ASD have used novel technologies, including eye tracking and electroencephalogram (EEG)/event-related potential methods, to study the infant neurocognitive predictors of later ASD diagnosis.[48] Several neurocognitive biomarkers have been identified in the first year of life. These biomarkers include differences in social response, such as a decline in eye fixation when viewing faces between ages 2 and 6 months[49]; reduced social orienting[50]; and a reduced neural response to dynamic gaze shifts from 6 months of age.[51] However, differences in nonsocial neurocognitive processes have also been associated with later ASD, including shorter fixation duration at 7 months of age[52] and a decline in attentional disengagement ability between 7 and 14 months.[53] Although no integrative theoretic account has achieved widespread acceptance, several models of emergent neurodevelopmental atypicality have been proposed.[54,55] Clinicians await the outcome of the translational work (which has now begun) before such technologies can be used in a reliable way to augment behavioral assessment of individual infants and toddlers to aid early diagnosis.

EARLY MANIFESTATIONS AND COURSE

Prospective infant sibling studies have elucidated early development in ASD by longitudinal tracking of infants at increased familial risk because of having an ASD-affected sibling. A major finding across these studies is that the rates of language, nonverbal cognition, and early social-communicative development in children show a marked deceleration in children with ASD. At 6 months of age, children who go on to have ASD have scores that do not significantly differ from those of typically developing infants at the group level in social function, nonverbal cognition, or preverbal language ability.[56] However, by 12 months, some measurable differences emerge,[57] with the first identifiable manifestations presenting as deficits in sensorimotor function and visual attention.[49,58,59] By 24 months, children with ASD score lower in most developmental domains,[59,60] highlighting a measurable decline across skills domains during the second year of life. The collective work from these studies, which include hundreds of children at increased risk of ASD, provides strong evidence that early atypical developmental trajectories serve as risk indicators of ASD.[61] Clinicians should therefore be prepared to assess core features of ASD as well as other delays and behavioral concerns in the infant and toddler period.

Social Communication Deficits

Among parents of children with ASD, roughly 30% to 40% have concerns about their child's development by the first year of life,[62] and the mean age of a child's initial presentation to a clinician is 18 months.[63] Children with more severe delays are likely to be referred earlier[16] and firstborn children, whose parents likely have less experience witnessing early child development, are often diagnosed later.[32]

The most common reason parents request evaluation is delayed speech and language development.[62,64] Receptive and expressive aspects of language can be affected and may vary substantially among children with ASD, consistent with the syndrome's inherent heterogeneity. Receptive language delays, which involve difficulties with comprehension, tend to be greater than expressive language delays in children with ASD.[65] Concerns over expressive language may include a failure or delay in achieving verbal language milestones, such as babbling or spoken words, as well as atypical vocalizations, including grunting or echolalia. For children with more intact speech abilities, parents may note frequent scripted phrases or unusual prosody.

Parents less commonly present with specific concerns about social development before the age of 3 years,[27] although deficits in social communication can be elicited. In retrospective studies, parents have reported concerns for poor social awareness, poor social understanding, lack of shared enjoyment in interactions, deficits in eye contact, and lack of interest in other children.[66,67] Analyses of videotapes of infants before an ASD diagnosis showed disturbances in early social behavior by 9 months of age, including looking at people infrequently, an absence of emotional expression, and poor social initiative.[68,69] In their studies of videotapes from 12-month-olds, Osterling and Dawson[70] observed that 4 features distinguished 91% of children with ASD from typically developing children:

1. Lack of pointing
2. Lack of showing objects or things to others

3. Infrequently looking at faces
4. Failure to respond to their own names being called

Other observations have included limited imitation, poor affect regulation, and reduced use of gestures.[71–73] These observations have contributed monumentally to a current generation of robust second-year-of-life screening tools with high positive predictive value.

During the preschool period, children with ASD may progress in some of these infant social milestones. For example, more basic joint attention behaviors have been shown to improve in children with ASD as they develop from a mental age of 18 months to 30 months.[74] Nevertheless, older preschoolers with ASD remain challenged by the social demands of increasingly sophisticated group interactions, which may bring them to teachers' attention once they enter a preschool setting.

Restricted Interests and Repetitive Behaviors

Children with ASD may show restricted interests and repetitive behaviors during infancy and early toddlerhood,[58] although these behaviors generally become prominent following the emergence of deficits in social communication skills.[22,75,76] These behaviors can be idiosyncratic and may involve extreme fixations, insistence on nonfunctional rituals, and distress with minor changes in the environment or schedule. Children may show odd attachments to toys, and their play may involve repeatedly lining things up rather than imaginative or narrative features.[76] Some children show motor stereotypies, such as odd hand and finger mannerisms, or visual stereotypies, in which, for example, they repeatedly fixate on looking at objects out of the corner of their eyes.

Sensory issues, now an aspect of the restricted, repetitive domain in DSM-5, are also observed in this age range.[77] Common examples are hypersensitivity to noise; tactile defensiveness; avoidance of certain food textures (often associated with a restricted diet); and hyposensitivity, such as a surprisingly high tolerance for pain. Other behavioral issues that are enriched but not specific to ASD include atypical reactivity, ranging from passivity to marked irritability. Sensory features and reactivity can show both extremes in the same child. Difficulty sleeping is also common.[67] The motor domain is affected as well, and many parents report toe-walking.[78,79]

Presentation of Regression

A subset of parents report a history of regression, whereby the child, who seemed to meet typical developmental milestones for the first 1 to 2 years of life, seems to lose previously acquired skills. Most cases occur between ages 13 and 18 months,[80–82] with loss of language being the most frequently reported feature.[80,83] Loss of social interest, interpersonal initiative, and basic social competencies, such as eye contact, have also been reported,[84] as well as reduced variety and interaction in play and loss of motor skills, although these are less common.[83,85,86] Regression was previously thought to be rare, but a review of 6 studies of clinical populations found a range of 22% to 50% in ASD,[87] a figure subsequently supported by several studies drawn from the general population.[88,89] Prognosis of regressive cases remains unclear (regression has been associated with lower IQ[84] but not consistently),[90] and several reports have observed an uneven profile of strengths and weaknesses related to autistic severity, IQ, and adaptive function.[91,92]

Evidence for seizures as a contributor to regressive ASD is mixed, because epilepsy is not observed in all cases.[78,79,93] Nevertheless, the recognized link between regression and ASD has made any history of regression a red flag for referral[94] and an indication for an EEG to rule out a comorbid seizure disorder. Further evaluation in such cases is also important to distinguish possible ASD from neurodegenerative conditions that present with regression, such as Rett syndrome.

INTERVENTION PLANNING

During infancy and early childhood, a stage of heightened neural plasticity, providers' first responsibility is to ensure the provision of appropriate developmental therapy to address the obstacles imposed by delays or deficiencies in reciprocal social behavior, motivation, social communication, and mental flexibility, which are inherent to the autistic syndrome, as well as the accompanying deficits in emotion regulation, attention, motor coordination, and cognition that accompany ASD in a plurality of patients. A review of the evidentiary base for early interventions that address these disparate domains of functioning is beyond the scope of this article, but there is an urgent need for rigorous studies to evaluate the impact of the relevant therapies, which include early intensive behavioral intervention (ie, applying principles of applied behavior analysis), speech and language therapy, augmentative communication, occupational therapy, physical therapy, parent training, and early childhood special education, each of which should be considered for its potential to enhance the development of every individual patient, along with appropriate neurologic and/or metabolic interventions as warranted by the patient's specific condition. Readers are referred to Zwaigenbaum and colleagues[95] for a recent review of early psychosocial and educational intervention in ASD. The entire intervention strategy for a child with ASD should prioritize language and communication, because the capacity to functionally communicate (whether through verbal language, sign, or augmentative communication methods) is, by far, the most important predictor of outcome and adaptation.

Children with ASD often show challenging behaviors, as well as medical and psychiatric comorbidities, which can profoundly affect quality of life for themselves and their families. Use of pharmacotherapy for disruptive behaviors and psychiatric comorbidities in young children should be preceded by a careful assessment of risks and benefits, and a fair appraisal of whether maladaptive behavior is context or environment specific (eg, much worse in the setting of child care than at home or vice versa), which raises important caveats to medication use and identifies opportunities for interventions that recapitulate the conditions of the more successful environment.

Mental health care providers can provide important psychosocial support to families as they confront the challenges of raising a child with ASD. Educating families about strategies for managing challenging behaviors in the home, critical evaluation of alternative treatments, or situations in which to obtain legal advocacy empowers families and promotes family-centered care. Physicians should also remind caregivers that their own well-being, which may be overlooked, is a priority of the treatment plan. By establishing a collaborative relationship, clinicians can effectively guide families in accessing appropriate resources, implementing comprehensive interventions, and developing an individualized treatment program that maximally capitalizes on a critical developmental window for improving outcomes in ASD.

SUMMARY

ASDs are neurodevelopmental disorders whose core features of impaired social communication and atypical repetitive behaviors and/or restrictions in range of interests emerge during the preschool period and carry significant and serious implications at successive stages of development. The ability to reliably identify most cases of the condition far earlier than the average age of diagnosis presents a novel opportunity for early intervention; however, the availability of such intervention is remarkably disparate across US communities and its impact is imperfectly understood. New waves of research on the efficacy of early intensive behavioral intervention, on genomic characterization of individual patients for personalized approaches to treatment, and on the development of novel therapies that target newly elucidated causal influences are poised, ultimately, to transform the clinical approach to these conditions in early childhood.

REFERENCES

1. American Psychiatric Association. Diagnostic and statistical manual of mental disorders: DSM-5. 5th edition. Washington, DC; 2013.
2. Constantino JN, Todorov A, Hilton C, et al. Autism recurrence in half siblings: strong support for genetic mechanisms of transmission in ASD. Mol Psychiatry 2013;18(2):137–8.
3. Constantino JN. Recurrence rates in autism spectrum disorders. JAMA 2014; 312(11):1154–5.
4. Fombonne E. Epidemiological surveys of autism and other pervasive developmental disorders: an update. J Autism Dev Disord 2003;33(4):365–82.
5. Developmental Disabilities Monitoring Network Surveillance Year 2010 Principal Investigators, Centers for Disease Control and Prevention (CDC). Prevalence of autism spectrum disorder among children aged 8 years - Autism and Developmental Disabilities Monitoring Network, 11 sites, United States, 2010. MMWR Surveill Summ 2014;63(2):1–21.
6. Bishop DV, Whitehouse AJ, Watt HJ, et al. Autism and diagnostic substitution: evidence from a study of adults with a history of developmental language disorder. Dev Med Child Neurol 2008;50(5):341–5.
7. Shattuck PT. The contribution of diagnostic substitution to the growing administrative prevalence of autism in US special education. Pediatrics 2006;117(4):1028–37.
8. Marrus N, Glowinski AL, Jacob T, et al. Rapid video-referenced ratings of reciprocal social behavior in toddlers: a twin study. J Child Psychol Psychiatry 2015; 56(12):1338–46.
9. Ronald A, Larsson H, Anckarsater H, et al. Symptoms of autism and ADHD: a Swedish twin study examining their overlap. J Abnorm Psychol 2014;123(2): 440–51.
10. Schaefer GB, Mendelsohn NJ, Professional Practice and Guidelines Committee. Clinical genetics evaluation in identifying the etiology of autism spectrum disorders: 2013 guideline revisions. Genet Med 2013;15(5):399–407.
11. Zecavati N, Spence SJ. Neurometabolic disorders and dysfunction in autism spectrum disorders. Curr Neurol Neurosci Rep 2009;9(2):129–36.
12. Constantino JN, Charman T. Gender bias, female resilience, and the sex ratio in autism. J Am Acad Child Adolesc Psychiatry 2012;51(8):756–8.
13. Jacquemont S, Coe BP, Hersch M, et al. A higher mutational burden in females supports a "female protective model" in neurodevelopmental disorders. Am J Hum Genet 2014;94(3):415–25.
14. Virkud YV, Todd RD, Abbacchi AM, et al. Familial aggregation of quantitative autistic traits in multiplex versus simplex autism. Am J Med Genet B Neuropsychiatr Genet 2009;150B(3):328–34.
15. Russell G, Steer C, Golding J. Social and demographic factors that influence the diagnosis of autistic spectrum disorders. Soc Psychiatry Psychiatr Epidemiol 2011;46(12):1283–93.

16. Daniels AM, Mandell DS. Explaining differences in age at autism spectrum disorder diagnosis: a critical review. Autism 2014;18(5):583–97.
17. Durkin MS, Maenner MJ, Meaney FJ, et al. Socioeconomic inequality in the prevalence of autism spectrum disorder: evidence from a U.S. cross-sectional study. PLoS One 2010;5(7):e11551.
18. Shattuck PT, Durkin M, Maenner M, et al. Timing of identification among children with an autism spectrum disorder: findings from a population-based surveillance study. J Am Acad Child Adolesc Psychiatry 2009;48(5):474–83.
19. Eaves LC, Ho HH. The very early identification of autism: outcome to age 4 1/2-5. J Autism Dev Disord 2004;34(4):367–78.
20. Lord C, Risi S, DiLavore PS, et al. Autism from 2 to 9 years of age. Arch Gen Psychiatry 2006;63(6):694–701.
21. Ozonoff S, Young GS, Landa RJ, et al. Diagnostic stability in young children at risk for autism spectrum disorder: a baby siblings research consortium study. J Child Psychol Psychiatry 2015;56(9):988–98.
22. Stone WL, Lee EB, Ashford L, et al. Can autism be diagnosed accurately in children under 3 years? J Child Psychol Psychiatry 1999;40(2):219–26.
23. Turner LM, Stone WL, Pozdol SL, et al. Follow-up of children with autism spectrum disorders from age 2 to age 9. Autism 2006;10(3):243–65.
24. van Daalen E, Kemner C, Dietz C, et al. Inter-rater reliability and stability of diagnoses of autism spectrum disorder in children identified through screening at a very young age. Eur Child Adolesc Psychiatry 2009;18(11):663–74.
25. Sutera S, Pandey J, Esser EL, et al. Predictors of optimal outcome in toddlers diagnosed with autism spectrum disorders. J Autism Dev Disord 2007;37(1): 98–107.
26. Rondeau E, Klein LS, Masse A, et al. Is pervasive developmental disorder not otherwise specified less stable than autistic disorder? A meta-analysis. J Autism Dev Disord 2011;41(9):1267–76.
27. Charman T, Baird G. Practitioner review: diagnosis of autism spectrum disorder in 2- and 3-year-old children. J Child Psychol Psychiatry 2002;43(3):289–305.
28. Warren Z, McPheeters ML, Sathe N, et al. A systematic review of early intensive intervention for autism spectrum disorders. Pediatrics 2011;127(5):e1303.
29. Frith U. Asperger and his syndrome. New York: Cambridge University Press; 1991.
30. Rutter M. Diagnosis and definition of childhood autism. J Autism Child Schizophr 1978;8(2):139–61.
31. McConachie H, Parr JR, Glod M, et al. Systematic review of tools to measure outcomes for young children with autism spectrum disorder. Health Technol Assess 2015;19(41):1–506.
32. Zwaigenbaum L, Bauman ML, Choueiri R, et al. Early identification and interventions for autism spectrum disorder: executive summary. Pediatrics 2015; 136(Suppl 1):S1–9.
33. Leyfer OT, Folstein SE, Bacalman S, et al. Comorbid psychiatric disorders in children with autism: interview development and rates of disorders. J Autism Dev Disord 2006;36(7):849–61.
34. Ventola P, Kleinman J, Pandey J, et al. Differentiating between autism spectrum disorders and other developmental disabilities in children who failed a screening instrument for ASD. J Autism Dev Disord 2007;37(3):425–36.
35. Constantino JN, Zhang Y, Abbacchi AM, et al. Rapid phenotyping of autism spectrum disorders: inclusion of direct observation in feasible paradigms for clinical assessment. Neuropsychiatry 2012;2(3):203–12.

36. Constantino JN. How continua converge in nature: cognition, social competence, and autistic syndromes. J Am Acad Child Adolesc Psychiatry 2009;48(2):97–8.

37. Kim YS, Leventhal BL. Genetic epidemiology and insights into interactive genetic and environmental effects in autism spectrum disorders. Biol Psychiatry 2015; 77(1):66–74.

38. Yuen RK, Thiruvahindrapuram B, Merico D, et al. Whole-genome sequencing of quartet families with autism spectrum disorder. Nat Med 2015;21(2):185–91.

39. Constantino JN, Zhang Y, Frazier T, et al. Sibling recurrence and the genetic epidemiology of autism. Am J Psychiatry 2010;167(11):1349–56.

40. Lyall K, Constantino JN, Weisskopf MG, et al. Parental social responsiveness and risk of autism spectrum disorder in offspring. JAMA Psychiatry 2014;71(8): 936–42.

41. Robinson E, Koenen KC, McCormick MC, et al. Evidence that autistic traits show the same etiology in the general population and at the quantitative extremes (5%, 2.5% and 1%). Arch Gen Psychiatry 2011;68(11):1113–21.

42. Jones EJH, Gliga T, Bedford R, et al. Developmental pathways to autism: a review of prospective studies of infants at risk. Neurosci Biobehav Rev 2014;39:1–33.

43. Moreno-De-Luca D, Moreno-De-Luca A, Cubells JF, et al. Cross-disorder comparison of four neuropsychiatric CNV loci. Curr Genet Med Rep 2014;2(3):151–61.

44. De Rubeis S, He X, Goldberg AP, et al. Synaptic, transcriptional and chromatin genes disrupted in autism. Nature 2014;515(7526):209–15.

45. Constantino JN, Charman T. Diagnosis of autism spectrum disorder: reconciling the syndrome, its diverse origins, and variation in expression. Lancet Neurol 2016;15(3):279–91.

46. Morris SM, Acosta MT, Garg S, et al. Disease burden and symptom structure of autism in neurofibromatosis type 1: a study of the International NF1-ASD Consortium Team (INFACT). JAMA Psychiatry 2016;73(12):1276–84.

47. Frazier TW, Youngstrom EA, Embacher R, et al. Demographic and clinical correlates of autism symptom domains and autism spectrum diagnosis. Autism 2014; 18(5):571–82.

48. Dawson G, Rogers S, Munson J, et al. Randomized, controlled trial of an intervention for toddlers with autism: the Early Start Denver Model. Pediatrics 2010; 125(1):e17–23.

49. Jones W, Klin A. Attention to eyes is present but in decline in 2-6-month-old infants later diagnosed with autism. Nature 2013;504(7480):427–31.

50. Chawarska K, Macari S, Shic F. Decreased spontaneous attention to social scenes in 6-month-old infants later diagnosed with autism spectrum disorders. Biol Psychiatry 2013;74(3):195–203.

51. Elsabbagh M, Mercure E, Hudry K, et al. Infant neural sensitivity to dynamic eye gaze is associated with later emerging autism. Curr Biol 2012;22(4):338–42.

52. Wass SV, Jones EJ, Gliga T, et al. Shorter spontaneous fixation durations in infants with later emerging autism. Sci Rep 2015;5:82–4.

53. Elsabbagh M, Fernandes J, Jane Webb S, et al. Disengagement of visual attention in infancy is associated with emerging autism in toddlerhood. Biol Psychiatry 2013;74(3):189–94.

54. Gliga T, Jones EJ, Bedford R, et al. From early markers to neuro-developmental mechanisms of autism. Dev Rev 2014;34(3):189–207.

55. Klin A, Shultz S, Jones W. Social visual engagement in infants and toddlers with autism: early developmental transitions and a model of pathogenesis. Neurosci Biobehav Rev 2015;50:189–203.

56. Ozonoff S, Iosif AM, Baguio F, et al. A prospective study of the emergence of early behavioral signs of autism. J Am Acad Child Adolesc Psychiatry 2010; 49(3):256–66.e1-e2.
57. Zwaigenbaum L, Bryson S, Rogers T, et al. Behavioral manifestations of autism in the first year of life. Int J Dev Neurosci 2005;23(2–3):143–52.
58. Rogers SJ. What are infant siblings teaching us about autism in infancy? Autism Res 2009;2(3):125–37.
59. Landa R, Garrett-Mayer E. Development in infants with autism spectrum disorders: a prospective study. J Child Psychol Psychiatry 2006;47(6):629–38.
60. Estes A, Zwaigenbaum L, Gu H, et al. Behavioral, cognitive, and adaptive development in infants with autism spectrum disorder in the first 2 years of life. J Neurodev Disord 2015;7(1):24.
61. Zwaigenbaum L, Bauman ML, Stone WL, et al. Early identification of autism spectrum disorder: recommendations for practice and research. Pediatrics 2015; 136(Suppl 1):S10–40.
62. De Giacomo A, Fombonne E. Parental recognition of developmental abnormalities in autism. Eur Child Adolesc Psychiatry 1998;7(3):131–6.
63. Howlin P, Asgharian A. The diagnosis of autism and Asperger syndrome: findings from a survey of 770 families. Dev Med child Neurol 1999;41(12):834–9.
64. Stone WL, Coonrod EE, Turner LM, et al. Psychometric properties of the STAT for early autism screening. J Autism Dev Disord 2004;34(6):691–701.
65. Bartak L, Rutter M, Cox A. A comparative study of infantile autism and specific development receptive language disorder. I. The children. Br J Psychiatry 1975;126:127–45.
66. Vostanis P, Smith B, Chung MC, et al. Early detection of childhood autism: a review of screening instruments and rating scales. Child Care Health Dev 1994; 20(3):165–77.
67. Young RL, Brewer N, Pattison C. Parental identification of early behavioural abnormalities in children with autistic disorder. Autism 2003;7(2):125–43.
68. Adrien JL, Lenoir P, Martineau J, et al. Blind ratings of early symptoms of autism based upon family home movies. J Am Acad Child Adolesc Psychiatry 1993; 32(3):617–26.
69. Maestro S, Muratori F, Cesari A, et al. Course of autism signs in the first year of life. Psychopathology 2005;38(1):26–31.
70. Osterling J, Dawson G. Early recognition of children with autism: a study of first birthday home videotapes. J Autism Dev Disord 1994;24(3):247–57.
71. Maestro S, Muratori F, Cavallaro MC, et al. Attentional skills during the first 6 months of age in autism spectrum disorder. J Am Acad Child Adolesc Psychiatry 2002;41(10):1239–45.
72. Volkmar F, Chawarska K, Klin A. Autism in infancy and early childhood. Annu Rev Psychol 2005;56:315–36.
73. Yirmiya N, Gamliel I, Shaked M, et al. Cognitive and verbal abilities of 24- to 36-month-old siblings of children with autism. J Autism Dev Disord 2007;37(2): 218–29.
74. Mundy P, Sigman M, Kasari C. Joint attention, developmental level, and symptom presentation in autism. Dev Psychopathol 1994;6(03):389–401.
75. Cox A, Klein K, Charman T, et al. Autism spectrum disorders at 20 and 42 months of age: stability of clinical and ADI-R diagnosis. J Child Psychol Psychiatry 1999; 40(5):719–32.

76. Moore V, Goodson S. How well does early diagnosis of autism stand the test of time? Follow-up study of children assessed for autism at age 2 and development of an early diagnostic service. Autism 2003;7(1):47–63.

77. Rogers SJ, Hepburn S, Wehner E. Parent reports of sensory symptoms in toddlers with autism and those with other developmental disorders. J Autism Dev Disord 2003;33(6):631–42.

78. Hoshino Y, Kaneko M, Yashima Y, et al. Clinical features of autistic children with setback course in their infancy. Jpn J Psychiatry Neurol 1987;41(2):237–45.

79. Tuchman RF, Rapin I. Regression in pervasive developmental disorders: seizures and epileptiform electroencephalogram correlates. Pediatrics 1997;99(4):560–6.

80. Goldberg WA, Osann K, Filipek PA, et al. Language and other regression: assessment and timing. J Autism Dev Disord 2003;33(6):607–16.

81. Kurita H. Infantile autism with speech loss before the age of thirty months. J Am Acad Child Psychiatry 1985;24(2):191–6.

82. Werner E, Dawson G. Validation of the phenomenon of autistic regression using home videotapes. Arch Gen Psychiatry 2005;62(8):889–95.

83. Siperstein R, Volkmar F. Brief report: parental reporting of regression in children with pervasive developmental disorders. J Autism Dev Disord 2004;34(6):731–4.

84. Rogers SJ, DiLalla DL. Age of symptom onset in young children with pervasive developmental disorders. J Am Acad Child Adolesc Psychiatry 1990;29(6): 863–72.

85. Davidovitch M, Glick L, Holtzman G, et al. Developmental regression in autism: maternal perception. J Autism Dev Disord 2000;30(2):113–9.

86. Ozonoff S, Williams BJ, Landa R. Parental report of the early development of children with regressive autism: the delays-plus-regression phenotype. Autism 2005; 9(5):461–86.

87. Fombonne E, Chakrabarti S. No evidence for a new variant of measles-mumps-rubella-induced autism. Pediatrics 2001;108(4):E58.

88. Hansen RL, Ozonoff S, Krakowiak P, et al. Regression in autism: prevalence and associated factors in the CHARGE study. Ambul Pediatr 2008;8(1):25–31.

89. Taylor B, Miller E, Lingam R, et al. Measles, mumps, and rubella vaccination and bowel problems or developmental regression in children with autism: population study. BMJ 2002;324(7334):393–6.

90. Short AB, Schopler E. Factors relating to age of onset in autism. J Autism Dev Disord 1988;18(2):207–16.

91. Richler J, Luyster R, Risi S, et al. Is there a 'regressive phenotype' of autism spectrum disorder associated with the measles-mumps-rubella vaccine? A CPEA study. J Autism Dev Disord 2006;36(3):299–316.

92. Wiggins LD, Rice CE, Baio J. Developmental regression in children with an autism spectrum disorder identified by a population-based surveillance system. Autism 2009;13(4):357–74.

93. Kobayashi R, Murata T. Setback phenomenon in autism and long-term prognosis. Acta Psychiatr Scand 1998;98(4):296–303.

94. Filipek PA, Accardo PJ, Baranek GT, et al. The screening and diagnosis of autistic spectrum disorders. J Autism Dev Disord 1999;29(6):439–84.

95. Zwaigenbaum L, Bauman ML, Choueiri R, et al. Early intervention for children with autism spectrum disorder under 3 years of age: recommendations for practice and research. Pediatrics 2015;136(Suppl 1):S60–81.

Feeding Disorders

Natalie Morris, MS[a,1], Rachel M. Knight, PhD[b], Teryn Bruni, PhD[c],
Laura Sayers, MA, CCC-SLP[d], Amy Drayton, PhD[e,*]

KEYWORDS

- Feeding disorders • Pediatrics • Interdisciplinary • Behavioral intervention
- Evidence-based treatment

KEY POINTS

- Pediatric feeding disorders are complex and require interdisciplinary treatment.
- Feeding disorders are unlikely to resolve without treatment, and early intervention prevents more severe feeding problems from developing.
- Feeding disorders among children with autism spectrum disorder are often overlooked because they usually do not present with impaired growth. However, they are at risk for significant nutritional deficits and potential long-term health issues resulting from extreme selective eating.
- There is significant empirical support for the use of behavioral therapy for pediatric feeding disorders.
- Other nonbehavioral treatments (eg, sensory integration, oral-motor exercises, play therapy, medication) currently lack empirical support.

INTRODUCTION

Feeding disorders, often seen in the first 1 to 3 years of life,[1] are multifaceted, frequently caused by a combination of medical, developmental, and behavioral factors. Although feeding disorders can vary in presentation, these difficulties significantly impact children's ability to grow and develop without intensive intervention. Prevalence estimates

Disclosure Statement: There are no commercial or financial conflicts of interest for any of the authors.
[a] Department of Pediatrics, C.S. Mott Children's Hospital, University of Michigan, Ann Arbor, MI, USA; [b] Department of Pediatrics, C.S. Mott Children's Hospital, University of Michigan Medical School, 1500 East Medical Center Drive, SPC 5718, D2240 MPB, Ann Arbor, MI 48109-5318, USA; [c] Department of Pediatrics, C.S. Mott Children's Hospital, University of Michigan Medical School, 1500 East Medical Center Drive, MPB D2214, Ann Arbor, MI 48109-5318, USA; [d] Department of Speech-Language Pathology, C.S. Mott Children's Hospital, University of Michigan, 1540 East Hospital Drive, C&W 12-658, Ann Arbor, MI 48109, USA; [e] Department of Pediatrics, C.S. Mott Children's Hospital, University of Michigan Medical School, D2232 MPB, 1500 East Medical Center Drive, SPC 5718, Ann Arbor, MI 48109-5718, USA
[1] Present address: 1720 Briarvista Way, Atlanta, GA 30329.
* Corresponding author.
E-mail address: adrayton@med.umich.edu

of feeding problems in the general population range from 3% to 10%,[2] but children most at risk are those who have experienced significant medical and developmental challenges. Up to 90% of children with an autism spectrum disorder (ASD)[3] and 70% to 90% of children who were born prematurely or have chronic medical issues[4] experience significant feeding difficulties. Feeding disorders have been associated with a variety of medical issues, including cardiac conditions, neuromuscular disorders, gastrointestinal disorders, chronic lung disease,[5–10] and food allergies.[5,11,12]

Some commonly reported feeding problems (**Table 1**) include a lack of independent self-feeding skills, limited intake related to food selectivity, disruptive mealtime behavior, and extreme food refusal.[1,13–15] For children with complex medical histories, extended physiologic discomfort and recurring medical procedures may be associated with painful eating or result in limited, delayed, or no early oral feeding experiences, thus hindering the child's opportunity to learn appropriate oral-motor skills required for eating. Children with such histories may engage in maladaptive feeding behaviors to avoid pain or discomfort. Other children may lack the appropriate oral-motor skills to efficiently accept, chew, and swallow food without gagging, choking, or vomiting—further reinforcing food refusal behaviors.[6,8] In many cases, even after the medical issue has been resolved, children may continue to refuse to eat because of the previous association between food and pain, resulting in a complex feeding presentation requiring intervention.

Children with ASD are 5 times more likely to have a feeding problem than those without ASD.[24] However, the feeding problems of many children with ASD are overlooked in light of their other developmental concerns and likely because selective eating patterns do not place the child at risk for compromised growth in the vast majority of cases (eg, failure to thrive, significant weight loss, and/or declining growth),[24] which typically initiates concern in traditional pediatric settings.[25–27]

Table 1
Common presentations of pediatric feeding disorders

Common Presentations	Examples
Lack of age-appropriate independent self-feeding skills and/or motivation to self-feed[1,13–15]	Unable to use utensils to scoop or pierce food Accepting food from caregiver but unwilling to eat if they have to self-feed
Extreme food selectivity that limits intake or nutrition[15–21]	Only eating certain foods that are a particular color, brand, temperature, shape, or texture
Extreme food refusal[1,15]	Extremely limited or no oral intake, sometimes requiring enteral feeding
Disruptive mealtime behavior[1,15]	"Need for sameness"—food prepared and presented in a specific way; refusing to sit at the table, throwing food,[22,23] crying, throwing tantrums, gagging, vomiting, hitting, spitting when presented with food
Inability to eat age-appropriate textures due to behavioral and/or oral-motor skill deficits	A 4-year-old who can only eat pureed foods A 2-year-old who only drinks formula and eats purees or dissolvable baby snack foods If presented with other textures, child might choke, gag, vomit
Inability to eat age-appropriate amounts of food (volume limiting)	Might request food, but only eat 1–2 bites despite not having eaten a significant amount of food all day
Only eating "snack foods"	Goldfish, pretzels, Cheetos, puffs, cereal

Children with ASD often demonstrate a strong preference for snack foods, processed foods, and starches with minimal intake of proteins, fruits, and vegetables,[26,27] leaving them at a greater risk for nutrient deficiencies and long-term medical complications.[28,29] Indeed, studies have found higher rates of vitamin and mineral deficiencies, including calcium, protein, vitamin B12, vitamin D, and vitamin A,[24,29] reduced bone cortical thickness,[30] obesity,[31-33] diabetes, cardiovascular disease,[33,34] and dyslipidemia.[33]

If unaddressed, pediatric feeding disorders are highly likely to persist into school age and adolescence, especially if the feeding problems started before the age of 12 months.[35,36] Given the negative outcomes, including delayed growth, malnutrition, cognitive deficits, developmental delays, behavior problems, social difficulties, medical procedures (eg, placement of a feeding tube), and poor academic achievement,[2,37-39] that are associated with chronic feeding issues, diagnosis and appropriate referral for empirically supported treatments are essential.

INTERDISCIPLINARY CARE

The multifaceted nature of feeding disorders (**Fig. 1**) necessitates the use of an interdisciplinary treatment model to effectively treat the physiologic, environmental, behavioral, and psychosocial correlates[40] related to the development and maintenance of feeding disorders. It is recommended that a team approach be used to individually tailor and modify the treatment package because developmental, medical, nutrition, skill-related, and behavioral factors change over time.[40] Health care professionals typically involved are from the following disciplines: medicine, psychology, nutrition, speech-language pathology, and occupational therapy (**Table 2**[1,40]).

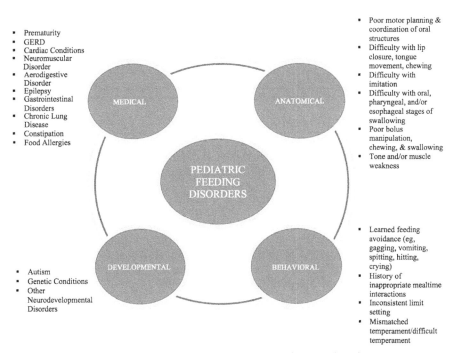

- Prematurity
- GERD
- Cardiac Conditions
- Neuromuscular Disorder
- Aerodigestive Disorder
- Epilepsy
- Gastrointestinal Disorders
- Chronic Lung Disease
- Constipation
- Food Allergies

MEDICAL

ANATOMICAL

PEDIATRIC FEEDING DISORDERS

DEVELOPMENTAL

BEHAVIORAL

- Poor motor planning & coordination of oral structures
- Difficulty with lip closure, tongue movement, chewing
- Difficulty with imitation
- Difficulty with oral, pharyngeal, and/or esophageal stages of swallowing
- Poor bolus manipulation, chewing, & swallowing
- Tone and/or muscle weakness

- Autism
- Genetic Conditions
- Other Neurodevelopmental Disorders

- Learned feeding avoidance (eg, gagging, vomiting, spitting, hitting, crying)
- History of inappropriate mealtime interactions
- Inconsistent limit setting
- Mismatched temperament/difficult temperament

Fig. 1. Factors influencing the development of pediatric feeding disorders. GERD, gastroesophageal reflux disease.

Table 2
Role of interdisciplinary team members

Professional	Role
Physician (may include pediatrician, gastroenterologist, allergist, and so forth)	• Monitors child's weight, addresses medical concerns
Psychologist	• Assesses the function of problem behavior, parent training, develops and implements intervention protocols, and guides and assists other team members with implementation of behavioral interventions • Development of treatment plans to address general behavior, sleep, and toileting concerns that may have impacted feeding
Speech and language pathologist	Assesses: • Physiologic function, trunk support, structural deformities (presence of tracheomalacia), tracheostomy tube/vent dependence, tracheoesophageal fistula, subglottic stenosis, and so forth • Hypersensitivity/hyposensitivity, jaw movements and symmetry, lip symmetry and closure, tongue symmetry and positioning, ankyloglossia, presence of normal or abnormal reflexes, tone of cheeks, shape of palate • Head and trunk control, facial muscular tone, symmetry of facial and oral structures, lingual protrusion, lateralization, and coordination, palate elevation and symmetry, condition of teeth, mastication, hypersensitivity • Cardiopulmonary changes, signs and symptoms of aspiration, gagging, expulsion, spitting up, nasal regurgitation, food refusal behaviors • Feeding/swallowing intervention, altered textures of foods or thickened liquids, compensatory strategies, instrumental assessment, collaboration with other providers
Dietitian	• Provide nutrition education, recommendations for calories goals, and guidance to team and family, monitor for weight loss, collect diet information from family
Occupational therapist	• Evaluates oral sensory, oral motor, and positioning aspects of the child; this may include recommending certain processes or utensils that promote safer feeding or more successful self-feeding[40]

An interdisciplinary approach in the treatment of feeding disorders is especially important because a difficulty in any one area can lead to an arrest in treatment progress.

REVIEW OF AVAILABLE TREATMENTS

Given the multifaceted nature of feeding disorders (ie, medical, behavioral, physiologic), several treatments have been developed. As a primary care physician or other referring physician, it can be difficult to know where to refer these high-need children. The following sections discuss treatments that are used for pediatric feeding disorders and highlight the current research on those approaches.

Behavioral Feeding

Behavioral feeding treatments are the most well-researched and empirically supported areas of feeding intervention.[2,15,26,41–43] Only 3 comparative effectiveness studies exist in the feeding disorder literature, and the results of those studies demonstrate better outcomes with behavior therapy. Behavior therapy resulted in markedly greater improvements in oral intake than did sensory integration therapy,[44] the sequential oral sensory approach,[45] or nutritional manipulation (ie, decreasing calories received enterally).[46]

Behavioral treatments begin with function-based assessments to identify the factors influencing the child's presentation, and treatment is modified based on the child's changing presentation in order to ensure the treatment is matching the underlying function of the behavior.[47] **Table 3** lists and describes empirically supported behavioral feeding techniques.

Sensory-Based and Oral-Motor Treatments

Sensory-based techniques, such as bouncing a child on a therapy ball, having a child play with food with his or her hands, oral stimulation using vibration, differently textured utensils, or hot or cold objects to "enhance sensory awareness,"[70] have not been studied empirically. These techniques are used in some of the interdisciplinary treatment programs described in the literature,[71–73] but there is currently no evidence that treatment using sensory-based techniques alone leads to improvement in oral intake.

A variety of oral-motor exercises (OMEs) have been described in the literature, including stretching, tapping, vibration, pressure, massage, stroking, blowing, cheek puffing, sucking, and other exercises of oral muscles, to change muscle tone and tongue movements, improve range of motion, and increase strength and endurance during oral feeding.[70,74,75] The Beckman Oral Motor Protocol is perhaps the most known oral-motor treatment program. Reviews of the literature found 3 studies that supported the use of OMEs to reduce tongue thrusting,[70] but no evidence of other benefits.[70,74]

Neuromuscular electrical stimulation (NMES, referred to commercially as VitalStim) has been used to treat swallowing problems and is hypothesized to work by strengthening and/or providing sensory stimulation to the muscles used when swallowing.[76] The only study (retrospective review with comparison group) examining the effectiveness of NMES in children found no improvements in swallow function over usual oral motor therapy in children with primary dysphagia.[77]

Nutritional Manipulation

Nutritional manipulation (also referred to as appetite manipulation or hunger provocation) involves an incremental yet relatively quick reduction of caloric intake over a prescribed time period aimed at triggering hunger.[78] Nutritional manipulation has been studied primarily in conjunction with other treatment techniques[72,78–85] with behavioral intervention the most commonly used. Variations in the format and intensity of the behavioral intervention, other treatment components used, duration of treatment, frequency of contact with health care professionals, rate of decrease in enteral feeds, degree of weight loss allowed, age of participants, time from treatment termination to final follow-up assessment, and methodological weaknesses (ie, primarily uncontrolled retrospective reviews) make drawing conclusions about how to use nutritional manipulation most effectively difficult. In fact, the reported success rates (ie, complete wean from enteral feeding) in the 2 studies that evaluated nutritional manipulation without additional treatment components differ dramatically from 6%[46] to 90.5%.[86]

Despite these variations and weaknesses, there are factors that tentatively appear to impact a child's success with nutritional manipulation techniques:

- *Age.* Studies identify different ages (range 12 months to 5 years) at which weaning is more likely to fail or require very extended treatment,[78,85,87,88] but the

Table 3
Empirically supported behavioral feeding techniques

Technique	Definition	Examples of Specific Treatment Techniques
Escape extinction[15,47–53]	Food refusal and disruptive behavior no longer results in escape/avoidance, which results in a decrease or elimination of refusal and disruptive behavior	• Holding a spoon near the child's mouth until the child accepts the bite instead of setting the spoon down when the child swats at it
Differential reinforcement of alternative behavior[2,42,47,54,55]	A consequence is provided contingent on the occurrence of a specific behavior, whereas the same consequence is withheld contingent on inappropriate behavior, resulting in an increase in the specific behavior and decreased rates of inappropriate behavior	• Talking and singing to a child after he or she swallows a bite rather than talking and singing to the child to try to get them to swallow the bite • Terminating a meal contingent on swallowing a specific number of bites rather than after the child engages in refusal behavior (eg, covering his or her mouth, spitting, swatting at the spoon)
Noncontingent attention[52]	Social attention is provided independent of behavior	• Talking and playing with the child throughout the meal both when he or she is engaged in the desired feeding-related behavior and when not
Systematic desensitization[1,56]	Gradual and repeated exposure to an aversive stimulus (eg, nonpreferred food) in the absence of an aversive event (eg, choking, gagging, emesis) to decrease refusal behaviors	• Holding the bottle where the infant can see it but sufficiently far away that he or she does not gag. Then, gradually moving the bottle progressively closer to his or her mouth • Touching a spoon progressively closer to the child's mouth
Stimulus fading[6,42,55,57–65]	Systematically modify a stimulus to closer approximate the desired stimulus	• Starting with a tiny bite of a nonpreferred food and gradually increasing the bite size • Gradually increasing the proportion of nonpreferred to preferred yogurt that is mixed together • Gradually adding more and larger lumps to purees
Simultaneous presentation[66–68]	The presentation of 2 foods at the same time	• Placing one piece of preferred and one piece of nonpreferred food on the same spoon
Flipped spoon[53,58,69]	In one motion, a spoon with puree is flipped at the midline of the child's tongue 180° and wiped toward the anterior portion of the mouth	
Other behavioral management strategies[1]		• Caregiver training • Structured mealtime • Child behavior management • Modeling

literature indicates that the younger the age of the child, the more likely treatment involving nutritional manipulation will be successful.

- *Prior history of successful oral feeding.* Children who have never been oral feeders are much less likely to respond to nutritional manipulation.[89]
- *Rapid and dramatic decreases in enteral feeding.* The groups with the smallest initial reductions in calories (10%–25%) reported lower rates of successful termination of enteral feeding.[46,82,85]
- *Availability of professional support.* The inpatient programs described in the literature[72,79,82–84] and a net-coaching program with 24/7 support available[86] reported higher rates of success in completely weaning children from enteral feeding than did the outpatient programs.[46,85] The higher rates of success when professional contact is more frequent or readily available may be related to 2 issues:
  - *Parental stress.* Children are expected to lose up to 15% of body weight[82] in response to nutritional manipulation. Dramatic weight loss is stressful for many parents[78,85] and can lead them to reengage in the enteral feeding process before the child has a chance to feel hunger cues associated with reduced energy intake and reassociate oral feeding with hunger satiation.
  - *Medical risk.* Health care professionals may think that it is safer to dramatically reduce fluid and calories when able to monitor the child very closely. The 2 outpatient programs reduced enteral feedings markedly slower (10%–25%)[46,85] than did the inpatient[72,79,82–84] and net-coaching program (50%–100%).[86]

Pharmacologic Management

Medical intervention, including pharmaceuticals, to address any source or sources of discomfort associated with feeding, such as gastroesophageal reflux or delayed gastric emptying, is essential. However, the number of studies investigating the use of medication to improve oral intake in children with feeding disorders is extremely limited, and with the exception of one, all of the studies that exist are not strong methodologically (**Table 4**).

Prevention

The following have been shown to facilitate the transition to oral feeding in infants who were unable to feed orally at birth for physical/medical reasons, such as prematurity:

- Nonnutritive sucking[94–96]
- Oral and perioral stimulation (both manual and patterned pulsating stimulation via a device)[70,97,98]
- Cue-based or "infant-driven" feeding in neonatal intensive care units[99–101]

The literature also supports the existence of sensitive periods of development during which certain feeding problems can be prevented by exposing children to different flavors and textures:

- *Advancing texture beyond smooth purees between the ages of 6 and 10 months* prevents chewing problems and refusal of table foods.[102–104]
- *Breast feeding* may reduce the risk of flavor selectivity during infancy[105–107] and childhood[108] by exposing children to a much wider variety of flavors than formula-fed infants.
- *Having children taste foods repeatedly (at least 10 times)*, even if the child does not initially like the taste, may help parents prevent flavor selectivity and increases the likelihood that children will eat a healthy variety of foods.[105,107,109]

Table 4
Summary of medication management literature

Medication	Study	Design	Results
Cyproheptadine	Mahachoklertwattana et al,[90] 2009	Randomized controlled trial (RCT)	Treatment group gained significantly more weight and height than the placebo control group
	Sant'Anna et al,[91] 2014	Retrospective chart review with comparison group of children who were prescribed cyproheptadine but did not adhere to or dropped out of treatment	Significant weight gain across time in children who took cyproheptadine but no significant differences in weight between the children who took cyproheptadine and those who did not
Megestrol	Davis et al,[80] 2009	Retrospective chart review	Specific contribution of megestrol to treatment effectiveness unclear because it was one element in a multicomponent treatment
Amitriptyline (to treat feeding-related pain)	Davis et al,[81] 2016	RCT	No significant contribution to the effectiveness of a multicomponent treatment
Fluoxetine	Celik et al,[92] 2007	Uncontrolled case report	Decrease in anxiety and fear during feeding was reported, but no data were collected. Nasogastric tube feeding was discontinued in the second month after medication began (in conjunction with behavior therapy)
Haloperidol	Celik et al,[92] 2007	Uncontrolled case report	No improvements reported
Risperidone	Berger-Gross et al,[93] 2004	Uncontrolled case report	Increased oral intake when added to a multicomponent intervention

To identify the number of treatment packages or approaches currently available to treat pediatric feeding disorders, the authors first conducted a generalized Internet search of "treatments for pediatric feeding disorders" and also examined the treatments mentioned on the Web site of a trusted feeding resource (Feeding Matters). This general search revealed 13 separate treatments, all of which claim to be effective

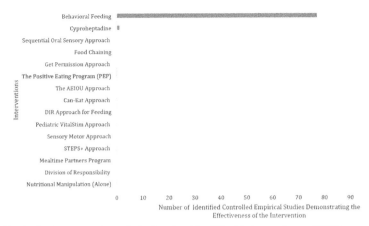

Fig. 2. Controlled, peer-reviewed studies for identified interventions. AEIOU, acceptance, exposure, independence, observation and understanding; STEPS, Supportive Treatment of Eating in PreschoolerS.

in the treatment of feeding disorders. The authors then sought to identify the number of controlled, peer-reviewed articles demonstrating support for the effectiveness of each separate identified therapy for feeding disorders by reviewing reference lists and conducting a comprehensive search of databases (PubMed, PsychInfo). A search of Google Scholar was also conducted in order to capture studies that may have been published outside of the medical or psychology literature. The search parameters included combinations of keywords reflective of the target population (feeding, pediatric feeding disorders, mealtime behaviors, food selectivity) and the name of the target intervention. **Fig. 2** highlights the stark discrepancy between the number of controlled, peer-reviewed studies supporting behavioral feeding treatments and the other treatments. From this graphical depiction, it is clear that at this time, only behavioral feeding currently has strong empirical support for treatment of feeding disorders.

SUMMARY

The purpose of this review was to outline common presentations of pediatric feeding disorders and the available treatment approaches.

Implications

The current review highlights several important practical implications surrounding assessment and treatment of pediatric feeding problems:

- Feeding disorders are multifaceted and require an interdisciplinary approach to evaluation and treatment.
- Feeding disorders among children with developmental disabilities are often overlooked because they usually do not present with impaired growth, despite significant nutritional deficits and the potential long-term health issues resulting from extreme selective eating.
- Early referral for empirically supported treatment is essential for improvement of feeding difficulties.
- Behavioral interventions should be at the core of interdisciplinary treatment packages given that they are the only empirically supported therapy for pediatric feeding disorders.

- Other nonbehavioral treatments (eg, sensory integration, OMEs, play therapy, medication) have limited empirical support and lack controlled studies demonstrating positive outcomes at this time.
- Given the high prevalence of pediatric feeding disorders, there is a need for more training of behavioral providers in academic programs to meet the needs of patients and families.

Future Research

More controlled research is needed to continue to move toward the effective treatment of pediatric feeding disorders. The following priorities are proposed:

- Given that many studies examine a variety of interdisciplinary, multicomponent treatments, future research is needed to examine the comparative effectiveness of specific components of treatment packages.
- Empirical support for nonbehavioral treatment techniques (eg, sensory-based, medication-based, nutritional manipulation alone) to treat feeding disorders is extremely limited. More controlled research demonstrating the efficacy of nonbehavioral treatment methods is necessary to support continued use of these methods in the treatment of pediatric feeding disorders.
- Although there are many controlled studies demonstrating the efficacy of behavioral techniques for feeding problems, most studies used experimental single-case design methods. More studies using a controlled randomized design across larger populations are needed to further validate the effectiveness and generalizability of behavioral interventions for pediatric feeding disorders.

REFERENCES

1. Silverman AH. Feeding disorders in infants and children behavioral management of feeding disorders of childhood. Nutr Metab 2015;66(5):33–42.
2. Kerwin ME. Empirically supported treatments in pediatric psychology: severe feeding problems. J Pediatr Psychol 1999;24(3):193–216.
3. Kodak T, Piazza CC. Assessment and behavioral treatment of feeding and sleeping disorders in children with autism spectrum disorders. Child Adolesc Psychiatr Clin N Am 2008;17(4):887–905.
4. Rudolph CD, Thompson Link D. Feeding disorders in infants and children. Pediatr Clin North Am 2002;49(1):97–112.
5. Haas A. Feeding disorders in food allergic children: current allergy and asthma reports. 2010. http://dx.doi.org/10.1007/s11882-010-0111-5.
6. Kerwin ME, Ahearn WH, Eicher PS, et al. The costs of eating: a behavioral economic analysis of food refusal. J Appl Behav Anal 1995;28(3):245–60.
7. Eicher PS. Feeding. In: Batshaw ML, editor. Children with disabilities. 4th edition. Baltimore (MD): Brookes Publishing Co; 1994. p. 621–41.
8. Morris SE, Klein MD. Pre-feeding skills: A comprehension resource for feeding development. 2nd edition. Tucson (AZ): Therapy Skill Builders; 1987. p. 59–94.
9. Iwata B, Riordan M, Wohl MK, et al. Pediatric feeding disorders: behavioral analysis and treatment. In: Accardo PJ, editor. Failure to thrive in infancy and early childhood. Baltimore (MD): University Park Press; 1982. p. 297–329.
10. Arvedson JC, Brodsky L. Pediatric swallowing and feeding: assessment and management. Thousand Oaks (CA): Singular Publishing; 1985. p. 157–208.
11. Pentiuk SP, Miller CK, Kaul A. Eosinophilic esophagitis in infants and toddlers. Dysphagia 2007;22(1):44–8.

12. Fortunato J, Scheimann A. Protein-energy malnutrition and feeding refusal secondary to food allergies. Clin Pediatr (Phila) 2008;47:496–9. Available at: http://cpj.sagepub.com/content/47/5/496.short. Accessed September 28, 2016.
13. Munk DD, Repp AC. Behavioral assessment of feeding problems of individuals with severe disabilities. J Appl Behav Anal 1994;27(2):241–50.
14. Sisson KA, Van Hasselt VB. Feeding disorders. In: Luiselli JK, editor. Behavioral medicine and developmental disabilities. NewYork: Springer; 1989. p. 45–73.
15. Sharp WG, Jaquess DL, Morton JF, et al. Pediatric feeding disorders: a quantitative synthesis of treatment outcomes. Clin Child Fam Psychol Rev 2010;13(4): 348–65.
16. Ahearn WH, Castine T, Nault K, et al. An assessment of food acceptance in children with autism or pervasive developmental disorder-not otherwise specified. J Autism Dev Disord 2001;31(5):505–11.
17. Bowers L. An audit of referrals of children with autistic spectrum disorder to the dietetic service. J Hum Nutr Diet 2002;15(2):141–4.
18. Collins MSR, Kyle R, Smith S, et al. Coping with the usual family diet: eating behaviour and food choices of children with Down's syndrome, autistic spectrum disorders or cri du chat syndrome and comparison groups of siblings. J Intellect Disabil 2003;7(2):137–55.
19. Cornish E. A balanced approach towards healthy eating in autism. J Hum Nutr Diet 1998;11(6):501–9.
20. Field D, Garland M, Williams K. Correlates of specific childhood feeding problems. J Paediatr Child Health 2003;39(4):299–304.
21. Schreck KA, Williams K, Smith AF. A comparison of eating behaviors between children with and without autism. J Autism Dev Disord 2004;34(4):433–8.
22. Rogers LG, Magill-Evans J, Rempel GR. Mothers' challenges in feeding their children with autism spectrum disorder: managing more than just picky eating. J Dev Phys Disabil 2012;24(1):19–33.
23. Curtin C, Hubbard K, Anderson SE, et al. Food selectivity, mealtime behavior problems, spousal stress, and family food choices in children with and without autism spectrum disorder. J Autism Dev Disord 2015;45(10):3308–15.
24. Sharp WG, Berry RC, McCracken C, et al. Feeding problems and nutrient intake in children with autism spectrum disorders: a meta-analysis and comprehensive review of the literature. J Autism Dev Disord 2013;43(9):2159–73.
25. Onis M. Assessment of differences in linear growth among populations in the WHO Multicentre Growth Reference Study. Acta Paediatr 2006;95:56–65. Available at: http://onlinelibrary.wiley.com/doi/10.1111/j.1651-2227.2006.tb02376.x/full. Accessed September 29, 2016.
26. Ledford JR, Gast DL. Feeding problems in children with autism spectrum disorders: a review. Focus Autism Other Dev Disabl 2006;21(3):153–66.
27. McElhanon BO, McCracken C, Karpen S, et al. Gastrointestinal symptoms in autism spectrum disorder: a meta-analysis. Pediatrics 2014;133(5):872–83.
28. Bandini LG, Anderson SE, Curtin C, et al. Food selectivity in children with autism spectrum disorders and typically developing children. J Pediatr 2010;157(2): 259–64.
29. Zimmer MH, Hart LC, Manning-Courtney P, et al. Food variety as a predictor of nutritional status among children with autism. J Autism Dev Disord 2012;42: 549–56.
30. Hediger M, England L, Molloy C, et al. Reduced bone cortical thickness in boys with autism or autism spectrum disorder. J Autism Dev Disord 2008;

38(5):848–56. Available at: http://link.springer.com/article/10.1007/s10803-007-0453-6. Accessed September 29, 2016.

31. Broder-Fingert S, Brazauskas K, Lindgren K, et al. Prevalence of overweight and obesity in a large clinical sample of children with autism. Acad Pediatr 2014; 14(4):408–14.

32. Curtin C, Anderson SE, Must A, et al. The prevalence of obesity in children with autism: a secondary data analysis using nationally representative data from the National Survey of Children's Health. BMC Pediatr 2010;10(1):1–5.

33. Croen LA, Zerbo O, Qian Y, et al. The health status of adults on the autism spectrum. Autism 2015;19(7):814–23.

34. Guh DP, Zhang W, Bansback N, et al. The incidence of co-morbidities related to obesity and overweight: a systematic review and meta-analysis. BMC Public Health 2009;9(1):88.

35. Babbitt R, Hoch T, Coe D, et al. Behavioral assessment and treatment of pediatric feeding disorders. Dev Behav Pediatr 1994;15:278–91. Available at: http://journals.lww.com/jrnldbp/Abstract/1994/08000/Behavioral_Assessment_and_Treatment_of_Pediatric.11.aspx. Accessed September 28, 2016.

36. Dahl M, Sundelin C. Feeding problems in an affluent society. Follow-up at four years of age in children with early refusal to eat. Acta Paediatr Scand 1992; 81(8):575–9. Available at: http://www.ncbi.nlm.nih.gov/pubmed/1392380.

37. Chatoor I. Feeding disorders in infants and toddlers: diagnosis and treatment. Child Adolesc Psychiatr Clin N Am 2002;11(2):163–83.

38. Benoit D. Feeding disorders, failure to thrive, and obesity. In: Zeanah CH, editor. Handbook of infant mental health. 3rd edition. New York: Guilford; 2009. p. 377–91.

39. Finney JW. Preventing common feeding problems in infants and young children. Pediatr Clin North Am 1986;33(4):775–88.

40. Edwards S, Davis AM, Ernst L, et al. Interdisciplinary strategies for treating oral aversions in children. J Parenter Enteral Nutr 2015;39(8):899–909.

41. Volkert V, Piazza C. Empirically supported treatments for pediatric feeding disorders. In: Sturmey P, Hersen M, editors. Handbook of evidence-based practice in clinical psychology, vol. 1. Hoboken (NJ): Wiley; 2012. p. 456–81.

42. Williams KE, Field DG, Seiverling L. Food refusal in children: a review of the literature. Res Dev Disabil 2010;31(3):625–33.

43. Lukens CT, Silverman AH. Systematic review of psychological interventions for pediatric feeding problems. J Pediatr Psychol 2014;39(8):903–17.

44. Addison L, Piazza C, Patel M, et al. A comparison of sensory integrative and behavioral therapies as treatment for pediatric feeding disorders. J Appl Behav Anal 2012;45(3):455–71.

45. Peterson KM, Piazza CC, Volkert VM. A comparison of a modified sequential oral sensory approach to an applied behavior-analytic approach in the treatment of food selectivity in children with autism spectrum disorder. J Appl Behav Anal 2016;49(3):485–511.

46. Benoit D, Wang EEL, Zlotkin SH. Discontinuation of enterostomy tube feeding by behavioral treatment in early childhood: a randomized controlled trial. J Pediatr 2000;137(4):498–503.

47. Piazza CC, Patel MR, Gulotta CS, et al. On the relative contributions of positive reinforcement and escape extinction in the treatment of food refusal. J Appl Behav Anal 2003;36(3):309–24.

48. Ahearn WH, Kerwin ML, Eicher PS, et al. An alternating treatments comparison of two intensive interventions for food refusal. J Appl Behav Anal 1996;29(3): 321–32.

49. Cooper LJ, Wacker DP, McComas JJ, et al. Use of component analyses to identify active variables in treatment packages for children with feeding disorders. J Appl Behav Anal 1995;28(2):139–53.

50. Hoch T, Babbitt RL, Coe DA, et al. Contingency contacting. Combining positive reinforcement and escape extinction procedures to treat persistent food refusal. Behav Modif 1994;18(1):106–28.

51. Patel MR, Piazza CC, Martinez CJ, et al. An evaluation of two differential reinforcement procedures with escape extinction to treat food refusal. J Appl Behav Anal 2002;35(4):363–74.

52. Reed GK, Piazza CC, Patel MR, et al. On the relative contributions of noncontingent reinforcement and escape extinction in the treatment of food refusal. J Appl Behav Anal 2004;37(1):27–42.

53. Sharp WG, Odom A, Jaquess DL. Comparison of upright and flipped spoon presentations to guide treatment of food refusal. J Appl Behav Anal 2012;45(1): 83–96. Volkert V, editor.

54. LaRue RH, Stewart V, Piazza CC, et al. Escape as reinforcement and escape extinction in the treatment of feeding problems. J Appl Behav Anal 2011; 44(4):719–35. Zarcone J, editor.

55. Sharp WG, Jaquess DL, Morton JF, et al. A retrospective chart review of dietary diversity and feeding behavior of children with autism spectrum disorder before and after admission to a day-treatment program. Focus Autism Other Dev Disabl 2011;26(1):37–48.

56. Siegel LJ. Classical and operant procedures in the treatment of a case of food aversion in a young child. J Clin Child Psychol 1982;11(2):167–72.

57. Seiverling L, Kokitus A, Williams K. A clinical demonstration of a treatment package for food selectivity. Behav Anal Today 2012;13(2):11–6.

58. Sharp WG, Harker S, Jaquess DL. Comparison of bite-presentation methods in the treatment of food refusal. J Appl Behav Anal 2010;43(4):739–43. Thompson R, editor.

59. Knox M, Rue HC, Wildenger L, et al. Intervention for food selectivity in a specialized school setting: teacher implemented prompting, reinforcement, and demand fading for an adolescent student with autism. Educ Treat Child 2012; 35(3):407–18.

60. Meier AE, Fryling MJ, Wallace MD. Using high-probability foods to increase the acceptance of low probability foods. J Appl Behav Anal 2012;45(1):149–53. Volkert V, editor.

61. Valdimarsdóttir H, Halldórsdóttir LÝ, SigurÐardóttir ZG. Increasing the variety of foods consumed by a picky eater: generalization of effects across caregivers and settings. J Appl Behav Anal 2010;43(1):101–5. Hanley GP, editor.

62. Luiselli JK, Ricciardi JN, Gilligan K. Liquid fading to establish milk consumption by a child with autism. Behav Interv 2005;20(2):155–63.

63. Patel MR, Piazza CC, Kelly L, et al. Using a fading procedure to increase fluid consumption in a child with feeding problems. J Appl Behav Anal 2001;34(3): 357–60.

64. Shore BA, Babbitt RL, Williams KE, et al. Use of texture fading in the treatment of food selectivity. J Appl Behav Anal 1998;31(4):621–33.

65. Mueller MM, Piazza CC, Patel MR, et al. Increasing variety of foods consumed by blending nonpreferred foods into preferred foods. J Appl Behav Anal 2004; 37(2):159–70.

66. Piazza CC, Patel MR, Santana CM, et al. An evaluation of simultaneous and sequential presentation of preferred and non-preferred food to treat food selectivity. J Appl Behav Anal 2002;35(3):259–70.

67. Kern L, Marder TJ. A comparison of simultaneous and delayed reinforcement as treatments for food selectivity. J Appl Behav Anal 1996;29(2):243–6.

68. Capaldi ED. Conditioned food preferences. In: Capaldi ED, editor. Why we eat what we eat: the psychology of eating. Washington, DC: American Psychological Association; 1996. p. 53–80.

69. Volkert VM, Vaz PC, Piazza CC, et al. Using a flipped spoon to decrease packing in children with feeding disorders. J Appl Behav Anal 2011;44(3):617–21.

70. Arvedson J, Clark H, Lazarus C, et al. Evidence-based systematic review: effects of oral motor interventions on feeding and swallowing in preterm infants. Am J Speech Lang Pathol 2010;19(4):321.

71. Angell A. Selective eaters and tactile sensitivity: a review of classification and treatment methods that address anxiety and support a child's need for a sense of control. Infant Child Adolesc Nutr 2010;2(5):299–303.

72. Brown J, Kim C, Lim A, et al. Successful gastrostomy tube weaning program using an intensive multidisciplinary team approach. J Pediatr Gastroenterol Nutr 2014;58(6):743–9.

73. Cornwell SL, Kelly K, Austin L. Pediatric feeding disorders: effectiveness of multidisciplinary inpatient treatment of gastrostomy-tube dependent children. Child Health Care 2010;39(3):214–31.

74. Lass NJ, Pannbacker M. The application of evidence-based practice to nonspeech oral motor treatments. Lang Speech Hear Serv Sch 2008;39(3): 408–21.

75. Manno CJ, Fox C, Eicher P, Kerwin M. Early oral-motor interventions for pediatric feeding problems: what, when and how. J Early Intensive Behav Interv 2005; 2(3):45–159.

76. Neuromuscular electrical stimulation in the treatment of dysphagia: a literature review. 2016. Available at: http://www.djoglobal.com/sites/default/files/pdfs/vitalstim/VS-Research-Summary.pdf. Accessed September 15, 2016.

77. Christiaanse ME, Mabe B, Russell G, et al. Neuromuscular electrical stimulation is no more effective than usual care for the treatment of primary dysphagia in children. Pediatr Pulmonol 2011;46(6):559–65.

78. Edwards S, Davis AM, Bruce A, et al. Caring for tube-fed children: a review of management, tube weaning, and emotional considerations. J Parenter Enteral Nutr 2015;40(5):616–22.

79. Byars KC, Burklow KA, Ferguson K, et al. A multicomponent behavioral program for oral aversion in children dependent on gastrostomy feedings. J Pediatr Gastroenterol Nutr 2003;37(4):473–80. Available at: http://journals.lww.com/jpgn/Abstract/2003/10000/A_Multicomponent_Behavioral_Program_for_Oral.14.aspx.

80. Davis AM, Bruce AS, Mangiaracina C, et al. Moving from tube to oral feeding in medically fragile nonverbal toddlers. J Pediatr Gastroenterol Nutr 2009;49(2): 233–6.

81. Davis AM, Dean K, Mousa H, et al. A randomized controlled trial of an outpatient protocol for transitioning children from tube to oral feeding: no need for amitriptyline. J Pediatr 2016;172:136–41.e2.

82. Hartdorff CM, Kneepkens CMF, Stok-Akerboom AM, et al. Clinical tube weaning supported by hunger provocation in fully-tube-fed children. J Pediatr Gastroenterol Nutr 2015;60(4):538–43.

83. Silverman AH, Kirby M, Clifford LM, et al. Nutritional and psychosocial outcomes of gastrostomy tube–dependent children completing an intensive inpatient behavioral treatment program. J Pediatr Gastroenterol Nutr 2013;57(5):668–72.

84. Trabi T, Dunitz-Scheer M, Kratky E, et al. Inpatient tube weaning in children with long-term feeding tube dependency: a retrospective analysis. Infant Ment Health J 2010;31(6):664–81.

85. Wright CM, Smith KH, Morrison J. Withdrawing feeds from children on long term enteral feeding: factors associated with success and failure. Arch Dis Child 2011;96(5):433–9.

86. Marinschek S, Dunitz-Scheer M, Pahsini K, et al. Weaning children off enteral nutrition by netcoaching versus onsite treatment: a comparative study. J Paediatr Child Health 2014;50(11):902–7.

87. Dunitz-Scheer M, Levine A, Roth Y, et al. Prevention and treatment of tube dependency in infancy and early childhood. Infant Child Adolesc Nutr 2009;1(2): 73–82.

88. Ishizaki A, Hironaka S, Tatsuno M, et al. Characteristics of and weaning strategies in tube-dependent children. Pediatr Int 2013;55(2):208–13.

89. Mason SJ, Harris G, Blissett J. Tube feeding in infancy: implications for the development of normal eating and drinking skills. Dysphagia 2005;20(1):46–61.

90. Mahachoklertwattana P, Wanasuwankul S, Poomthavorn P, et al. Short-term cyproheptadine therapy in underweight children: effects on growth and serum insulin-like growth factor-I. J Pediatr Endocrinol Metab 2009;22(5):425–32.

91. Sant'Anna AM, Hammes PS, Porporino M, et al. Use of cyproheptadine in young children with feeding difficulties and poor growth in a pediatric feeding program. J Pediatr Gastroenterol Nutr 2014;59(5):674–8.

92. Celik G, Diler RS, Tahiroglu AY, et al. Fluoxetine in posttraumatic eating disorder in 2-year-old twins. J Child Adolesc Psychopharmacol 2007;17(2):233–6.

93. Berger-Gross P, Coletti DJ, Hirschkorn K, et al. The effectiveness of risperidone in the treatment of three children with feeding disorders. J Child Adolesc Psychopharmacol 2004;14(4):621–7.

94. Bingham PM, Ashikaga T, Abbasi S. Prospective study of non-nutritive sucking and feeding skills in premature infants. Arch Dis Child Fetal Neonatal Ed 2010; 95(3):194–200.

95. Davis A, Kennedy C. Meta analysis: effects of interventions on premature infants. J Perinat Neonatal Nurs 2000;14(3):62–77. Available at: http://journals. lww.com/jpnnjournal/Abstract/2000/12000/Meta_Analysis__Effects_of_Interventions_on.6.aspx.

96. Pinelli J, Symington AJ. Non-nutritive sucking for promoting physiologic stability and nutrition in preterm infants. In: Pinelli J, editor. Cochrane database of systematic reviews. Chichester (United Kindom): John Wiley & Sons, Ltd; 2005. http://dx.doi.org/10.1002/14651858.CD001071.pub2.

97. Barlow SM, Lee J, Wang J, et al. Frequency-modulated orocutaneous stimulation promotes non-nutritive suck development in preterm infants with respiratory distress syndrome or chronic lung disease. J Perinatol 2014;34(2):136–42.

98. Fucile S, Gisel E, Lau C. Effect of an oral stimulation program on sucking skill maturation of preterm infants. Dev Med Child Neurol 2005;47(3):158–62.

99. Jadcherla SR, Peng J, Moore R, et al. Impact of personalized feeding program in 100 NICU infants: pathophysiology-based approach for better outcomes. J Pediatr Gastroenterol Nutr 2012;54(1):62–70.

100. Kirk AT, Alder SC, King JD. Cue-based oral feeding clinical pathway results in earlier attainment of full oral feeding in premature infants. J Perinatol 2007; 27(9):572–8.

101. Puckett B, Grover V, Holt T, et al. Cue-based feeding for preterm infants: a prospective trial. Am J Perinatol 2008;25(10):623–8.

102. Strologo Dello L, Principato F, Sinibaldi D, et al. Feeding dysfunction in infants with severe chronic renal failure after long-term nasogastric tube feeding. Pediatr Nephrol 1997;11(1):84–6.

103. Gisel EG. Effect of food texture on the development of chewing of children between six months and two years of age. Dev Med Child Neurol 2008;33(1): 69–79.

104. Northstone K, Emmett P, Nethersole F. The effect of age of introduction to lumpy solids on foods eaten and reported feeding difficulties at 6 and 15 months. J Hum Nutr Diet 2001;14(1):43–54.

105. Forestell CA, Mennella JA. Early determinants of fruit and vegetable acceptance. Pediatrics 2007;120(6):1247–54.

106. Gerrish CJ, Mennella JA. Flavor variety enhances food acceptance in formula-fed infants. Am J Clin Nutr 2001;73(6):1080–5. Available at: http://www.ncbi.nlm.nih.gov/pubmed/11382663. Accessed September 28, 2016.

107. Sullivan SA, Birch LL. Infant dietary experience and acceptance of solid foods. Pediatrics 1994;93(2):271–7.

108. Galloway AT, Lee Y, Birch LL. Predictors and consequences of food neophobia and pickiness in young girls. J Am Diet Assoc 2003;103(6):692–8.

109. Birch LL, McPhee L, Shoba BC, et al. What kind of exposure reduces children's food neophobia?: looking vs. tasting. Appetite 1987;9(3):171–8.

Sleep Disorders

Assessment and Treatment in Preschool-Aged Children

Amy Licis, MD, MSCI

KEYWORDS

- Sleep • Preschool • Sleep disorders • Sleep deprivation • Pediatric sleep

KEY POINTS

- Obtaining sufficient good-quality sleep optimizes behavior and cognitive functioning in preschool-aged children.
- Several sleep disorders are prevalent in preschoolers, including insomnia, obstructive sleep apnea, parasomnias, and restless legs syndrome.
- The quality of sleep obtained during the preschool age may have effects on long-term mental health.

INTRODUCTION

Sleep disorders are common in preschoolers, defined generally as ages 3 to 5 years. Sleep of poor quality or insufficient duration can cause issues with behavior and learning. Several psychiatric disorders are comorbid with sleep disorders, and the relationship is likely bidirectional. It is possible that sleep disorders in the preschool age may contribute to long-term mental health issues. This article reviews normal sleep and sleep disorders seen in preschoolers.

SLEEP IN THE PRESCHOOL YEARS

Sleep is an evolving process, changing in duration and pattern as children grow and develop. Children may develop sleep issues in certain stages of development, sometimes resolving in other stages of development, and sometimes persisting. Sleep during the preschool years is distinct, differing from infant and toddler sleep and also from the sleep of school-aged children. Sleep disorders may either resolve or emerge during the preschool years.

There are no conflicts of interest to disclose and no funding sources.
Department of Neurology, Washington University School of Medicine, Campus Box 8111, 660 South Euclid Avenue, St Louis, MO 63110, USA
E-mail address: licisa@wustl.edu

NORMAL SLEEP IN THE PRESCHOOL YEARS

According to a consensus statement of the American Academy of Sleep Medicine, the recommended sleep duration for children aged 3 to 5 years in order to optimize health is 10 to 13 hours in a 24-hour period, including naps.[1] Sleeping less than the recommended amount may increase the likelihood of attention, behavior, and learning problems, and may have medical consequences such as an increased risk of accidents, injuries, hypertension, obesity,[2] diabetes, and depression.[1] There is some evidence that short sleep duration in childhood may also increase the likelihood of obesity in adulthood.[3] Sleeping in excess of the recommended amount may also be associated with worse mental health and an increased risk of hypertension, diabetes, and obesity.[1,2] Acute sleep restriction has been shown to be associated with increased caloric intake in preschoolers, and chronic sleep restriction may contribute to obesity.[4]

The National Sleep Foundation Sleep in America Poll is an annual poll assessing the prevalence of sleep issues in the American population. The 2004 poll specifically focused on children and included the preschool years. The 2004 poll participants were n = 1473 parents/caregivers of children aged newborn to 10 years.[5] Participants tended to be female (72% were the mother or stepmother of the child), married (91%), white (89%), with some college education (74%), employed (71%), and with a median household income of $57,500.[5] The poll assessed n = 387 preschoolers, in whom 10.2% of caregivers perceived problematic sleep. Sleep onset latency was reported at a mean of 17.4 minutes (standard deviation, 16.7 minutes), 35.6% reported at least 1 night waking, and a mean sleep duration of 9.6 hours (standard deviation, 1.5).[5]

The 2004 National Sleep Foundation Sleep in America Poll further characterized sleep conditions for preschool participants. Findings for preschoolers included the presence of a consistent bedtime routine for 93% of participants.[5] Reading was a part of the bedtime routine for 57.9% and parents were present at bedtime for 45.7% of preschoolers.[5] Problematic sleep behaviors were identified, including a late bedtime (defined as after 9 PM) in 53%.[5] Televisions were present in the bedrooms of 30% of preschoolers, and 27.1% of preschoolers drank at least 1 caffeinated beverage per day regularly.[5] Evidence shows that proper sleep routines may be associated with measures of good-quality sleep. A consistent bedtime routine correlated with earlier bedtimes, shorter sleep onset latency, reduced night wakings, and increased sleep duration in a parent-completed questionnaire study of n = 10,085 children (parents in Australia–New Zealand, Canada, China, Hong Kong, India, Japan, Korea, Malaysia, Philippines, Singapore, Thailand, United Kingdom, and the United States completed the Brief Infant/Child Sleep Questionnaire).[6]

Most preschoolers take naps. The most common nap duration in nappers aged 2 to 6 years is 2 hours.[7] Although most children 3 to 4 years old nap, nap rates decreased with increasing age. A minority of children 5 to 6 years old nap, and by age 7 years nearly all children have stopped napping.[7] Napping may facilitate learning in preschoolers by providing more frequent opportunities for the memory consolidation that occurs with sleep. A study by Kurdziel and colleagues[8] examined learning with and without daytime napping in preschool-aged children. Preschoolers performed a visuospatial memory task similar to the game Memory, and then either napped or played quietly without napping and recall was assessed 30 minutes after the nap and also the following morning, 24 hours after the task. When napping occurred, the children showed greater recall both at the postnap and 24-hour time points, whereas there was significant long-term forgetting when they did not nap. As children age, the facilitation in learning with napping is less evident. Napping in children 9 to

12 years old does not seem to improve learning any more than obtaining adequate sleep at night improves learning.[9]

Sleep timing is regulated by environmental cues, sleep drive, and individual variations in internal circadian rhythms, some of which may be genetically determined.[10] Chronotype, or tendency to an early, typical, or late preferred sleep schedule, has an overall heritability of around 50%, with environmental factors accounting for about 50% of the difference in sleep timing among individuals.[11] There is an overall trend toward morningness in young children.[10] In one study of n = 7826 children 3 to 5 years old attending preschools and daycares in Japan, parents completed the Children's Chronotype Questionnaire and the prevalences of morning types, neither, and evening types were 31.6%, 55.9%, and 10.0% of children, respectively.[12] Preschool children with a delayed preferred sleep schedule are more likely to have a nocturnal sleep deficit during the weekdays than children with an early or typical preferred sleep schedule, with longer sleep durations on the weekend.[12] There is some evidence that sleep deprivation from circadian rhythm malalignment may increase risk of depression.[10]

Sleep deprivation is becoming increasingly common in preschoolers, perhaps in part related to the effect of scheduling pressures on limiting sleep time. In a study of n = 297 families with children 5 to 6 years old, parent-reported short sleep duration (<9 hours, in about 9.6% of the sample) on the Sleep Disturbance Scale was related to inattention (adjusted odds ratio, 4.70; 95% confidence interval [CI], 1.58–14.00) and internalizing behaviors (adjusted odds ratio, 3.84; 95% CI, 1.32–11.21) on the parent-completed Child Behavior Checklist.[13]

SLEEP DISORDERS

Sleep disorders are fairly prevalent in preschoolers. It is estimated that as much as 25% of preschool children may have sleep issues.[14] A study of n = 995 Norwegian 4-year-olds assessed by caregiver interview showed that the overall sleep disorder rate was 19.2% (rates of insomnia were 16.6%, nightmare disorder 2.2%, and sleepwalking disorder 0.7%).[15] A common sleep issue in the preschool age that is not necessarily pathologic is nocturnal enuresis. Primary nocturnal enuresis has been described in about 9% to 14% of children 5 to 6 years old, decreasing in prevalence to about 5% of 10-year-olds.[16] Nocturnal enuresis is generally considered problematic if it occurs more than once per month.[17] Enuresis may be associated with obstructive sleep apnea (OSA), with the association being strongest for girls with severe OSA.[17]

Nightmares are common in the preschool ages, but frequent nightmares are not necessarily common, reported in 2% to 4% of children 29 months to 6 years old and a peak occurring at 41 months (3.9%).[18] Preschoolers with nightmare disorder were more likely to have symptoms of generalized anxiety disorder than preschoolers without problematic nightmares.[15]

Preschoolers sometimes develop behavioral sleep issues such as longer sleep latencies or refusal to sleep alone. When preschoolers were followed longitudinally across the next 6 years until school age (9–13 years), long sleep onset latency and refusal to sleep alone were significant independent predictors of depression and anxiety severity in children.[19] Problematic sleep is more likely when sleep hygiene is poor. A late bedtime correlates with a longer sleep latency and shorter total sleep time, whereas children requiring parental presence for sleep onset to occur tend to have more night wakings.[5] Shorter total sleep time was obtained when a consistent bedtime routine was lacking, a television was present in the bedroom, and regular caffeine consumption occurred.[6] Insomnia is fairly common in preschoolers, with problems in initiating or maintaining sleep present in perhaps as much as 15% to 30%.[5,20] Preschoolers with insomnia were more likely to have symptoms of generalized anxiety disorder, separation anxiety, and specific phobias than children without insomnia.[15]

Medical or psychiatric conditions such as asthma, medication use, restless legs, or anxiety can contribute to insomnia in children.[20] Insomnia is highly prevalent in children with neurodevelopmental issues, occurring in 30% to 80% of children with significant cognitive impairment of various causes.[20] Many complex issues may produce the high rate of insomnia in children with neurodevelopmental issues, including underlying abnormalities in the sleep-wake cycle and circadian rhythms, hypersensitivity to environmental factors, comorbid medical conditions such as epilepsy, and side effects of medications used to treat comorbid conditions.[14,20]

Treatment strategies for insomnia in preschoolers can include psychotherapy and medications. A task force appointed by the American Academy of Sleep Medicine found that across n = 52 studies examined, 80% of children treated with behavioral therapy for insomnia showed clinically significant improvement that was maintained at least for 3 to 6 months.[21] In particular, there was strong support for unmodified extinction (approach of not providing parental attention unless physical needs are present) and preventive parent education regarding habits conducive to sleep. In addition, there is evidence of efficacy with graduated extinction (approach of gradual withdrawal of parental attention unless physical needs are present), bedtime routines, and scheduled awakenings.[21]

Medications to aid in sleep onset are not well studied in children in general but can be considered if needed as an adjunct to behavioral strategies. Most children with insomnia do not require medications. Melatonin is a naturally occurring hormone secreted by the pineal gland, binding to receptors in the suprachiasmatic nucleus in the hypothalamus. Small doses of melatonin (eg, 0.5 mg) taken 5 to 7 hours before bedtime may help treat circadian rhythm disorder through a phase-shifting effect and larger doses (eg, 3–5 mg) taken closer to bedtime may help insomnia through a hypnotic effect.[20] Clonidine is commonly used for childhood insomnia and has some data suggesting efficacy, but there is a narrow therapeutic index.[20] Sedating antidepressants can be considered if concurrent mood issues exist.[20] Benzodiazepines act on gamma-aminobutyric acid (GABA) A receptors to shorten sleep latency, increase total sleep time, and improve sleep maintenance and anxiety. However, because of the risk of habituation, short-term use is preferred when possible.[20] The efficacy of nonbenzodiazepine receptor agonists, which bind selectively to GABA A receptor complexes, is not clear in young children, including the short-term agents zaleplon and zolpidem and long-term agents zolpidem-extended-release and eszopiclone.[20]

OSA is an important sleep disorder during the preschool age. Diagnostic criteria for pediatric OSA (adapted from the International Classification of Sleep Disorders, third edition)[22,23]:

Criteria A and B must be met:

A. The presence of 1 or more of the following:
  1. Snoring
  2. Labored, paradoxic, or obstructed breathing during the child's sleep
  3. Sleepiness, hyperactivity, behavioral problems, or learning problems
B. Sleep study shows 1 or more of the following:
  1. One or more obstructive apneas, mixed apneas, or hypopneas, per hour of sleep

2. A pattern of obstructive hypoventilation, defined as at least 25% of total sleep time with hypercapnia ($Paco_2$ >50 mm Hg) in association with 1 or more of the following:
   a. Snoring
   b. Flattening of the inspiratory nasal pressure waveform
   c. Paradoxic thoracoabdominal motion[22,23]

OSA is found in about 1% to 5% of children, most common in ages 2 to 6 years, in part caused by the tonsillar hypertrophy that is often present at this age.[24]

With regard to evaluation and treatment of OSA, revised guidelines of the American Academy of Pediatrics recommend that:

1. All children/adolescents should be screened for snoring.
2. Polysomnography should be performed in children/adolescents with snoring and symptoms/signs of OSA; if polysomnography is not available, then alternative diagnostic tests or referral to a specialist for more extensive evaluation may be considered.
3. Adenotonsillectomy is recommended as the first-line treatment of patients with adenotonsillar hypertrophy.
4. High-risk patients should be monitored as inpatients postoperatively.
5. Patients should be reevaluated postoperatively to determine whether further treatment is required. Objective testing should be performed in patients who are high risk or have persistent symptoms/signs of OSA after therapy.
6. Continuous positive airway pressure is recommended as treatment if adenotonsillectomy is not performed or if OSA persists postoperatively.
7. Weight loss is recommended in addition to other therapy in patients who are overweight or obese.
8. Intranasal corticosteroids are an option for children with mild OSA in whom adenotonsillectomy is contraindicated or for mild postoperative OSA.[24]

OSA has been shown to adversely affect areas of cognitive function such as vigilance, verbal learning, attention, executive function, and memory.[25–29] OSA has been associated with deficits in behavior and emotional regulation.[27] Possible pathophysiologic mechanisms that may contribute to behavioral deficits include hypoxia secondary to obstructive apneas/hypopneas and/or disrupted sleep architecture from frequent arousals during sleep.[27]

Parasomnias occur frequently in early childhood. Sleepwalking involves walking and possibly other complex behaviors initiated during partial arousals from slow wave sleep, including disorientation, incomplete response to questions, and anterograde and retrograde memory impairment.[23,30] Sleep terrors involve partial arousals from slow wave sleep and may include screaming, manifestations of fear, and sometimes inconsolable crying.[23,30] A study of n = 1940 children in Quebec found that night terrors peaked in prevalence at 1.5 years (34.4% of children; 95% CI, 32.3%–36.5%), and sleepwalking peaked in prevalence at 10 years (13.4%; 95% CI, 11.3%–15.5%).[30] During the preschool ages, sleep terrors and sleepwalking were common in this study. There was a 21% prevalence for night terrors at age 3 years and 13% prevalence at age 5 years, and a 2.6% prevalence for sleepwalking at 3 years and 5% prevalence at 5 years.[30] Sleepwalkers are more likely than nonsleepwalkers to complain of sleepiness, fatigue, insomnia, depressive and anxiety symptoms, and altered quality of life.[31] If sleepwalking events are frequent or dangerous, treatment can be considered. Improvement in sleepwalking can be induced by reducing the cause of sleep fragmentation, such as by treating OSA, if present. The most frequently used medication is clonazepam, with a response rate of about 73.7%, as described in a case series of n = 103 patients.[32,33]

The International Restless Legs Syndrome Study Group defined consensus diagnostic criteria for pediatric restless legs syndrome (RLS) in 2013, as:

1. An urge to move the legs, usually but not always accompanied by or thought to be caused by uncomfortable and unpleasant sensations in the legs.
2. The urge to move the legs and any accompanying unpleasant sensations begin or worsen during periods of rest or inactivity such as lying down or sitting.
3. The urge to move the legs and any accompanying unpleasant sensations are partially or totally relieved by movement, such as walking or stretching, at least as long as the activity continues.
4. The urge to move the legs and any accompanying unpleasant sensations during rest or inactivity only occur or are worse in the evening or night than during the day.
5. The occurrence of the above features is not solely accounted for as symptoms primary to another medical or a behavioral condition (eg, myalgia, venous stasis, leg edema, arthritis, leg cramps, positional discomfort, habitual foot tapping).[34]

The prevalence of RLS has not been well characterized in the preschool age group, but has been characterized in a large-scale study involving slightly older children. In the United States and United Kingdom, n = 10,523 families completed an Internet-based questionnaire, revealing that criteria for definite RLS were met by 1.9% of children 8 to 11 years old.[35] Parents of children 8 to 11 years old retrospectively reported the age of onset as less than 5 years old in 15%, 5 to 7 years old in 63%, and 8 years old or older in 22%[35] Restless legs symptoms are likely often mistaken for growing pains in preschoolers, especially if the key historical information about worsening with rest and amelioration with movement is not assessed. Growing pains are often present more in the late afternoon and evening hours, like restless legs symptoms, and are common in the preschool age group. A history of presumed growing pains was retrospectively more common in children with restless legs symptoms than in those without restless legs symptoms (80.6% vs 63.2%).[35] Periodic limb movements are frequent in children with restless leg symptoms. More than 5 periodic limb movements per hour have been reported in 63% to 74% of children with RLS (normal, <5 per hour for children).[36,37]

Psychiatric disorders are common in children with RLS, with 49.5% of children with RLS reporting a negative effect on mood, a lack of energy (40.8%), and an inability to concentrate on schoolwork/work (40.0%).[35] In a study of n = 374 children with RLS, attention-deficit/hyperactivity disorder (ADHD) was found in 25% of patients, mood disturbances in 29.1% of patients, anxiety disorders in 11.5% of patients, and behavioral disturbances in 10.9% of patients.[38] ADHD was more common in boys, and mood disturbances were more common in girls.[38] Iron deficiency is frequent in children with RLS. The rate of iron deficiency seems to be higher in children with ADHD and RLS (n = 6, 20.7%) than in children with ADHD but without RLS (n = 1, 1.7%; $P = .005$).[39]

SLEEP ISSUES IN CHILDREN WITH PSYCHIATRIC DIAGNOSES

Sleep issues are highly prevalent in children with psychiatric diagnoses, especially depression, anxiety, and ADHD. Up to 75% of children with depression may have some degree of insomnia[20] and up to 16% may have hypersomnia.[40] Children with anxiety are likely to have sleep issues, with 88% reporting at least 1 sleep issue, most commonly insomnia, nightmares, and reluctance/refusal to sleep alone.[41] Perhaps as many as one-third of children with ADHD have RLS.[39] Preschoolers with ADHD seem to have worse sleep quality than preschoolers without ADHD as measured by actigraphy, including increased nocturnal activity with more restless sleep (activity index, 31.57 vs 25.74; $P<.05$), more night-to-night variability for sleep time (56.44 vs 32.79; $P<.01$), and more waking episodes (mean 1.34 vs 0.98 per night; $P<.05$).[42] A meta-analysis of 9 articles (N = 246) found that stimulants were associated with long sleep latencies in children with ADHD. This effect was less evident when children were taking the stimulants for a longer duration and took less frequent dosing.[43]

HEALTH DISPARITIES

Behaviors that promote sleep, including a regular bedtime, reading at bedtime, and falling asleep in bed, were more common in the high-socioeconomic-status group compared with the low-socioeconomic-status group in a study of n = 84 3-year-old children.[44] Reasons cited for not following good sleep hygiene included inability and inconvenience.[44] Members of minority and low-income populations disproportionately have an inadequate duration of sleep and poor-quality sleep, possibly contributing to a range of disparities of health conditions, including cardiovascular disease.[45]

SUMMARY/DISCUSSION

Sleep issues seen during the preschool ages include insomnia, OSA, parasomnias, and RLS. Sleep disorders seem to exacerbate mood and attention disturbances. Treatment of sleep issues is important for long-term mental health. Referral to a pediatric sleep specialist can be considered whether the sleep issue seems complex or simple. A pediatric sleep appointment is especially suggested if the preschooler's sleep issue is not improving over multiple visits or if the child or family seems to be particularly affected. Evaluation by a pediatric sleep specialist may be helpful when a child has significant sleepiness, intractable insomnia, problematic or frequent parasomnias, restless leg symptoms, frequent awakenings during sleep, or persistent or severe OSA. Referrals can also be placed for sleep issues that seem to be straightforward but for which additional guidance is sought.

REFERENCES

1. Paruthi S, Brooks LJ, D'Ambrosio C, et al. Recommended amount of sleep for pediatric populations: a consensus statement of the American Academy of Sleep Medicine. J Clin Sleep Med 2016;12(6):785–6.
2. Wang F, Liu H, Wan Y, et al. Sleep duration and overweight/obesity in preschool-aged children: a prospective study of up to 48,922 children of the Jiaxing birth cohort. Sleep 2016;39(11):2013–9.
3. Patel SR, Hu FB. Short sleep duration and weight gain: a systematic review. Obesity (Silver Spring) 2008;16(3):643–53.
4. Mullins EN, Miller AL, Cherian SS, et al. Acute sleep restriction increases dietary intake in preschool-age children. J Sleep Res 2017;26(1):48–54.
5. Mindell JA, Meltzer LJ, Carskadon MA, et al. Developmental aspects of sleep hygiene: findings from the 2004 National Sleep Foundation sleep in America poll. Sleep Med 2009;10(7):771–9.
6. Mindell JA, Li AM, Sadeh A, et al. Bedtime routines for young children: a dose-dependent association with sleep outcomes. Sleep 2015;38(5):717–22.
7. Weissbluth M. Naps in children: 6 months-7 years. Sleep 1995;18(2):82–7.
8. Kurdziel L, Duclos K, Spencer RM. Sleep spindles in midday naps enhance learning in preschool children. Proc Natl Acad Sci U S A 2013;110(43):17267–72.

9. Backhaus J, Hoeckesfeld R, Born J, et al. Immediate as well as delayed post learning sleep but not wakefulness enhances declarative memory consolidation in children. Neurobiol Learn Mem 2008;89(1):76–80.

10. Adan A, Archer SN, Hidalgo MP, et al. Circadian typology: a comprehensive review. Chronobiol Int 2012;29(9):1153–75.

11. Barclay NL, Eley TC, Parsons MJ, et al. Monozygotic twin differences in non-shared environmental factors associated with chronotype. J Biol Rhythms 2013; 28(1):51–61.

12. Doi Y, Ishihara K, Uchiyama M. Epidemiological study on chronotype among pre-school children in Japan: prevalence, sleep-wake patterns, and associated factors. Chronobiol Int 2016;33:1340–50.

13. Paavonen EJ, Porkka-Heiskanen T, Lahikainen AR. Sleep quality, duration and behavioral symptoms among 5-6-year-old children. Eur Child Adolesc Psychiatry 2009;18(12):747–54.

14. Wiggs L. Sleep problems in children with developmental disorders. J R Soc Med 2001;94(4):177–9.

15. Steinsbekk S, Berg-Nielsen TS, Wichstrøm L. Sleep disorders in preschoolers: prevalence and comorbidity with psychiatric symptoms. J Dev Behav Pediatr 2013;34(9):633–41.

16. Wen JG, Wang QW, Chen Y, et al. An epidemiological study of primary nocturnal enuresis in Chinese children and adolescents. Eur Urol 2006;49(6):1107–13.

17. Su MS, Li AM, So HK, et al. Nocturnal enuresis in children: prevalence, correlates, and relationship with obstructive sleep apnea. J Pediatr 2011;159(2):238–42.

18. Simard V, Nielsen T, Tremblay R, et al. Longitudinal study of bad dreams in preschool-aged children: prevalence, demographic correlates, risk and protective factors. Sleep 2008;31(1):62–70.

19. Whalen DJ, Gilbert KE, Barch DM, et al. Variation in common preschool sleep problems as an early predictor for depression and anxiety symptom severity across time. J Child Psychol Psychiatry 2017;58(2):151–9.

20. Owens JA, Mindell JA. Pediatric insomnia. Pediatr Clin North Am 2011;58(3): 555–69.

21. Mindell JA, Kuhn B, Lewin DS, et al, American Academy of Sleep Medicine. Behavioral treatment of bedtime problems and night wakings in infants and young children. Sleep 2006;29(10):1263–76.

22. Zuconni M, Ferri R. Assessment of sleep disorders and diagnostic procedures: classification of sleep disorders. In: Bassetti C, Dogas Z, Philippe Peigneux P, editors. Sleep medicine textbook. Regensburg (Germany): European Sleep Research Society (ESRS); 2014. p. 97–100.

23. American Academy of Sleep Medicine. International classification of sleep disorders. 3rd edition. Darien (IL): American Academy of Sleep Medicine; 2014.

24. Marcus CL, Brooks LJ, Draper KA, et al, American Academy of Pediatrics. Diagnosis and management of childhood obstructive sleep apnea syndrome. Pediatrics 2012;130(3):576–84.

25. Beebe DW. Neurobehavioral morbidity associated with disordered breathing during sleep in children: a comprehensive review. Sleep 2006;29(9):1115–34.

26. Adams N, Strauss M, Schluchter M, et al. Relation of measures of sleep-disordered breathing to neuropsychological functioning. Am J Respir Crit Care Med 2001;163(7):1626–31.

27. Berry DT, Webb WB, Block AJ, et al. Nocturnal hypoxia and neuropsychological variables. J Clin Exp Neuropsychol 1986;8(3):229–38.

28. Quan SF, Archbold K, Gevins AS, et al. Long-term neurophysiologic impact of childhood sleep disordered breathing on neurocognitive performance. Southwest J Pulm Crit Care 2013;7(3):165–75.
29. de Carvalho LB, do Prado LB, Ferrreira VR, et al. Symptoms of sleep disorders and objective academic performance. Sleep Med 2013;14(9):872–6.
30. Petit D, Pennestri MH, Paquet J, et al. Childhood sleepwalking and sleep terrors: a longitudinal study of prevalence and familial aggregation. JAMA Pediatr 2015; 169(7):653–8.
31. Lopez R, Jaussent I, Scholz S, et al. Functional impairment in adult sleepwalkers: a case-control study. Sleep 2013;36(3):345–51.
32. Cochen De Cock V. Sleepwalking. Curr Treat Options Neurol 2016;18(2):6.
33. Attarian H, Zhu L. Treatment options for disorders of arousal: a case series. Int J Neurosci 2013;123(9):623–5.
34. Picchietti DL, Bruni O, de Weerd A, et al. International restless Legs Syndrome Study Group (IRLSSG). Pediatric restless legs syndrome diagnostic criteria: an update by the International Restless Legs Syndrome Study Group. Sleep Med 2013;14(12):1253–9.
35. Picchietti D, Allen RP, Walters AS, et al. Restless legs syndrome: prevalence and impact in children and adolescents–the Peds REST study. Pediatrics 2007;120(2): 253–66.
36. Picchietti DL, Rajendran RR, Wilson MP, et al. Pediatric restless legs syndrome and periodic limb movement disorder: parent–child pairs. Sleep Med 2009; 10(8):925–31.
37. Muhle H, Neumann A, Lohmann-Hedrich K, et al. Childhood-onset restless legs syndrome: clinical and genetic features of 22 families. Mov Disord 2008;23(8): 1113–21.
38. Pullen SJ, Wall CA, Angstman ER, et al. Psychiatric comorbidity in children and adolescents with restless legs syndrome: a retrospective study. J Clin Sleep Med 2011;7(6):587–96.
39. Oner P, Dirik EB, Taner Y, et al. Association between low serum ferritin and restless legs syndrome in patients with attention deficit hyperactivity disorder. Tohoku J Exp Med 2007;213(3):269–76.
40. Ryan ND, Puig-Antich J, Ambrosini P, et al. The clinical picture of major depression in children and adolescents. Arch Gen Psychiatry 1987;44(10):854–61.
41. Alfano CA, Ginsburg GS, Kingery JN. Sleep-related problems among children and adolescents with anxiety disorders. J Am Acad Child Adolesc Psychiatry 2007;46(2):224–32.
42. Melegari MG, Vittori E, Mallia L, et al. Actigraphic sleep pattern of preschoolers with ADHD. J Atten Disord 2016. [Epub ahead of print].
43. Kidwell KM, Van Dyk TR, Lundahl A, et al. Stimulant medications and sleep for youth with ADHD: a meta-analysis. Pediatrics 2015;136(6):1144–53.
44. Jones CH, Ball H. Exploring socioeconomic differences in bedtime behaviours and sleep duration in English preschool children. Infant Child Dev 2014;23(5): 518–31.
45. Jackson CL, Redline S, Emmons KM. Sleep as a potential fundamental contributor to disparities in cardiovascular health. Annu Rev Public Health 2015;36: 417–40.

Setting the Stage for Collaboration and Future Directions

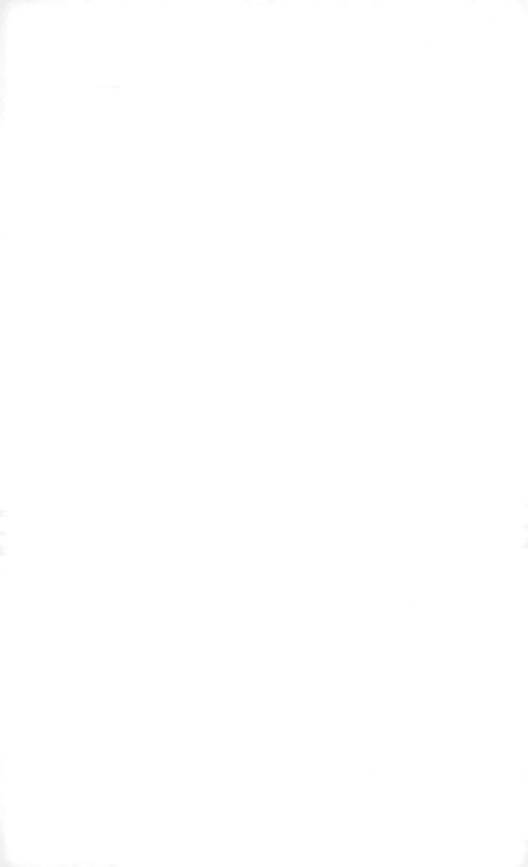

Partnerships with Primary Care for the Treatment of Preschoolers

Sheila M. Marcus, MD*, Nasuh M. Malas, MD, MPH,
Joanna M. Quigley, MD, Katherine L. Rosenblum, PhD,
Maria Muzik, MD, MS, Dayna J. LePlatte-Ogini, MD,
Paresh D. Patel, MD, PhD

KEYWORDS

- Preschool mental health • Integrated care • Collaborative care • Telepsychiatry

KEY POINTS

- This article informs the reader about access issues in child psychiatry and how access impacts the appropriate diagnosis and treatment of preschool children.
- The article presents a model for a collaborative care program in Michigan (Michigan Child Collaborative Care Program [MC3]), which is a program providing phone-based and telepsychiatric consultation in primary care in 40 counties in the state of Michigan.
- The article describes demographic and diagnostic data from preschool children referred to the MC3 program.

BACKGROUND

The first years of life provide a critical window to promote healthy social and emotional development across the life span,[1] and systems of care that support the cognitive and emotional development in early childhood can play a crucial role in addressing issues that have both quality-of-life and cost implications. Early detection of preschool mental health begins in the primary care setting.[2] Primary care physicians (PCPs) work closely with families in early childhood administering regularly scheduled well-child visits, treating illnesses common to preschoolers, and supporting families with regard to infant behavioral regulation, sleep, and nutrition. PCPs are ideally suited to identify risk factors for preschool behavioral disorders. Although infants and

Disclosure: This program is funded by The Health and Human Services Department of Centers for Medicare and Medicaid Services (MA No. 20170199-00) and The Michigan State of Health and Human Service (MA No. 20170199-00). Past funding has also included The Mary Meader Foundation (G009566) and The Ravitz Foundation (G007220).
Department of Psychiatry, University of Michigan, 4250 Plymouth Road, Ann Arbor, MI 48109, USA
* Corresponding author.
E-mail address: smmarcus@med.umich.edu

toddlers may exhibit externalizing behavioral problems ranging from social to developmental delays, these children are less likely to be identified by their parents, who may perceive these problems as developmentally appropriate or transient.[3,4] Thus, the burden of identification falls on PCPs who may have a window of opportunity to identify social and developmental delays, perturbation of the parent-child relationship, or trauma.

Despite frequent visits to primary care, most youths with mental health conditions do not receive care for their conditions.[5–8] Chronic stress and adverse life events can have a toxic effect on the developing young brain.[9,10] Failure to detect and treat psychiatric conditions in early childhood can undermine social and academic development and may negatively impact relational security.[11–14] Preschool children are even less likely than older children to be identified for treatment; when identified, only about half attend treatment.[15] There are important psychosocial barriers (such as poverty) as well as practical barriers (childcare, transportation) that disproportionately impact access to care for young children.[16] Therefore, it is imperative that PCPs have access to behavioral health expertise and support, ideally through trained clinicians who can partner with the PCP and families to provide education and collaborate on referrals for mental health resources in the community that are feasible for the family.

PCPs s are often willing to treat mild behavioral health conditions, particularly in rural areas,[17–21] but report discomfort treating more complex conditions,[22] including those in early childhood. PCPs can often recognize and appreciate the high frequency of common behavioral conditions in their practice, the difference between normal development and psychopathology, and the value of psychotherapeutic intervention for behavioral psychopathology. This recognition is critical for families, as PCP recommendations are the best predictor of parents seeking further care for preschool behavior problems.[23]

Medical silos, time constraints inherent in PCP visits, limited numbers of child mental health providers, and limited care coordination between medical and behavioral health conditions have been linked to the undertreatment of mental health conditions. For high-risk children, PCPs note lack of access to child psychiatric care either due to long waits or lack of available providers. This failure of the systems of care leaves young children at risk for devastating long-term outcomes, including increased health care utilization, poor academic outcomes, and later mental health issues.[24]

The emerging evidence about integrated care strategies and economic scaffolding provided through the Affordable Care Act has enabled many PCP offices to employ an embedded behavioral health consultant (BHC). This BHC is usually a master's level social worker who assists with assessment, local mental health referrals, provision of mental health education, and brief behavioral therapy, often using techniques of motivational interviewing and behavioral activation to increase engagement of patients and families. In a 2012 study, BHC involvement was shown to result in high levels of parental satisfaction, enhanced access to behavioral services, and improved behavioral outcomes in children with mental health conditions.[25] In most of these integrated programs, however, there is no child psychiatric involvement, which is related both to availability and expense.

Infant and early childhood psychiatrists are individuals trained in highly specialized assessments of preschoolers, including a developmentally appropriate, relationally sensitive evaluation of common disorders (autism and other developmental disorders, anxiety, trauma, disruptive behavioral disorders) as well as the parent-child dyad. Access to child psychiatrists familiar with preschool mental health is markedly poor because of the overwhelming demand for services. This problem is further compounded by the scarcity of child psychiatry training programs with specific clinical expertise in early childhood, further straining the demand for infant and early childhood psychiatrists.

INCREASING ACCESS TO EARLY CHILDHOOD MENTAL HEALTH CARE

Many academic child psychiatry programs are developing regional and state partnerships with PCPs to improve access to psychiatric care in underserved communities. Both the American Academy of Pediatrics and the American Academy of Child and Adolescent Psychiatry endorse such programs to improve access to mental health care in high-risk regions of the country. These programs provide embedded and remote access to specialty child psychiatrists and may include embedded BHCs. In areas with greater access to academic centers, the programs may offer select face-to-face evaluations for diagnostically complex youths. Relative to traditional specialty services, these programs are economical and connect PCPs with a regional team of mental health specialists who provide remote consultations and refer the most complex patients to more intense mental health treatment. For those youths with mild-moderate mental health conditions, the PCP determines the treatment plan and provides ongoing prescribing with backup consultation from the psychiatrist. For young children, most commonly, recommendations are for behavioral treatments, which can be facilitated through a regional BHC. Currently, there is a major national initiative through the National Network of Child Psychiatry Access Programs (www.nncpap.org) to promote the use of such consultation programs for children and adolescents served in community-based practices with limited access to mental health specialists. There are now 30 consultation programs nationally with improved access to psychiatric care demonstrated in 2 states with rigorous evaluations.[26–28] The ability of these programs to deliver subspecialized care to very young children is impacted by the presence of psychiatrists specifically trained in early childhood within the regions where they are located.

TELEPSYCHIATRY AND CHILDREN

Telepsychiatry is a promising approach that has been used to improve access to mental health clinicians. A cost-effective delivery, it provides video linkages between patients and specialists who are geographically distant. It is acceptable to patients and feasible in most settings and improves remote access to mental health clinicians.[29] Several studies have demonstrated that telepsychiatry can be successful in a variety of settings and patient populations, including patients with developmental disabilities[30] and patients in rural settings.[31] Although most of the literature centers on adult patients, telepsychiatry has been useful for children as young as 3 years old.[32] Literature reviews demonstrate no difference in acceptance of telepsychiatry from in-person assessments,[33] and parents report a positive experience noting both improvements in access and satisfaction with care received during the consultations.[34] In a randomized control trial in which patients were assessed both in person and using telepsychiatry, there were no significant differences in the diagnosis and treatment recommendations between the two assessment processes.[35]

OVERVIEW: THE MICHIGAN CHILD COLLABORATIVE CARE PROGRAM

The Michigan Child Collaborative Care Program (MC3) is a consultation program providing phone-based mental health consultations to PCPs and telepsychiatry (videoconferencing) evaluations to patients and families in 40 counties in Michigan. It is funded through state, federal, and private dollars to enhance integration of mental health services to youths and pregnant and postpartum women.

MC3 provides both virtual and colocated services to high-risk patients without access to child and perinatal psychiatrists. PCPs in private offices, federally qualified health centers, rural health centers, and school-based health centers have been enrolled in each county. There are no payer restrictions, and the program serves youths aged 0 to 26 years as well as pregnant and postpartum women of all ages. The program funds Community Mental Health–affiliated BHCs who are assigned by region to provide coverage to primary care practices. The BHCs facilitate phone consultations that link PCPs with child and perinatal psychiatrists. They are responsible for locating and connecting patients and families with local mental health resources. For complex cases requiring a more comprehensive diagnostic assessment, the BHC will facilitate a telepsychiatry consultation. In larger practices, the BHCs are embedded part-time and are available onsite for referrals, psychoeducation, motivational interviewing, and connecting families with local mental health resources. In select practices, the BHCs are also available to work with PCPs to triage and refer those patients with positive screens for autism. BHCs assist in determining which children require further evaluation using the Autism Diagnostic Observation Scale (ADOS) and help PCPs negotiate the labyrinth of behavioral assessments and services necessary for children newly diagnosed with autism. As part of the services offered through MC3, BHCs work closely with clinic and practice leadership to integrate MC3 into their clinical workflow so that screening, assessment, and MC3 consultation, as necessary, are tailored to the needs of a particular clinical environment.

Phone consultations are most commonly real-time consultations requested by the PCPs, most often for guidance related to diagnosis or medication management. Responses from child and perinatal psychiatrists typically occur within 2 to 4 hours (Monday–Friday, 8 AM–5 PM). PCPs will often determine which cases in their following day might require phone consultation and arrange consultation before the next office visit to maximize efficiency. In phone consultations, only initials and dates of birth are provided without exchange of identifying protected health information. These phone consultations usually take 20 to 30 minutes, including the clinician conversation and necessary documentation. Data gathered at the time of the phone consultation include the child's initials; date of birth; presenting concerns; current and past psychotropic use; brief illness course; current psychotherapies; previous diagnostic/screening evaluations; need for hospitalization, including suicidality assessment; and rapid overview of parenting behavior/psychosocial strain and trauma. This consultation may also include a brief review of pertinent medical and family history. This information is collected and uploaded by the BHC who alerts the psychiatrist to the waiting consult by page or instant message. The psychiatrist is then able to access this information remotely, engage the PCP in a conversation to further gather any additional pertinent history, and respond to the PCP query regarding diagnostic evaluation, psychotherapy, pharmacotherapy, and pursuing additional school-based services or community mental health resources. Following the phone consultation, the child psychiatrist will pull in information gathered from the PCP and BHC into a standardized documentation template on a secure, internal electronic medical record and provide brief documentation on the contents of the call, the assessment, and subsequent recommendations. This document is then provided to the PCP by the BHC within 24 hours of the call.

Another option for consultation is a group case consultation format allowing providers to review multiple cases in a scheduled hour. These reviews are conducted via video and telephonic conference for groups of PCPs, nurse practitioners, physician assistants, and trainees. One advantage of this model is that it enhances group learning so that evidence-based guidelines can be standardized within a group practice. It also fosters greater relationship building with the child psychiatrist.

For those patients who require repeat consultations or who are diagnostically challenging, the BHC, child psychiatrist, and PCP may make a joint decision for a telepsychiatric visit. In these cases, the BHC obtains consent for telepsychiatric evaluation from the parent or legal guardian. Most telepsychiatric consultations can be arranged within 2 weeks. Typically, the interview is conducted similarly to a face-to-face interview, with a parent interview, a separate child interview depending on the age of the child, and observation of the parent-child interaction as elaborated later. Following the visit, a copy of the consultation note is faxed to the PCP.

POPULATION DEMOGRAPHICS

Michigan is a diverse state with large urban and rural underserved areas. The southeast region is urban, with the automotive industry having a significant presence as one of the chief employers in the area. Other regions of Michigan are rural, with farming and tourism dominating the economy. About 1 in 4 children in Michigan grow up in poverty. State estimates suggest 53,000 children have an incarcerated parent and about 190,000 have a parent with a significant mental illness. In 2014, there were 21,049 substantiated cases of childhood neglect involving 30,953 children; 38% of these children were younger than 4 years.[36] Many of these high-risk youths have no access to child psychiatrists, and in most counties in Michigan there are no child psychiatrists. The prevalence of child psychiatrists by geography is shown in **Fig. 1**.[37]

Telepsychiatry Preschool Assessment

The University of Michigan has a clinic, the Infant and Early Childhood Clinic (IECC), dedicated to evaluations of preschool children that served as a model for the telepsychiatric

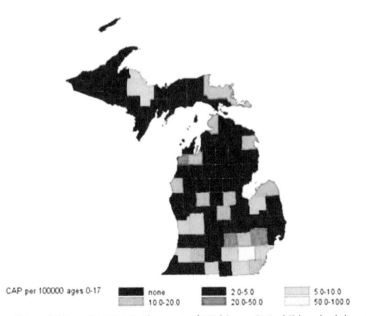

Fig. 1. Practicing child psychiatrists in the state of Michigan. CAP, child and adolescent psychiatrist. (*From* Holzer CE. American Academy of Child & Adolescent Psychiatry. Available at: http://www.aacap.org/aacap/Advocacy/Federal_and_State_Initiatives/Workforce_Maps/Michigan.aspx. Accessed August 31, 2016; with permission.)

assessment. In IECC, a comprehensive parent interview is conducted and relational qualities are assessed using several questions from the Working Model of The Child Interview (Zeanah CH, Benoit D, Barton M. Working model of the child interview, unpublished work, 1986). Following the interview, there is an observational assessment of parent-child interaction using a modification of structured interactive tasks (Crowell Problem Solving Procedure[38]) and child attachment assessment via the Strange Situation. Parents also complete standard normed questionnaires to assess child behavior problems (Infant-Toddler Social and Emotional Assessment[39]; Child Behavioral Check List [CBCL][40]), social communication (Social Communication Questionnaire [SCQ][41]), and trauma (Trauma Symptom Checklist for Young Children [TSCYC][42]).

A variation of the protocol outlined earlier for the IECC is used for all telepsychiatric visits for young children. Before the telepsychiatry clinic visit, the BHC orients the parent to the visit and collects survey information, including the CBCL,[40] the SCQ,[41] and a general Health History Questionnaire. An interview with parents is conducted eliciting the standard components of a psychiatric assessment including chief complaint, present illness, medical, birth/developmental, social and family history. During the parent interview, a small set of selected questions from the Working Model of the Child Interview[38] were chosen, such as the following: Tell me about your child's personality, what he or she likes. Give me 3 words or phrases that describe your relationship with your child. Give me an example so that I can understand why you chose this word. Often the BHC will take the child into an adjacent waiting area to play during part of the interview to allow parents to have privacy while communicating sensitive information. Following the interview, observational assessments of the child using structured tasks are obtained and commonly include a free-play task, cleanup task, and emotional-drawing task.[38]

The telepsychiatry evaluation allows for a comprehensive evaluation of the child and enables the clinician to observe parent-child interaction to determine the quality of the parent-child dyad. Elements of the preschool mental status examination can be easily assessed via telepsychiatry using the modified Crowell procedure, including frustration tolerance, attention, concentration, language, mood/affect, gross cognitive capabilities, eye contact (with parent), social relatedness, and social referencing. Additionally, qualities of the parent-child relationship, including the degree to which the parent scaffolds the child in a challenging task, the parent's capacity to coregulate the child, the level of support/delight expressed versus intrusiveness or hostility, and the general qualities of the parent-child dance can all be viewed during the telepsychiatric interview. The telepsychiatric interview is not videotaped; the entire session is completed in about 90 minutes, as in live evaluations. Recommendations are shared with the parent and the BHC; the PCP is then called with pharmacotherapy recommendations (if any), psychotherapy, and general diagnostic considerations. During the parent recommendations, parenting strengths, acknowledgment of the child's challenging behavior (and how recommended interventions will help), and evidence of the importance of the parent-child relationship are shared with the parent and the BHC.

RESULTS: DATA FROM THE MICHIGAN CHILD COLLABORATIVE CARE PROGRAM
Primary Care Providers

MC3 was initially launched in May 2012. As of May 2016, the program has enrolled 894 primary care clinicians in 40 counties in Michigan. The program is working with 19 community mental health regions and 5 school-based programs. A survey of PCP satisfaction (N = 33) suggested high rates of satisfaction, with 85% "strongly agreeing" and 12% "agreeing" with the following question: "I felt more confident that I could effectively treat this child's behavior problems as a result of this consultation."

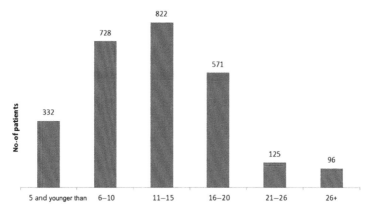

Fig. 2. Age distribution (MC3 consultations, all ages).

Patient Referrals: All Ages

There were 2676 unique patient referrals for all services. Youth patients ranged in age from 0 to 26 years with perinatal patients aged up to 43 years. Preschool children represented about 12.4% of the total patient referrals. The age distribution of the overall group is shown in **Fig. 2**. Of the patients referred, 98% had no contact with psychiatrists at the time of the consultation.

Patient Referrals: Preschool Children

There were 92 preschool children (aged from newborn through the end of their fifth year) who were presented to the child psychiatrist for phone consultation in the period from May 2012 to May 2016. **Fig. 3** is a graph of an age distribution of these youths. Of the total consultations, 66 (72%) were male and 26 (28%) were female.

The following diagnoses were considered by the psychiatrists (**Fig. 4**).

Attention-deficit/hyperactivity disorder (ADHD) and disruptive behavioral disorders were the most common presumptive diagnoses that the PCP discussed with the child psychiatrist. Frequently, with further exploration of the history and presentation with the PCP, the differential diagnosis was expanded to include anxiety (with externalizing symptoms), posttraumatic stress disorder (PTSD) or traumatic stress reaction, and autism spectrum disorder. These diagnoses often suggested a deeper explanatory model for the child's disruptive behavior. Parent-child relational issues were also surfaced (but not always specified diagnostically). PCPs anecdotally noted that the conversations prompted them to widen their perspective and consider questions about *why* a child was acting this way versus how he was behaving. Features of autism

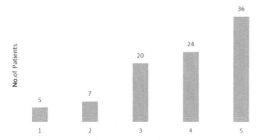

Fig. 3. Age distribution (MC3 consultations, preschool).

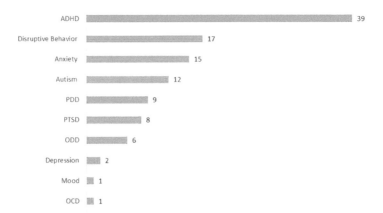

Fig. 4. Diagnostic considerations (MC3 consultations, preschool). ADHD, attention-deficit/ hyperactivity disorder; CAPP, child and adolescent psychiatrist; OCD, obsessive-compulsive disorder; ODD, oppositional defiant disorder; PDD, pervasive developmental delay; PTSD, post-traumatic stress disorder.

spectrum disorder (ASD) were commonly discussed; in 36% of the consultations, the need for further testing with the ADOS was reviewed with the PCP. Although initially not presenting trauma as a presenting concern, 21% of all preschool youths were identified as having a potential history of trauma, abuse, or neglect during the phone consultation with the child psychiatrist.

Pharmacotherapy in Preschoolers

Of the 92 preschool children discussed in phone consultation, 21 (23%) were on at least one psychotropic prescription at the time of the initial MC3 consult. There was an average of 1.95 prescriptions per patient (**Fig. 5**). Stimulants were most commonly prescribed, followed by alpha agonists and atypical neuroleptics.

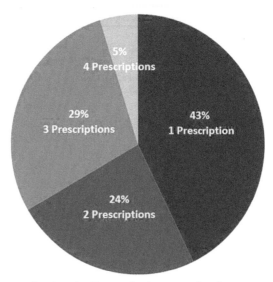

Fig. 5. Prescription medications (MC3 consultations, preschool).

Referrals to Behavioral Health Consultant for Preschoolers

There was a total of 264 patients, aged 0 to 5 years, referred for BHC services. Most of these patient queries (36%) centered on referral information and parenting/behavioral management support. In some cases, there were several reasons for the referral; thus, the percentages total greater than 100% (**Fig. 6**A). Noteworthy is the concern regarding escalating disruptive behavior, often reflecting parents' helplessness in managing the behavior, relational concerns, trauma, and in some cases autistic traits in the child. Some of these concerns would be referred on to higher level of care (community mental health) or to MC3 psychiatric consultation to assist with diagnostic clarification and for treatment planning. Although psychotherapy resources were very commonly requested, the BHCs reported frustration in finding these resources, especially in more rural areas. Specific psychotherapy resources (trauma-informed psychotherapy for young children, developmentally relationally informed psychotherapy

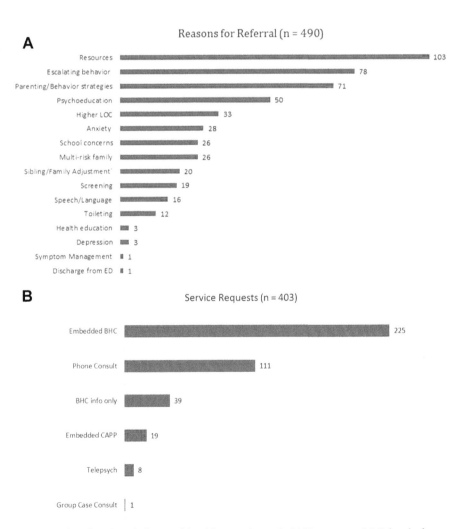

Fig. 6. (*A, B*) Referrals to behavioral health consultants in MC3 program. LOC, level of care.

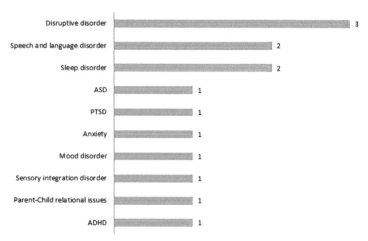

Fig. 7. Telepsychiatric consultations in MC3 program.

services) were likewise challenging to find. This challenge was compounded by the challenges of negotiating coverage for services with private insurance providers or patients deemed noneligible for infant mental health services.

Telepsychiatry Summary (Ages 0–5 Years)

There were 8 telepsychiatric consultations for patients 5 years of age or younger.

Seven unique patients, 5 male and 2 female, were served in this time period. One patient (14%) was 2 years old, 4 were 3 years old (57%), 1 was 4 years old (14%) at first consultation and 5 years old at the second consultation, and 1 was 5 years old (14%) at the time of consultation. Three patients had Medicaid health insurance (43%), whereas 4 patients had commercial health insurance (57%) (**Fig. 7**).

As with the phone consultations, those children with disruptive behavior disorders were often diagnosed with co-occurring anxiety, traumatic, language, sensory, or mood disorders.

SUMMARY

There is a significant shortage of child psychiatrists, particularly those with expertise in preschool children. Collaborative care programs, such as MC3, which allow for PCP phone consultation and patient telepsychiatric consultations with child psychiatrists, allow preschool children access to this expertise. PCPs report high levels of satisfaction with this service and feel more confident in managing children within their practices as a result of the program. Preschoolers are most frequently referred to BHCs and child psychiatrists in the MC3 for diagnostic clarification, referral information, and pharmacotherapy expertise. A significant percentage (23%) of preschoolers are on medication at the time of the phone consultation. ADHD and nonspecific disruptive behaviors are the most common diagnoses considered for these youths and may be driving pharmacotherapy decisions. In 21% of the preschool phone consultations, trauma was surfaced as a potential contributor to the child's behavior. The introduction of this possibility changed the treatment algorithm for these youths. The MC3 consultation can assist further diagnostic clarification and assist PCPs in developing a more nuanced approach to the diagnosis and management of these children.

Commonly, the preschool children referred for telepsychiatric consultation were complex, and the presenting disruptive behaviors were often likely to be attributed to undiagnosed anxiety, autism spectrum, parent-child relational disorders, trauma, or a combination of these factors. PCPs very appropriately used BHCs to assist in finding mental health referral resources, particularly psychotherapy, for young children. BHCs report frustration in finding appropriate trauma-informed, evidence-based programs for young children; additional programmatic research to improve both remote and in-person training in evidence-based therapies will be essential to provide alternatives to pharmacotherapy for young children and to maximize clinical outcomes in this population.

ACKNOWLEDGMENTS

The authors would like to acknowledge Richard R. Dopp, MD, Anne Kramer, LMSW, Erin Hughes-Krieger, LMSW, Jane Spinner, MSW, MBA, and Elizabeth Tengelitsch, PhD, for their assistance with this article.

REFERENCES

1. National Research Council (US) and Institute of Medicine (US) Committee on Integrating the Science of Early Childhood Development. From neurons to neighborhoods: the science of early childhood development. In: Shonkoff JP, Phillips DA, editors. Washington, DC: National Academies Press; 2000. Available at: http://www.ncbi.nlm.nih.gov/books/NBK225557/. Accessed September 22, 2016.
2. Heckman JJ, Masterov DV. The productivity argument for investing in young children. Cambridge (MA): National Bureau of Economic Research; 2007. Available at: http://www.nber.org/papers/w13016. Accessed September 22, 2016.
3. Glascoe FP. Parents' evaluation of developmental status: how well do parents' concerns identify children with behavioral and emotional problems? Clin Pediatr (Phila) 2003;42(2):133–8.
4. Ellingson KD, Briggs-Gowan MJ, Carter AS, et al. Parent identification of early emerging child behavior problems: predictors of sharing parental concern with health providers. Arch Pediatr Adolesc Med 2004;158(8):766–72.
5. Jaycox LH, Stein BD, Paddock S, et al. Impact of teen depression on academic, social, and physical functioning. Pediatrics 2009;124(4):e596–605.
6. A 14-month randomized clinical trial of treatment strategies for attention-deficit/hyperactivity disorder. The MTA Cooperative Group. Multimodal Treatment Study of Children with ADHD. Arch Gen Psychiatry 1999;56(12):1073–86.
7. Merikangas KR, He J, Burstein M, et al. Service utilization for lifetime mental disorders in U.S. adolescents: results of the National Comorbidity Survey-Adolescent Supplement (NCS-A). J Am Acad Child Adolesc Psychiatry 2011;50(1):32–45.
8. Merikangas KR, He J-P, Brody D, et al. Prevalence and treatment of mental disorders among US children in the 2001-2004 NHANES. Pediatrics 2010;125(1):75–81.
9. Dong M, Anda RF, Felitti VJ, et al. The interrelatedness of multiple forms of childhood abuse, neglect, and household dysfunction. Child Abuse Negl 2004;28(7):771–84.
10. Edwards VJ, Holden GW, Felitti VJ, et al. Relationship between multiple forms of childhood maltreatment and adult mental health in community respondents: results from the adverse childhood experiences study. Am J Psychiatry 2003;160(8):1453–60.

11. Ghandour RM, Kogan MD, Blumberg SJ, et al. Mental health conditions among school-aged children: geographic and sociodemographic patterns in prevalence and treatment. J Dev Behav Pediatr 2012;33(1):42–54.

12. Costello EJ, Mustillo S, Erkanli A, et al. Prevalence and development of psychiatric disorders in childhood and adolescence. Arch Gen Psychiatry 2003;60(8): 837–44.

13. Kim WJ. American Academy of Child and Adolescent Psychiatry Task Force on Workforce Needs. Child and adolescent psychiatry workforce: a critical shortage and national challenge. Acad Psychiatry 2003;27(4):277–82.

14. Berdahl TA, Friedman BS, McCormick MC, et al. Annual report on health care for children and youth in the United States: trends in racial/ethnic, income, and insurance disparities over time, 2002-2009. Acad Pediatr 2013;13(3):191–203.

15. Godoy L, Carter AS, Silver RB, et al. Mental health screening and consultation in primary care: the role of child age and parental concerns [corrected]. J Dev Behav Pediatr 2014;35(5):334–43.

16. Office of the Surgeon General (US), Center for Mental Health Services (US), National Institute of Mental Health (US). Mental health: culture, race, and ethnicity: a supplement to mental health: a report of the surgeon general. Rockville (MD): Substance Abuse and Mental Health Services Administration (US); 2001. Available at: http://www.ncbi.nlm.nih.gov/books/NBK44243/. Accessed October 10, 2016.

17. Brown JD, Wissow LS. Discussion of sensitive health topics with youth during primary care visits: relationship to youth perceptions of care. J Adolesc Health 2009; 44(1):48–54.

18. Garbutt JM, Leege E, Sterkel R, et al. Providing depression care in the medical home: what can we learn from ADHD? Arch Pediatr Adolesc Med 2012;166(7): 672–3.

19. Stensrud TL, Mjaaland TA, Finset A. Communication and mental health in general practice: physicians' self-perceived learning needs and self-efficacy. Ment Health Fam Med 2012;9(3):201–9.

20. Zuckerbrot RA, Cheung AH, Jensen PS, et al, GLAD-PC Steering Group. Guidelines for adolescent depression in primary care (GLAD-PC): I. Identification, assessment, and initial management. Pediatrics 2007;120(5):e1299–1312.

21. Cheung AH, Zuckerbrot RA, Jensen PS, et al. Guidelines for adolescent depression in primary care (GLAD-PC): II. Treatment and ongoing management. Pediatrics 2007;120(5):e1313–26.

22. Stein REK, Horwitz SM, Storfer-Isser A, et al. Do pediatricians think they are responsible for identification and management of child mental health problems? Results of the AAP periodic survey. Ambul Pediatr 2008;8(1):11–7.

23. Fanton JH, MacDonald B, Harvey EA. Preschool parent-pediatrician consultations and predictive referral patterns for problematic behaviors. J Dev Behav Pediatr 2008;29(6):475–82.

24. Dunlap G, Strain PS, Fox L, et al. Prevention and intervention with young children's challenging behavior: perspectives regarding current knowledge. Behav Disord 2006;32(1):29–45.

25. Kolko DJ, Campo JV, Kilbourne AM, et al. Doctor-office collaborative care for pediatric behavioral problems: a preliminary clinical trial. Arch Pediatr Adolesc Med 2012;166(3):224–31.

26. Kilbourne AM, Spinner J, Kramer A, et al. Sustainable lifelines: supporting integrated behavioral health services for children and adolescents in the accountable care era. American Journal of Managed Care 2014;20(12):26–32.

27. Sarvet B, Gold J, Bostic JQ, et al. Improving access to mental health care for children: the Massachusetts Child Psychiatry Access Project. Pediatrics 2010; 126(6):1191–200.
28. Hilt RJ, Romaire MA, McDonell MG, et al. The partnership access line: evaluating a child psychiatry consult program in Washington State. JAMA Pediatr 2013; 167(2):162–8.
29. Myers KM, Vander Stoep A, McCarty CA, et al. Child and adolescent telepsychiatry: variations in utilization, referral patterns and practice trends. J Telemed Telecare 2010;16(3):128–33.
30. Szeftel R, Federico C, Hakak R, et al. Improved access to mental health evaluation for patients with developmental disabilities using telepsychiatry. J Telemed Telecare 2012;18(6):317–21.
31. Pignatiello A, Teshima J, Boydell KM, et al. Child and youth telepsychiatry in rural and remote primary care. Child Adolesc Psychiatr Clin N Am 2011;20(1):13–28.
32. Lau ME, Way BB, Fremont WP. Assessment of SUNY Upstate Medical University's child telepsychiatry consultation program. Int J Psychiatry Med 2011;42(1): 93–104.
33. Diamond JM, Bloch RM. Telepsychiatry assessments of child or adolescent behavior disorders: a review of evidence and issues. Telemed J E Health 2010; 16(6):712–6.
34. Pesämaa L, Ebeling H, Kuusimäki M-L, et al. Videoconferencing in child and adolescent telepsychiatry: a systematic review of the literature. J Telemed Telecare 2004;10(4):187–92.
35. Elford R, White H, Bowering R, et al. A randomized, controlled trial of child psychiatric assessments conducted using videoconferencing. J Telemed Telecare 2000;6(2):73–82.
36. The Michigan Department of Health and Human Services. Children's protective services 2014 trends report summary. Flint (MI): The Michigan Department of Health and Human Services; 2014.
37. Holzer CE. Michigan: practicing child and adolescent psychiatrists 2012 [online image]. 2013. Available at: http://www.aacap.org/aacap/Advocacy/Federal_and_State_Initiatives/Workforce_Maps/Michigan.aspx. Accessed August 31, 2016.
38. Sprang G, Craig C. Crowell problem solving procedure: a psychometric analysis of a laboratory measure of the caregiver–child relationship. Child Adolesc Ment Health 2015;20(4):202–9.
39. Carter AS, Briggs-Gowan MJ. Infant-toddler social and emotional assessment. San Antonio (TX): Harcourt; 2006.
40. Achenbach TM, Edelbrock C. Manual for the child behavior checklist and 1991 profile. Burlington (VT): University of Vermont Department of Psychiatry; 1991.
41. Rutter M, Bailey A, Lord C. The social communication questionnaire: manual. Los Angeles (CA): Western Psychological Services; 2003.
42. Briere J, Johnson K, Bissada A, et al. The trauma symptom checklist for young children (TSCYC): reliability and association with abuse exposure in a multi-site study. Child Abuse Negl 2001;25(8):1001–14.

The Future of Preschool Prevention, Assessment, and Intervention

Jim Hudziak, MD*, Christopher Archangeli, MD

KEYWORDS

- Preschool • Children • Brain health • Wellness • Mindfulness • Exercise • Music
- Nutrition

KEY POINTS

- Promoting brain health improves the emotional-behavioral health of all children, can prevent problems in children at risk, and can alter the trajectory of children already suffering.
- The environment shapes the structure and function of the developing brain, so promoting brain health requires cultivation of healthy environments at home, school, and in the community.
- Promoting brain health requires assessing and treating the entire family and equipping parents with the principles of parent management training.
- Clinicians should incorporate wellness prescriptions for nutrition, physical activity, mindfulness, and music into work with families.

INTRODUCTION

This article presents neuroscience that establishes that it is possible to promote brain health as a pathway to

- Improving emotional-behavioral and general medical health in all children.
- Preventing the development of emotional-behavioral problems in those at very high risk.
- Staying and reversing the toll of pre-existing emotional-behavioral problems in children who are already suffering.

Added to the extant neuroscience data, it presents health promotion prescriptions that the authors believe are the future of brain and body health. The goal is to promote the argument that building healthy brains in young children promotes

Disclosure: The authors have nothing to disclose.
Division of Child Psychiatry, University of Vermont Medical Center, University of Vermont College of Medicine, 1 South Prospect Street, Burlington, VT 05401, USA
* Corresponding author.
E-mail address: James.Hudziak@uvm.edu

healthy bodies, families, and communities. The article provides examples of how these interventions are interrelated and must be integrated into a family-based model.

Early Childhood Brain Development: from Infinity to Beyond

Modern neuroscience, genetics, epigenetics, and public health research has presented the tantalizing possibility that it can now be said with relative certainty that much (certainly not all) is understood about why some children struggle and others soar. Although it is an oversimplification, it can now be suggested that it is possible to understand how environmental factors, both negative and positive, influence the genome or epigenome, which in turn influence the structure and function of the brain and thus human thoughts, actions, and behaviors.

Equally important is the supposition that thoughts, actions, and behaviors are responsible for the arc of human development, again in both positive and negative arcs. Why are some children able to calm themselves, smile, play, engage, and learn with ease; whereas others follow paths of pan-dysregulation, expressing impairment in attentional, mood regulatory, and cognitive domains? For much of the past 50 years, clinicians and researchers have been on a hunt for causal influences on why children suffer, with little attention paid to the causal influences on why children succeed.

The relatively simple idea that building healthy brains in young children requires healthy environments (family, school, communities) is difficult to ignore. It is clear that children raised in adversity, particularly those who face multiple adverse events,[1] are probabilistically at greater risk to struggle from all of the negative outcomes of adulthood, including psychopathologic conditions, drug abuse, hypertension, diabetes, obesity, and the cancers. It is also clear that some children are able to rise above the toll of adversity and achieve great things; however, these exceptions do little to dim the light that healthy environments lead to healthy outcomes.

Unlike adults, who have some influence as to what environment they will live in (eg, partners, jobs, lifestyles, food), children, particularly those in the preschool age group, have almost no choice. Keep in mind, little kids do not get to choose their parents, whether or not they have siblings, where they live, what or how much they can eat, whether or not they are loved or neglected, and in whose care they will be entrusted. In many ways, early life is simply a reaction to the environmental influences to which a child is exposed. Understanding the dynamic process in how the environment influences the genome (epigenome), which then influences the structure and function of the developing brain and subsequent cognitive and emotional health, is central to understanding how best to promote healthy brain development in preschool children. A key and obvious starting point is to help the parents of the child present a protective, healthy brain-developing environment for their child. Second, is to collaborate in developing high-quality childcare and preschool settings to build on (and sadly in some cases, undo) the influences of the home environment on the child. Taken together, promoting positive home and preschool environments can be best considered as the targets for assuring that all is being done to help little ones develop to their potential.

Family-Based Health Promotion

The lead author has previously published on the importance of seeing families as the unit of health promotion and illness prevention for young children.[2] This article specifically addresses some of the salient issues of early brain development and provides examples of prescribed health-promoting strategies for the preschool period. The specific health-promoting strategies addressed are nutrition, physical activity, mindfulness, music, and parent training (touching briefly on the role parents can have in improving sleep and encouraging reading). The central thesis is that each of these promotes general healthy brain development in young children, diminishes the engagement in negative behaviors by the family, and on a day-to-day basis can improve emotional health and lead a child and family to wellness. Throughout this article are examples of how wellness domains affect each other. For example, increased physical activity improves sleep and improved sleep lowers risk for obesity.[3] For most interventions, evidence is provided supporting their use in both children and parents (adults with or at risk for psychopathologic complications). This multimodal approach may have synergistic effects on patient outcome and the authors believe that the child psychiatrist is uniquely qualified to develop and execute such a comprehensive treatment plan.

Wellness Prescriptions

In the authors' center and in our applied work in pediatric settings, preschool, and school settings all the way through the college period,[4] as well as in obstetrics or gynecology settings, we prescribe to our patients and families these wellness interventions. We have included these recommendations at the end of each section.

UNDERSTANDING THE DEVELOPING BRAIN

The preschool period, which the authors define as conception to age 5, is the most pivotal period of brain development. Neurogenesis, synaptogenesis, and apoptosis occur more rapidly during this period than in any other. Large-scale projects, such as the Human Connectome Project, have led to substantial advances in the understanding of the structure and function of the brain. Glasser and colleagues[5] recently identified 180 distinct brain regions, including 97 which were completely novel. Although large studies of the adult brain remain essential to progress in neuroscience, work to understand the developing brain is equally essential, such as that of Kim and colleagues,[6] who published new measures of cortical development in a sample of children 6 to 24 months of age.

In step with colleagues studying normal brain development, others are making great progress in describing the exquisite sensitivity of the brain to environmental influences. Research on the prenatal environment shows profound effects of maternal psychopathologic states on the structure of a child's brain. Prenatal anxiety affects hippocampal development.[7] Maternal depression leads to alterations in right amygdala microstructure in newborns[8] and cortical thickness in late childhood.[9] Specific molecular exposures are even being related to functional outcomes. Howland and colleagues[10] found exposure to placental corticotropin-releasing hormone is associated with elevated internalizing symptoms at age 5 years, and low internalizing and externalizing problems at age 5 years predicts mental toughness at age 14.[11]

In infancy and early childhood, the home environment continues to affect the developing brain. Luby and colleagues[12] have linked maternal support with the trajectory of hippocampal development throughout the preschool period. Larger hippocampal volume is associated with a combination of high maternal support and less preschool depression, whereas a smaller hippocampus is associated with combination of low maternal support and severe preschool depression.[13] Researchers have also demonstrated the effects of poverty on brain development, leading to smaller white and cortical gray matter volumes, as well as smaller hippocampal and amygdala volumes.[14] Lawson and colleagues[15] demonstrated that parental education predicts cortical thickness in the right anterior cingulate cortex and left superior frontal gyrus of children. Again, these findings of environmental influences on structure have corresponding evidence of structure on functional outcome. Ducharme and colleagues[16] showed relationships between impulsive aggression in healthy children and the structure of the striatum and right anterior cingulate cortex. Attention-deficit/hyperactivity disorder (ADHD) is characterized by a delay in cortical maturation.[17] A finding confirmed when Ducharme and colleagues[18] showed decreased regional cortical thickness and thinning rate are associated with inattention symptoms in healthy children. Anxious or depressed symptoms have been linked to right ventromedial prefrontal cortical thickness maturation in healthy children[19] and right anterior insula volume has been shown to predict subsequent depression diagnosis 1.5 years later.[20] The evidence base for environmental effects on brain development and the effects of altered brain development on emotional-behavioral outcomes is growing rapidly.

NUTRITION
Parental Influences

Nutrition interventions should be used throughout the preschool period, should target all family members, and may enhance other wellness interventions. Starting prenatally, maternal obesity is linked to autism spectrum disorders, ADHD, anxiety, depression, schizophrenia, and eating disorders in offspring.[21] At the same time, maternal stress hormones (potentially reflective of untreated psychopathologic conditions) seem to increase risk for obesity in offspring.[22] Abnormal eating behaviors are regularly established by preschool age, lead to high rates of children both underweight and overweight, and are influenced by parents.[23] Increased structure of meal time and responsive feeding (not restricting or pressuring a child to eat) are associated with more desirable eating behaviors.[24] Families will make healthier eating choices, such as increasing vegetable consumption and decreasing soda consumption, when incentivized.[25]

Nutrition, Mental Health, and Specific Interventions

A systematic review completed by O'Neil and colleagues[26] of 12 epidemiologic studies revealed a consistent relationship between unhealthy dietary patterns and poorer mental health in children and adolescents, and healthy diets with better mental health. Lopresti[27] reviewed the evidence for specific nutrient treatment of pediatric depression and found the following evidence: positive support for omega-3 polyunsaturated fatty acids (PUFAs) in 2 trials; however, 1 was open label and the other had a small sample size. Vitamin C adjunct to fluoxetine significantly decreased depressive symptoms in a small, 6-month, double-blind, placebo-controlled trial. Studies yielded some positive results for mood with vitamin D, zinc, iron, and B-vitamin supplementation; however, these tended to be less methodologically robust. S-adenosyl- methionine is supported via case report only. Among naturally derived and dietary interventions for ADHD, essential fatty acids are the most studied.[28] A Cochrane review did not demonstrate an improvement in ADHD symptoms with PUFA in ADHD but did demonstrate improvements in the studies that were specific to omega-3/6 PUFA.[29] Although a Cochrane review of PUFA in learning disorders revealed only 2 studies with inconclusive evidence,[30] a Swedish double-blind, placebo-controlled, randomized controlled trial (RCT) showed omega fatty acids were associated with improved reading outcomes in mainstream children.[31]

Taken collectively, these studies show benefits of good nutrition from the prenatal period onward, and it provides evidence for interconnectedness of parental nutrition and eating behavior with child nutrition and eating behavior. Finally, there is also evidence that psychopathologic conditions can contribute to eating abnormalities. Pieper and Laugero[32] demonstrated that preschool children with lower executive function are more vulnerable to eating in the absence of hunger. Practically, this evidence informs the authors' strong recommendations that patients and their families work toward a healthier diet.

Wellness Prescription

Eat structured meals together as a family. Meditate for 2 minutes before and after. Provide your child with 5 meals a day: large breakfast, 10 AM snack, lunch, 3 PM snack, and family dinner. Meals and snacks should be based on fruits and vegetables; include sources of omega-3 fatty acids, such as fish; and probiotic Greek yogurt should be considered (given the growing evidence of the role of the gut-microbiota-brain axis on neuropsychiatric disorders[33]).

PHYSICAL ACTIVITY
Correlates of Physical Activity in Children

Low levels of leisure time physical activities in adolescent girls predict poor mental health in adulthood.[34] Sport participation was positively associated with emotional wellbeing independently of sex, social class, and health status in a cohort study of 16-year-olds.[35] Physical activity incorporated into a school curriculum led to lower levels of conduct and hyperactivity problems in girls when compared with control schools.[36] A cross-sectional study of Chinese adolescents demonstrated physical activity improved mental wellness and the effect seemed to be mediated by developing resilience.[37]

Physical Activity Effects on Psychopathologic Conditions

Cerrillo-Urbina and colleagues[38] conducted a systematic review of exercise in children with ADHD and found 8 RCTs that met their inclusion criteria. One of these was a yoga program that showed improvement in core ADHD symptoms. They performed a meta-analysis of the remaining 7 studies, which were aerobic exercise programs. These programs demonstrated moderate to large effect sizes on core symptoms, including attention (standardized mean difference [SMD] 0.84), hyperactivity (SMD 0.56), and impulsivity (SMD 0.56); and related symptoms, including anxiety (SMD 0.66), executive function (SMD 0.58), and social disorders (SMD 0.59).

Carter and colleagues[39] recently published a systematic review of 11 trials on exercise (all included either aerobic, resistance, or strength exercises) in children with depression. Eight of the studies were used in a meta-analysis that showed moderate overall effect in reducing depressive symptoms and, in trials with exclusively clinical samples, moderate effect (SMD 0.43) on depressive symptoms with lower levels of heterogeneity. Aerobic exercise as short as 10 minutes has demonstrated improved impulsivity and affect among children with behavioral problems (with 72% of the sample already taking medications).[40] Our own group demonstrated that 4 or more days of exercise per week led to a 23% reduction in suicidal ideation and attempts among bullied students.[41]

Factors Affecting Physical Activity in Children

A Brazilian sample of 328 children whose physical activity was measured with actigraphy found that maternal employment, travel mode to school, and having a television in the bedroom were correlated with physical activity levels.[42] An Irish sample demonstrated social factors (activities with friends, popularity) were associated with physical activity, whereas individual factors (body mass index, access to play space) were associated with screen time.[43] A Canadian sample of children 7 to 14 years of age examined the role of outdoor time and found that each additional hour spent outdoors was associated with 7.0 more minutes of moderate-to-vigorous physical activity, 13 fewer minutes of sedentary time, 762 more steps, and lower odds of negative psychosocial outcomes.[44] Physical activity is associated with better mental health in children and adolescents, and is effective in treating symptoms of ADHD and depression. Moving forward, clinicians will need to incorporate this in practice via individual recommendations, such as removing a television from the bedroom, and through advocacy for access to play space and the outdoors, as well as physical activity in schools. Although these studies were in children older than preschoolers, they may inform the need to incorporate at earlier ages.

Wellness Prescription

Thirty-five minutes of moderate physical activity every day for the whole family are advised. Where possible, families should find activities they enjoy doing together to provide natural positive reinforcement. Additionally, television should be removed from the bedroom and screen time limits enforced (see later discussion).

MINDFULNESS

Mindfulness is an intervention that has been the subject of great public interest and increasing scientific inquiry over recent years. Some work is being done to understand the relationship between brain structure and mindfulness. Adolescents with naturally higher levels of mindfulness demonstrated less thinning of the left anterior insula over a 3-year period.[45] However, the greater question remains how to use mindfulness interventions to shape the brain and, in turn, behavior.

Mindfulness in Schools

Mindfulness practice is being used successfully in schools. Sibinga and colleagues[46] studied a mindfulness-based stress reduction intervention compared with a health education program in 300 middle school children. This RCT showed significantly lower levels of somatization, depression, negative affect, negative coping, rumination, self-hostility, and post-traumatic symptoms compared with control. These effects do not seem limited to older children because a pilot study of mindfulness training in primary schools by Vickery and colleagues[47] showed that children 7 to 9 years of age like mindfulness and wish to continue the practice. Additionally, they found that, relative to controls, the intervention group had decreased negative affect and increased meta-cognition as reported by their teachers. An RCT of a 12-week mindfulness-based Kindness Curriculum was studied in 68 public preschool children, demonstrating improvements in social competence and higher report card grades in areas of learning, health, and social-emotional development.[48] Mindfulness interventions have shown profound effects in older children, studies in younger children show that they like it, and even preschool children have seen positive effects from the practice.

Effects in Clinical Populations

Mindfulness interventions are being studied for specific disorders in children; however, this data is less methodologically robust. A small 8-week mindfulness intervention trial showed positive results for ADHD.[49] In the near future, more robust randomized clinical trial data will be available because RCTs evaluating meditation versus medication[50] and family-based mindfulness for ADHD[51] are under way. Mindfulness interventions are showing promise in other disorders as well. A pilot study of mindfulness-based stress reduction for Tourette syndrome and chronic tic disorders showed improvement in tic severity and tic-related impairment in 59% of the subjects.[52] Mindful parenting decreased aggression and increased social behavior in case studies of children with developmental disabilities.[53]

Mindfulness in the Family

Mindfulness interventions hold such great promise because they can be used throughout the family and affect a child's trajectory at many crucial developmental periods. An RCT of 80 pregnant women comparing mindfulness-integrated cognitive behavioral therapy with treatment as usual showed significantly lower anxiety and depression scores in the group receiving mindfulness-integrated cognitive behavioral therapy.[54] This finding is especially encouraging given the previously described role of maternal depression and anxiety on child brain development. Smalley and colleagues[55] compared adults with ADHD to controls and found adults with ADHD to be less mindful and less self-directed. This study suggests that mindfulness might improve symptoms of ADHD in adults and, given the high heritability of ADHD, these adults are the parents of the clinician's patients. Finally, mindfulness has great potential to be used in conjunction with parent training. An 8-week mindful parent training trial of 70 parent–child dyads showed decreases in both child and parental psychopathologic conditions.[56]

Wellness Prescription

Meditate for 5 sessions of 2 to 3 minutes daily. Meditate together as a family. Once parents have developed a meditation practice, they can begin teaching the basics of belly-breathing and focusing on the breath to even very young children.

MUSIC

A systematic review by Carr and colleagues[57] of music therapy suggests effectiveness in addressing a range of symptoms in adults with psychiatric illness. In children and adolescents with serious health conditions, Mrázová and Celec[58] evaluated 28 RCTs of music interventions.[58] Twenty-three of the 28 studies indicated significant positive effects of the interventions, typically on socioemotional outcomes; for example, pain, procedure-related distress, anxiety, and depressive symptoms. Treurnicht Naylor and colleagues[59] reviewed 17 RCTs (only 5 overlapping with Mrázová and Celec[58]) that had mixed results but significant improvements in the 4 studies that looked at mostly young children. Music therapy showed differential effects on cingulate and prefrontal cortex when used as an aid to neurorestoration in children with severe neurologic conditions.[60] Hudziak and colleagues[61] suggest that playing a musical instrument is associated with more rapid cortical maturation within areas responsible for motor planning and coordination, visuospatial ability, and emotion and impulse regulation. Kraus and colleagues[62] demonstrated that children in at-risk, impoverished, auditory environments who are exposed to music training through the Harmony Project develop stronger encoding of speech and increased reading scores. Future work will help us fine-tune recommendations for music interventions and examine areas such as dosage because some work has already been done showing a dose-response relationship in music therapy for adults with serious mental disorders.[63]

Listening to music in pregnant women is associated with decreased stress and anxiety, and improved sleep quality, again demonstrating the interrelatedness of these wellness interventions and their family-wide effects.[64]

Wellness Prescription

The authors advise learning how to play an instrument and playing it 1 hour a day for 2 years. Listen to music together as a family and consider incorporating classical composers such as Bach because there is some evidence suggesting benefits on heart-rate variability.[65]

PARENT TRAINING

Dretzke and colleagues[66] conducted a systematic review and meta-analysis of 57 RCTs and found significant improvements in outcomes as measured by parents (SMD 0.67) and independently (SMD 0.44). They determined that there was insufficient evidence to determine the relative effectiveness of different approaches to delivering parenting programs. This builds on prior work by Maughan and colleagues,[67] who performed a meta-analytic review of 79 clinical trials with families of children and adolescents. They reported the efficacy of behavioral parent training interventions specifically for 3-year-olds to 5-year-olds. Although the number of studies was not reported, the effect size of the intervention on children's behavior problems for studies with between-subjects designs was moderate (SMD 0.40) and large for studies with within-subject designs (SMD 0.75). Dishion and colleagues[68] demonstrated that a 3-session assessment and feedback intervention (Family Check-Up Intervention) that involves assessment of parent–child interactions from the perspective of behavioral parent training and gives parents feedback about the results of their assessment using motivational enhancement strategies was effective in population-wide prevention trials.

Moving forward, it is expected that interventions will continue to be scaled as Sourander and colleagues[69] did when they conducted a parallel-group randomized clinical trial of Internet-assisted parent training in Finland. A population of 4656 children was screened and 464 parents of 4-year-old children were randomized to an intervention group or an educational control. The intervention was an 11-session Internet-based parent training program with weekly telephone coaching. Child Behavior Checklist data at 12 month follow-up showed the intervention group had significant improvement compared with controls in externalizing problems (effect size 0.34), internalizing problems (effect size 0.35), and total problems (effect size 0.37). The authors also expect that interventions will continue to be validated in regard to other emotional and behavioral problems, such as depression, in preschoolers. Luby and colleagues[70] have piloted studies of parent-child interaction therapy for depression in this population with positive results thus far.

Parenting Choices (Sleep, Screen Time, and Reading)

Bedtime problems and night awakenings are prevalent in young children, with cross-sectional estimates of 20% to 30%. Mindell and colleagues[71] reviewed 52 intervention trials conducted with parents of young children for children's sleep. Behavioral parenting interventions and parental education interventions produced significant reductions in children's bedtime resistance and night-waking in 49 of the 52 trials and, on average, 82% of subjects showed improvement. These trials occurred in the general population and tested behavioral interventions targeting parenting practices (eg, soothing bedtime routines, ignoring noncompliant behavior, and consistency). Chaput and Dutil[3] reviewed the contribution of poor sleep to obesity in adolescents and found that multiple systematic reviews and meta-analyses demonstrate increased risk for obesity with poor sleep, with increased risk for the shortest durations. Furthermore, they characterize the interrelatedness of sleep with many of the domains discussed. Aerobic activity and diet can improve sleep quality and poor sleep can reduce physical activity due to fatigue and increased food intake. Additionally, screen time has been shown to disrupt sleep. In addition to its effects on physical activity and sleep, television exposure increases the incidence and the persistence of externalizing problems in preschool children.[72] Santisteban and colleagues[73] demonstrated that reading mediated lower risk for aggression in both boys and girls. A recent RCT of a combined parent training and shared reading intervention showed significant improvement in parenting behaviors, child behaviors, and language development of the children in the intervention group.[74]

Wellness Prescription

All parents should be educated on the principles of parent management training. Children with sleep disturbances should engage in behavioral interventions around sleep. Screen time should be limited and shared reading encouraged. The authors recommend a 1:1 ratio of minutes spent reading to minutes of screen time allowed.

SUMMARY

The future of prevention and treatment of emotional and behavioral problems in the preschool population is centered on growing knowledge of the developing brain and how shaping the home environment through supporting family health, and shaping the school environment by supporting community health, can modify the trajectory of young children's lives. The first step in this journey is adopting a family-based approach as a discipline in which strengths and weaknesses of parents are assessed; partnership is created via motivational interviewing to build on their strengths; and, when needed, parents accept care for their own emotional-behavioral needs. Through parent training for all parents, clinicians can help assure that the knowledge, skills, and attitudes necessary to raise healthy children are widely disseminated. By identifying and treating existing emotional-behavioral, substance use, and general medical problems in parents, clinicians can contribute to better overall parental health and place parents in a better place to actualize the lessons in parent training. When parents are doing well, they will be able to learn more easily and apply these lessons in their children's lives.

The real power of this approach is the day-to-day benefit of working with parents of young children in prescriptive health promotion. Not only do these prescriptions bring families closer together (exercising together, meditating together, eating, reading, producing music together), the emerging neuroscience literature provides evidence that each of these improves overall general cognitive and emotional-behavioral health. This article provided several examples of such prescriptions and advised health care professionals to encourage and incentivize parents to follow these paths with the goal of working as a team to build healthier preschool brains and, it is hoped, alter the arc of possibilities for all children. Healthy diets, regular exercise, adequate sleep, regular reading, mindful meditation practiced by parents and children, learning an instrument, and several different forms of parent training are all promising avenues for addressing the needs of this population. Improvement in an area can synergistically lead to improvement in other areas, supporting the authors' recommendation that as many of these interventions as possible should be used in creating a comprehensive treatment plan.

Although much of this research is in its infancy, or perhaps in its preschool years, alternative approaches such as medication are of questionable overall benefit and have not been lauded as potential avenues for positive brain development. Last, and perhaps most importantly, prescriptive health promotion for preschool children and families carries the added benefit of bringing positive benefits to all on a daily basis. Each day that a child enjoys is a good day.

The authors argue that taking an approach of health promotion, illness prevention, and family-based intervention will help all children and families. This approach has the potential to help those who are well achieve new strategies for raising healthy children. This approach has the potential to prevent at-risk children and families from developing emotional-behavioral and general medical problems. Finally, this approach has the potential to assist those already struggling with severe emotional-behavioral problems a new way to bring positive strategies into their lives. The authors believe this is the future of child psychiatry.

REFERENCES

1. Felitti VJ, Anda RF, Nordenberg D, et al. Relationship of childhood abuse and household dysfunction to many of the leading causes of death in adults. The Adverse Childhood Experiences (ACE) Study. Am J Prev Med 1998;14:245–58.
2. Hudziak J, Ivanova MY. The Vermont family based approach: family based health promotion, illness prevention, and intervention. Child Adolesc Psychiatr Clin N Am 2016;25:167–78.
3. Chaput J-P, Dutil C. Lack of sleep as a contributor to obesity in adolescents: impacts on eating and activity behaviors. Int J Behav Nutr Phys Act 2016;13:103.
4. Hudziak J, Chung W W. The transitional age brain: the best of times and the worst of times. Child Adolesc Psychiatr Clin N Am 2017;26(2):157–75.
5. Glasser MF, Coalson TS, Robinson EC, et al. A multi-modal parcellation of human cerebral cortex. Nature 2016;536:171–8.
6. Kim SH, Lyu I, Fonov VS, et al. Development of cortical shape in the human brain from 6 to 24 months of age via a novel measure of shape complexity. Neuroimage 2016;135:163–76.
7. Qiu A, Rifkin-Graboi A, Chen H, et al. Maternal anxiety and infants' hippocampal development: timing matters. Transl Psychiatry 2013;3:e306.
8. Rifkin-Graboi A, Bai J, Chen H, et al. Prenatal maternal depression associates with microstructure of right amygdala in neonates at birth. Biol Psychiatry 2013; 74:837–44.
9. Sandman CA, Buss C, Head K, et al. Fetal exposure to maternal depressive symptoms is associated with cortical thickness in late childhood. Biol Psychiatry 2015;77:324–34.
10. Howland MA, Sandman CA, Glynn LM, et al. Fetal exposure to placental corticotropin-releasing hormone is associated with child self-reported internalizing symptoms. Psychoneuroendocrinology 2016;67:10–7.
11. Sadeghi Bahmani D, Hatzinger M, Gerber M, et al. The origins of mental toughness - prosocial behavior and low internalizing and externalizing problems at age 5 predict higher mental toughness scores at age 14. Front Psychol 2016;7:1221.
12. Luby JL, Belden A, Harms MP, et al. Preschool is a sensitive period for the influence of maternal support on the trajectory of hippocampal development. Proc Natl Acad Sci U S A 2016;113:5742–7.

13. Luby JL, Barch DM, Belden A, et al. Maternal support in early childhood predicts larger hippocampal volumes at school age. Proc Natl Acad Sci U S A 2012;109: 2854–9.
14. Luby J, Belden A, Botteron K, et al. The effects of poverty on childhood brain development: the mediating effect of caregiving and stressful life events. JAMA Pediatr 2013;167:1135–42.
15. Lawson GM, Duda JT, Avants BB, et al. Associations between children's socio-economic status and prefrontal cortical thickness. Dev Sci 2013;16:641–52.
16. Ducharme S, Hudziak JJ, Botteron KN, et al. Right anterior cingulate cortical thickness and bilateral striatal volume correlate with child behavior checklist aggressive behavior scores in healthy children. Biol Psychiatry 2011;70:283–90.
17. Shaw P, Eckstrand K, Sharp W, et al. Attention-deficit/hyperactivity disorder is characterized by a delay in cortical maturation. Proc Natl Acad Sci U S A 2007;104:19649–54.
18. Ducharme S, Hudziak JJ, Botteron KN, et al. Decreased regional cortical thickness and thinning rate are associated with inattention symptoms in healthy children. J Am Acad Child Adolesc Psychiatry 2012;51:18–27.e2.
19. Ducharme S, Albaugh MD, Hudziak JJ, et al. Anxious/depressed symptoms are linked to right ventromedial prefrontal cortical thickness maturation in healthy children and young adults. Cereb Cortex 2014;24:2941–50.
20. Belden AC, Barch DM, Oakberg TJ, et al. Anterior insula volume and guilt: neuro-behavioral markers of recurrence after early childhood major depressive disorder. JAMA Psychiatry 2015;72:40–8.
21. Edlow AG. Maternal obesity and neurodevelopmental and psychiatric disorders in offspring. Prenat Diagn 2017;37(1):95–110.
22. Stout SA, Espel EV, Sandman CA, et al. Fetal programming of children's obesity risk. Psychoneuroendocrinology 2015;53:29–39.
23. Jansen PW, Roza SJ, Jaddoe VW, et al. Children's eating behavior, feeding practices of parents and weight problems in early childhood: results from the population-based Generation R Study. Int J Behav Nutr Phys Act 2012;9:130.
24. Finnane JM, Jansen E, Mallan KM, et al. Mealtime structure and responsive feeding practices are associated with less food fussiness and more food enjoyment in children. J Nutr Educ Behav 2016;49(1):11–8.e1.
25. Bowling AB, Moretti M, Ringelheim K, et al. Healthy Foods, Healthy Families: combining incentives and exposure interventions at urban farmers' markets to improve nutrition among recipients of US federal food assistance. Health Promot Perspect 2016;6:10–6.
26. O'Neil A, Quirk SE, Housden S, et al. Relationship between diet and mental health in children and adolescents: a systematic review. Am J Public Health 2014;104: e31–42.
27. Lopresti AL. A review of nutrient treatments for paediatric depression. J Affect Disord 2015;181:24–32.
28. Ahn J, Ahn HS, Cheong JH, et al. Natural product-derived treatments for attention-deficit/hyperactivity disorder: safety, efficacy, and therapeutic potential of combination therapy. Neural Plast 2016;2016:132042.
29. Gillies D, Sinn JK, Lad SS, et al. Polyunsaturated fatty acids (PUFA) for attention deficit hyperactivity disorder (ADHD) in children and adolescents. Cochrane Database Syst Rev 2012;(7):CD007986.
30. Tan ML, Ho JJ, Teh KH. Polyunsaturated fatty acids (PUFAs) for children with specific learning disorders. Cochrane Database Syst Rev 2016;(9):CD009398.

31. Johnson M, Fransson G, Östlund S, et al. Omega 3/6 fatty acids for reading in children: a randomized, double-blind, placebo-controlled trial in 9-year-old mainstream schoolchildren in Sweden. J Child Psychol Psychiatry 2016;58: 83–93.

32. Pieper JR, Laugero KD. Preschool children with lower executive function may be more vulnerable to emotional-based eating in the absence of hunger. Appetite 2013;62:103–9.

33. Petra AI, Panagiotidou S, Hatziagelaki E, et al. Gut-microbiota-brain Axis and its effect on neuropsychiatric disorders with suspected immune dysregulation. Clin Ther 2015;37:984–95.

34. Hoegh Poulsen P, Biering K, Andersen JH. The association between leisure time physical activity in adolescence and poor mental health in early adulthood: a prospective cohort study. BMC Public Health 2016;16:3.

35. Steptoe A, Butler N. Sports participation and emotional wellbeing in adolescents. Lancet 1996;347:1789–92.

36. Bunketorp Käll L, Malmgren H, Olsson E, et al. Effects of a curricular physical activity intervention on Children's school performance, wellness, and brain development. J Sch Health 2015;85:704–13.

37. Ho FKW, Louie LHT, Chow CB, et al. Physical activity improves mental health through resilience in Hong Kong Chinese adolescents. BMC Pediatr 2015;15:48.

38. Cerrillo-Urbina AJ, García-Hermoso A, Sánchez-López M, et al. The effects of physical exercise in children with attention deficit hyperactivity disorder: a systematic review and meta-analysis of randomized control trials. Child Care Health Dev 2015;41:779–88.

39. Carter T, Morres ID, Meade O, et al. The effect of exercise on depressive symptoms in adolescents: a systematic review and meta-analysis. J Am Acad Child Adolesc Psychiatry 2016;55:580–90.

40. Bowling AB, Haneuse SJ, Miller DP, et al. Duration of aerobic exercise and effects on self-regulation among children with behavioral health disorders: 2294 board #4 June 2, 3: 15 PM - 5: 15 pm. Med Sci Sports Exerc 2016;48:639.

41. Sibold J, Edwards E, Murray-Close D, et al. Physical activity, sadness, and suicidality in bullied US adolescents. J Am Acad Child Adolesc Psychiatry 2015;54: 808–15.

42. de Moraes Ferrari GL, Matsudo V, Barreira TV, et al. Correlates of moderate-to-vigorous physical activity in Brazilian children. J Phys Act Health 2016;1–35. http://dx.doi.org/10.1123/jpah.2015-0666.

43. Garcia JM, Healy S, Rice D. The individual, social, and environmental correlates of physical activity and screen time in Irish children: growing up in Ireland study. J Phys Act Health 2016;13:1–28.

44. Larouche R, Garriguet D, Gunnell KE, et al. Outdoor time, physical activity, sedentary time, and health indicators at ages 7 to 14: 2012/2013 Canadian Health Measures Survey. Health Rep 2016;27:3–13.

45. Friedel S, Whittle SL, Vijayakumar N, et al. Dispositional mindfulness is predicted by structural development of the insula during late adolescence. Dev Cogn Neurosci 2015;14:62–70.

46. Sibinga EMS, Webb L, Ghazarian SR, et al. School-based mindfulness instruction: an RCT. Pediatrics 2016;137(1):e20152532.

47. Vickery CE, Dorjee D. Mindfulness training in primary schools decreases negative affect and increases meta-cognition in children. Front Psychol 2015;6:2025.

48. Flook L, Goldberg SB, Pinger L, et al. Promoting prosocial behavior and self-regulatory skills in preschool children through a mindfulness-based Kindness Curriculum. Dev Psychol 2015;51:44–51.

49. van der Oord S, Bögels SM, Peijnenburg D. The effectiveness of mindfulness training for children with ADHD and mindful parenting for their parents. J Child Fam Stud 2012;21:139–47.

50. Meppelink R, de Bruin EI, Bögels SM. Meditation or Medication? Mindfulness training versus medication in the treatment of childhood ADHD: a randomized controlled trial. BMC Psychiatry 2016;16:267.

51. Lo HHM, Wong SYS, Wong JYH, et al. The effect of a family-based mindfulness intervention on children with attention deficit and hyperactivity symptoms and their parents: design and rationale for a randomized, controlled clinical trial (Study protocol). BMC Psychiatry 2016;16:65.

52. Reese HE, Vallejo Z, Rasmussen J, et al. Mindfulness-based stress reduction for tourette syndrome and chronic tic disorder: a pilot study. J Psychosom Res 2015; 78:293–8.

53. Singh NN, Lancioni GE, Winton AS, et al. Mindful parenting decreases aggression and increases social behavior in children with developmental disabilities. Behav Modif 2007;31:749–71.

54. Yazdanimehr R, Omidi A, Sadat Z, et al. The effect of mindfulness-integrated cognitive behavior therapy on depression and anxiety among pregnant women: a randomized clinical trial. J Caring Sci 2016;5:195–204.

55. Smalley SL, Loo SK, Hale TS, et al. Mindfulness and attention deficit hyperactivity disorder. J Clin Psychol 2009;65:1087–98.

56. Meppelink R, de Bruin EI, Wanders-Mulder FH, et al. Mindful parenting training in child psychiatric settings: heightened parental mindfulness reduces parents' and Children's psychopathology. Mindfulness 2016;7:680–9.

57. Carr C, Odell-Miller H, Priebe S. A systematic review of music therapy practice and outcomes with acute adult psychiatric in-patients. PLoS One 2013;8.

58. Mrázová M, Celec P. A systematic review of randomized controlled trials using music therapy for children. J Altern Complement Med 2010;16:1089–95.

59. Treurnicht Naylor K, Kingsnorth S, Lamont A, et al. The effectiveness of music in pediatric healthcare: a systematic review of randomized controlled trials. Evid Based Complement Altern Med 2011;2011:464759.

60. Bringas ML, Zaldivar M, Rojas PA, et al. Effectiveness of music therapy as an aid to neurorestoration of children with severe neurological disorders. Front Neurosci 2015;9:427.

61. Hudziak JJ, Albaugh MD, Ducharme S, et al. Cortical thickness maturation and duration of music training: health-promoting activities shape brain development. J Am Acad Child Adolesc Psychiatry 2014;53:1153–61, 1161.e1–2.

62. Kraus N, Hornickel J, Strait DL, et al. Engagement in community music classes sparks neuroplasticity and language development in children from disadvantaged backgrounds. Front Psychol 2014;5:1403.

63. Gold C, Solli HP, Krüger V, et al. Dose-response relationship in music therapy for people with serious mental disorders: systematic review and meta-analysis. Clin Psychol Rev 2009;29:193–207.

64. Liu Y-H, Lee CS, Yu C-H, et al. Effects of music listening on stress, anxiety, and sleep quality for sleep-disturbed pregnant women. Women Health 2016;56: 296–311.

65. Chuang C-Y, Han W-R, Li P-C, et al. Effect of long-term music therapy intervention on autonomic function in anthracycline-treated breast cancer patients. Integr Cancer Ther 2011;10:312–6.

66. Dretzke J, Davenport C, Frew E, et al. The clinical effectiveness of different parenting programmes for children with conduct problems: a systematic review of randomised controlled trials. Child Adolesc Psychiatry Ment Health 2009;3:7.

67. Maughan DR, Christiansen E, Jenson WR, et al. Behavioral parent training as a treatment for externalizing behaviors and disruptive behavior disorders: a meta-analysis. Sch Psychol Rev 2005;34:267–86.

68. Dishion TJ, Shaw D, Connell A, et al. The family check-up with high-risk indigent families: preventing problem behavior by increasing parents' positive behavior support in early childhood. Child Dev 2008;79:1395–414.

69. Sourander A, McGrath PJ, Ristkari T, et al. Internet-assisted parent training intervention for disruptive behavior in 4-year-old children: a randomized clinical trial. JAMA Psychiatry 2016;73:378–87.

70. Luby J, Lenze S, Tillman R. A novel early intervention for preschool depression: findings from a pilot randomized controlled trial. J Child Psychol Psychiatry 2012;53:313–22.

71. Mindell JA, Kuhn B, Lewin DS, et al. Behavioral treatment of bedtime problems and night wakings in infants and young children. Sleep 2006;29:1263–76.

72. Verlinden M, Tiemeier H, Hudziak JJ, et al. Television viewing and externalizing problems in preschool children: the Generation R Study. Arch Pediatr Adolesc Med 2012;166:919–25.

73. Santisteban C, Alvarado JM, Recio P. Evaluation of a Spanish version of the Buss and Perry aggression questionnaire: some personal and situational factors related to the aggression scores of young subjects. Personal Individ Differ 2007;42:1453–65.

74. Chacko A, Fabiano GA, Doctoroff GL, et al. Engaging fathers in effective parenting for preschool children using shared book reading: a randomized controlled trial. J Clin Child Adolesc Psychol 2017. [Epub ahead of print].

Index

Note: Page numbers of article titles are in **boldface** type.

A

ABC. *See* Attachment and Biobehavioral Catch-Up (ABC)
ADHD. *See* Attention deficit hyperactivity disorder (ADHD)
Affect
   in mental health assessment of young children, 445–446
Anxiety
   sleep disorders in preschoolers with, 592–593
Anxiety disorders
   ASD *vs.,* 559
   in preschoolers, **503–506, 511–514** *See also* Preschooler(s), anxiety
      disorders in
Appearance
   in mental health assessment of young children, 445
ARC. *See* Attachment, regulation, and competency (ARC)
ASDs. *See* Autism spectrum disorders (ASDs)
Attachment, **455–476**. *See also* Attachment disorder
   assessment of, 462–465
   described, 455–457
   developmental process and, 457–458
   development of, 458–460
   fostering of
      evidence-based therapeutic interventions in, 465–470
         ABC, 468–469
         Mom Power, 469
         MTP, 465, 468
         video feedback, 468
   individual differences in, 460
   introduction, 455–457
   pharmacotherapy and, 470
   psychological function and, 460–461
   significantly disturbed
      clinical aspects of
         Circle of Security framework in assessing, 466–467, 469
Attachment, regulation, and competency (ARC)
   in trauma management in very young children, 485
Attachment and behavioral catch-up
   in trauma management in very young children, 483, 485
Attachment and Biobehavioral Catch-Up (ABC)
   in fostering attachment, 468–469
Attachment disorder(s), **455–476**. *See also* Attachment
   described, 455–457, 462

Attachment (*continued*)
    introduction, 455–457
Attention deficit hyperactivity disorder (ADHD)
    ASD *vs.,* 559
    causes of, 524
    described, 523–524
    in preschoolers, **523–538**
        introduction, 523–525
        sleep disorders and, 592–593
        treatment of, 525–534
            COPE in, 527–529
            emotion regulation in, 527
            evidence-based behavioral intervention in, 525–527
            evidence-based combination behavioral and pharmacologic therapy
                in, 532–534
            evidence-based nonpharmacologic approaches in, 525–530
            evidence-based pharmacologic therapy in, 530–532
            exercise in, 532–534
            neurofeedback in, 529–530
            NFPP in, 526–527
            nutrition in, 532–534
            PBT in, 525–527
            sleep in, 532–534
            Triple P in, 526
    symptoms of, 524
Autism. *See also* Autism spectrum disorders (ASDs)
    early origins of, **555–570**
    introduction, 555–556
Autism spectrum disorders (ASDs), **555–570**
    course of, 563–565
    diagnosis of
        causation and impending revolution in, 562–563
        clinical assessment in, 558–559
        criteria in, 557
        current process for, 557–562
        differential diagnosis in, 559–560
        early childhood, 556–557
        standardized measures of symptom burden in, 560–562
    differential diagnosis of, 559–560
    early manifestations of, 563–565
    early origins of, **555–570**
    epidemiology of, 556–557
    feeding problems associated with, 572–573
    intervention planning in, 565
    introduction, 555–556
    regression associated with, 564–565
    restricted interest in, 564
    social communication deficits in, 563–564
    symptom burden in
        standardized measures of, 560–562

B

Behavior(s)
    challenging
        ID–related, 542–543
        language disorders–related, 547–548
    in mental health assessment of young children, 445
    repetitive
        in ASDs, 564
Behavioral feeding
    in feeding disorders management, 574–575
Brain development
    in early childhood, 612
    understanding, 613–614
Brain health
    in preschoolers, **611–624**
        family-based health promotion and, 612–613
        introduction, 611–613
        mindfulness and, 616–617
        music and, 617–618
        nutrition and, 614–615
        parent training and, 618–619
        physical activity and, 615–616

C

Caregiver-child interaction
    in mental health assessment of young children, 446–447
CBT. *See* Cognitive behavioral therapy (CBT)
CD. *See* Conduct disorder (CD)
Challenging behaviors
    ID–related, 542–543
    language disorders–related, 547–548
Child mental health
    implications for, 413
Child-parent psychotherapy
    in trauma management in very young children, 485
Children. *See also* Preschooler(s); *specific age groups, e.g.,* Newborn(s)
    young
        mental health assessment of, **441–454** *See also* Young children, mental
            health assessment of
    0-6 years old
        DBDs in, **491–502** *See also* Disruptive behavior disorders (DBDs), in
            children 0-6 years old
Circle of Security framework
    in fostering attachment, 466–467, 469
Cognitive behavioral therapy (CBT)
    trauma-focused
        in trauma management in very young children, 485

Communication
   social
      in ASDs
         deficits of, 563–564
Community Parent Education Program (COPE)
   in ADHD management in preschoolers, 527–529
Conduct disorder (CD)
   described, 491–492
   in preschoolers
      prevalence of, 491
COPE. *See* Community Parent Education Program (COPE)
Crowell parent-child interaction procedure
   in mental health assessment of young children, 478

D

DBDs. *See* Disruptive behavior disorders (DBDs)
Depression
   in preschoolers, **503–522** *See also* Preschooler(s), depression in
   sleep disorders in preschoolers with, 592–593
Development
   in mental health assessment of young children, 446
   trauma effects on
      in very young children, 478–479
Development process
   attachment and, 457–458
Diagnostic Infant Preschool Assessment (DIPA)
   in mental health assessment of young children, 449
DIPA. *See* Diagnostic Infant Preschool Assessment (DIPA)
Disability(ies)
   intellectual, **539–543** *See also* Intellectual disability (ID)
Disruptive behavior disorders (DBDs). *See also* Oppositional defiant disorder
   (ODD); *specific types, e.g.,* Conduct disorder (CD)
   ASD *vs.,* 559
   in children 0-6 years old, **491–502**
      assessment of, 495–496
      comorbidity associated with, 492
      described, 491–492
      environmental risk factors for, 492–494
      genetic risk factors for, 494
      introduction, 491–492
      neuroimaging of, 494–495
      neuropsychological profiles and neurophysiologic correlates, 495
      treatment of, 496–497

E

Early childhood
   ASD diagnosis in, 556–557
   brain development in, 612

Early childhood mental health, **411–426**
    implications for, 413
    introduction, 411–412
Early childhood mental health assessment
    contexts of, 441–442
Emotion regulation
    in ADHD management in preschoolers, 527
Evidence-based behavioral intervention
    in ADHD management in preschoolers, 525–527
Evidence-based combination behavioral and pharmacologic therapy
    in ADHD management in preschoolers, 532–534
Evidence-based pharmacologic therapy
    in ADHD management in preschoolers, 530–532
Exercise
    in ADHD management in preschoolers, 532–534

F

Family-based health promotion, 612–613
Feeding disorders, **571–586**
    ASDs and, 572–573
    introduction, 571–573
    management of
        behavioral feeding in, 574–575
        interdisciplinary care in, 573–574
        nutritional manipulation in, 575–577
        oral-motor treatments in, 575
        pharmacologic, 577
        sensory-based techniques in, 575
    prevention of, 577–579

I

ID. *See* Intellectual disability (ID)
Incredible years (IY)
    in trauma management in very young children, 485
Infant(s)
    temperament of
        newborn assessment and, 432–434
Intellectual disability (ID), **539–543**
    ASD *vs.,* 559
    challenging behaviors related to, 542–543
    characteristics of, 540
    comorbidity associated with, 542–543
    developmental progress with
        promotion of, 543
    differential diagnosis of, 541
    evaluation of, 541
    introduction, 539
    management of, 542–543

Intellectual (*continued*)
    future directions in, 550
    prevalence of, 540–541
Internalizing disorders
    in preschoolers
        research on, 504–506
Interview(s)
    structured diagnostic
        in mental health assessment of young children, 448–449
IY. *See* Incredible years (IY)

L

Language delay
    language disorders *vs.*, 544–545
Language disorders, **543–550**
    challenging behavior associated with, 547–548
    comorbidities associated with, 547–548
    described, 543–544
    differential diagnosis of, 547
    evaluation of, 545–547
    language delay *vs.*, 544–545
    late talkers *vs.*, 544–545
    management of, 548–549
        future directions in, 550
    prevalence of, 543
Late talkers
    language disorders *vs.*, 544–545

M

Maternal mental health
    introduction, 411–412
MC3. *See* Michigan Child Collaborative Care Program (MC3)
Medication(s)
    in feeding disorders management, 577
Mental health
    early childhood, **411–426** *See also* Early childhood mental health
    maternal
        introduction, 411–412
    of preschoolers
        partnerships with primary care for, **597–609** *See also* Preschool mental health,
            partnerships with primary care for
Mental health assessment
    of young children, **441–454** *See also* Young children, mental health assessment of
Mental status examination
    in mental health assessment of young children, 445–446
Michigan Child Collaborative Care Program (MC3), 599–606
    data from, 602–606
        patient referrals
            all ages, 603

preschoolers, 603–604
PCPs, 602
pharmacotherapy in preschoolers, 604
referrals to behavioral health consultant, 605–606
telepsychiatry summary, 606
overview of, 599–601
population demographics of, 601–602
telepsychiatry preschool assessment in, 601–602
Mindfulness
brain health in preschoolers related to, 616–617
Mom Power
in fostering attachment, 469
Mood
in mental health assessment of young children, 445–446
Mothers and Toddlers Program (MTP)
in fostering attachment, 465, 468
MTP. *See* Mothers and Toddlers Program (MTP)
Music
brain health in preschoolers related to, 617–618

N

Neonatal neurobehavioral assessment, **427–440**
clinical implications of, 437
described, 428–429
introduction, 427–428
neurobiological framework of, 429–432
socioemotional impairments in infants related to, 434–435
temperament in infants related to, 432–434
Neurobehavioral assessment
neonatal, **427–440** *See also* Neonatal neurobehavioral assessment
Neurofeedback
in ADHD management in preschoolers, 529–530
Newborn(s)
assessment of, 428–436 *See also* Neonatal neurobehavioral assessment
New Forest Parenting Programme (NFPP)
in ADHD management in preschoolers, 526–527
NFPP. *See* New Forest Parenting Programme (NFPP)
Nightmares
in preschoolers, 589
Nutrition
in ADHD management in preschoolers, 532–534
brain health in preschoolers related to, 614–615
Nutritional manipulation
in feeding disorders management, 575–577

O

Obstructive sleep apnea (OSA)
in preschoolers, 589–591
ODD. *See* Oppositional defiant disorder (ODD)

Oppositional defiant disorder (ODD)
    described, 491–492
    in preschoolers
        prevalence of, 491
Oral-motor treatments
    in feeding disorders management, 575
OSA. See Obstructive sleep apnea (OSA)

P

PAPA. See Preschool Age Psychiatric Assessment (PAPA)
Parasomnias
    in preschoolers, 591–592
Parent behavior training (PBT)
    in ADHD management in preschoolers, 525–527
Parent-child interaction therapy (PCIT)
    in trauma management in very young children, 485
Parent-report measures
    in mental health assessment of young children, 449
Parent training
    brain health in preschoolers related to, 618–619
Partnerships with primary care
    for preschool mental health, **597–609** See also Preschool mental health,
        partnerships with primary care for
PBT. See Parent behavior training (PBT)
PCIT. See Parent-child interaction therapy (PCIT)
PCPs. See Primary care physicians (PCPs)
Pharmacotherapy
    attachment and, 470
Physical activity
    brain health in preschoolers related to, 615–616
Pregnancy
    psychiatric disorders during, 411–412
        future directions related to, 418–419
        incidence of, 412–413
        prevalence of, 412–413
        screening for, 413–417
            barriers and facilitators to, 415–417
            instruments in, 415
        psychosocial assessment during, 417–418
Preschool Age Psychiatric Assessment (PAPA)
    in mental health assessment of young children, 449
Preschooler(s)
    ADHD in, **523–538** See Attention deficit hyperactivity disorder (ADHD), in preschoolers
    anxiety disorders in, **503–506, 511–514**
        assessment of, 511–512
        case study, 513–514
        prevalence of, 512
        risk factors for, 512–513
        treatment of, 513
    brain health in, **611–624** See also Brain health, in preschoolers

CD in
    prevalence of, 491
depression in, **503–511**
    assessment of, 506
    course of, 507
    factors associated with, 507–509
    introduction, 503–504
    neurobiological correlates of, 509–510
    prevalence of, 507
    treatment of, 510–511
internalizing disorders in
    research on, 504–506
mental health of
    partnerships with primary care for, **597–609** See also Preschool mental health,
        partnerships with primary care for
normal sleep in, 588–589
ODD in
    prevalence of, 491
sleep disorders in, **587–595** See also Sleep disorders, in preschoolers
Preschool internalizing disorders
    research on, 504–506
Preschool mental health
    partnerships with primary care for, **597–609**
        background of, 597–599
        in increasing access early childhood mental health, 599
        MC3 in, 599–606 See also Michigan Child Collaborative Care Program (MC3)
        telepsychiatry in, 599
            MC3, 601–602, 606
Primary care physicians (PCPs)
    in preschool mental health, **597–609** See also Preschool mental health, partnerships
        with primary care for
Psychiatric disorders
    during pregnancy, 411–412 See also Pregnancy, psychiatric disorders during
Psychological function
    attachment and, 460–461

R

Regression
    ASDs and, 564–565
Repetitive behaviors
    in ASDs, 564
Restless legs syndrome (RLS)
    in preschoolers, 592
Restricted interests
    in ASDs, 564
RLS. See Restless legs syndrome (RLS)

S

Sensory-based techniques
    in feeding disorders management, 575

Sleep
    in ADHD management in preschoolers, 532–534
    normal
        in preschoolers, 588–589
    in preschool years, 587
Sleep apnea
    obstructive
        in preschoolers, 589–591
Sleep disorders
    in preschoolers, **587–595**
        health disparities associated with, 593
        introduction, 587
        nightmares, 589
        OSA, 589–591
        parasomnias, 591–592
        prevalence of, 589
        with psychiatric diagnoses, 592–593
        RLS, 592
Social communication
    in ASDs
        deficits of, 563–564
Socioemotional impairments
    in childhood
        neonatal assessment and, 434–435
Specific language impairment
    ASD *vs.,* 559
Speech
    in mental health assessment of young children, 445
SSP. *See* Strange situation procedure (SSP)
Strange situation procedure (SSP), 460
Structured diagnostic interviews
    in mental health assessment of young children, 448–449

T

Talker(s)
    late
        vs. language disorders, 544–545
Telepsychiatry
    in preschool mental health, 599
Telepsychiatry preschool assessment
    in MC3, 601–602, 606
TF-CBT. *See* Trauma-focused cognitive behavioral therapy (TF-CBT)
Thought content
    in mental health assessment of young children, 446
Thought process
    in mental health assessment of young children, 446
Trauma
    very young children exposed to, **477–490**
        assessment of, 480–481
        clinical consequences, 479–480

    developmental effects, 478–479
    interventions for, 481–486
      ARC, 485
      attachment and behavioral catch-up, 483, 485
      child-parent psychotherapy, 485
      IY, 485
      PCIT, 485
      TF-CBT, 485
      trauma-informed systems, 481–483
    introduction, 477–479
    prevalence of, 477–478
    protective factors and resilience, 480
Trauma-focused cognitive behavioral therapy (TF-CBT)
    in trauma management in very young children, 485
Triple P
    in ADHD management in preschoolers, 526

V

Video feedback
    in fostering attachment, 468

W

WMCI. *See* Working Model of the Child Interview (WMCI)
Working Model of the Child Interview (WMCI)
    in mental health assessment of young children, 448

Y

Young children
    mental health assessment of, **441–454**
      contexts of, 441–442
      developmentally specific context, 442
      diagnostic systems, 442
      formulation in, 452
      introduction, 441–442
      mental status examination in, 445–446
      observation of caregiver-child interaction in, 446–447
      process of, 443–444
        patient history in, 443–444
        planning for appointment in, 443
      structured assessment tools in, 447–452
        Crowell parent-child interaction procedure, 478
        DIPA, 449
        laboratory evaluation, 449, 452
        PAPA, 449
        parent-report measures, 449
        structured diagnostic interviews, 448–449
        WMCI, 448
      unstructured observations in, 444–447
    trauma effects on, **477–490** *See also* Trauma, impact on very young children

Moving?

Make sure your subscription moves with you!

To notify us of your new address, find your **Clinics Account Number** (located on your mailing label above your name), and contact customer service at:

Email: journalscustomerservice-usa@elsevier.com

800-654-2452 (subscribers in the U.S. & Canada)
314-447-8871 (subscribers outside of the U.S. & Canada)

Fax number: 314-447-8029

Elsevier Health Sciences Division
Subscription Customer Service
3251 Riverport Lane
Maryland Heights, MO 63043

*To ensure uninterrupted delivery of your subscription, please notify us at least 4 weeks in advance of move.

Printed and bound by CPI Group (UK) Ltd, Croydon, CR0 4YY

07/10/2024

01040500-0005